Principles of Cancer Genetics

Fred Bunz

Principles of Cancer Genetics

Second Edition

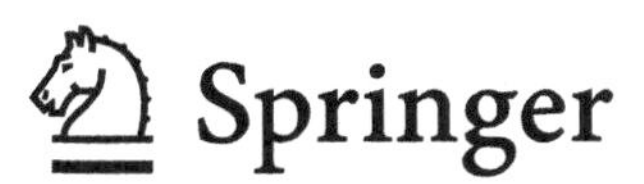

Fred Bunz
The Johns Hopkins University
Baltimore, Maryland, USA

ISBN 978-94-017-7482-6 ISBN 978-94-017-7484-0 (eBook)
DOI 10.1007/978-94-017-7484-0

Library of Congress Control Number: 2016931289

Springer Dordrecht Heidelberg New York London

Printed on acid-free paper

Springer Science+Business Media B.V. Dordrecht is part of Springer Science+Business Media (www.springer.com)

Preface to the Second Edition

Cancer is caused by alterations to the genome. To understand the nature of these alterations is to grasp the essence of cancer. The eight years that have passed since the publication of the first edition of this text have seen an unprecedented deluge of new information as to the genetic basis of cancer in nearly all of its forms. The specific genes that cause most common types of cancer have now been conclusively identified. These mutant genes have illuminated basic pathways and regulatory networks that control cell growth. The identification of cancer genes and the elucidation of their respective functions in cells and tissues have revolutionized our view of tumors and how they grow. These advances have also guided our efforts to improve cancer detection and to devise new modes of cancer therapy.

This book is aimed at advanced undergraduates who have completed introductory courses in genetics, biology, and biochemistry and medical students. There are several excellent texts that provide an overview of cancer biology and genetics, including *The Biology of Cancer*, by Weinberg and *The Genetic Basis of Human Cancer*, by Vogelstein and Kinzler. In contrast to these comprehensive texts, this modest book is focused on the genes that underlie the most common cancers. Attention is primarily devoted to cancer genes and the application of evolutionary theory to explain why the cell clones that harbor cancer genes tend to expand. Areas of controversy are avoided, in favor of firmly established concepts. This book does not delve into tumor pathobiology beyond what is required to understand the role of genetic alterations in neoplastic growth. For students with a general interest in cancer, this book will provide an accessible overview. For students contemplating future study in the fields of clinical oncology or cancer research, this book will be suitable as a primer. *Principles of Cancer Genetics* is intended not to replace existing texts but to complement them.

I am indebted to my teachers. The mentors I encountered in the course of my career have largely taught by example. Sanford Simon generously provided me with my first undergraduate laboratory experience at Stony Brook University. Bruce Stillman, the supervisor of my doctoral research at Cold Spring Harbor, introduced me to molecular biology and biochemistry as tools for rigorous cancer research. At Johns Hopkins, Bert Vogelstein and Ken Kinzler have provided a model of incisive thinking, dedication, fearlessness, generosity, and friendship that everyone should attempt to emulate. I am also indebted to my students, who continue to challenge me in every way and fuel me with their energy and determination.

A career in science is filled with ups and downs, and so I've been lucky to have good company on my personal journey of discovery. My wife Karla has been a steadfast source of inspiration, as well as a wellspring of unconditional love and patience. And my children, Zoe and Milo, fill me with a sense of wonder.

To all of these people, I will be forever grateful.

Baltimore, MD, USA
September 2015

Fred Bunz

Contents

Chapter 1
The Genetic Basis of Cancer

The Cancer Gene Theory

The human body is composed of about 200 different types of cells that organize into a multitude of tissues. Cancers can arise from nearly all of these cell populations. What we casually refer to as cancer is actually a diverse spectrum of human diseases. The most common cancers in adults are *carcinomas*, derived from epithelial cells that line body cavities and glands. *Sarcomas* arise from the mesenchymal tissues that form the connective tissues of the body. Melanomas, retinoblastomas, neuroblastomas and glioblastomas are derived from pigmented cells of the skin, dividing cells in the ocular retina, immature peripheral neurons and neural support cells known as glia, respectively. Lymphomas and leukemias, sometimes referred to as the 'liquid tumors', arise in the tissues that give rise to lymphoid and blood cells. All of these diseases will be collectively referred to as 'cancer' throughout this book. The rationale for this simplification is that all of these diverse diseases have a single root cause.

Cancers have many contributory factors and diverse clinical manifestations. Nonetheless, there is an elemental concept that underlies this complexity: *Cancer is caused by altered genes*. In recent decades, scientists have developed powerful tools to study the human genome in detail, and to systematically pinpoint and examine the genetic alterations that trigger the formation and growth of tumors. From decades of productive study, a theory has emerged that is both illuminating and highly useful. Throughout this text, the assembled principles of cancer genetics will be referred to as *the cancer gene theory*. The cancer gene theory has provided a framework for understanding how both hereditary and environmental factors contribute to cancers. As will be described in the chapters that follow, this powerful theory has informed new strategies for cancer risk assessment, detection and treatment.

The discovery that cancer is a genetic disease stands as one of the great triumphs of medical science. To put the importance of the cancer gene theory and its potential impact on public health in perspective, it may be useful to consider another epochal

F. Bunz, *Principles of Cancer Genetics*, DOI 10.1007/978-94-017-7484-0_1

theory that preceded it: *the germ theory*. There are several notable similarities between infectious diseases and cancers in terms of how they were perceived by physicians of the early nineteenth century. Both types of diseases were common and fearsome ailments, shrouded in mystery and superstition. The underlying mechanism for each was essentially a black box. Both kinds of diseases were attributed to many different causes and were generally resistant to available forms of treatment.

The studies of Louis Pasteur and his contemporaries in the mid nineteenth century led to the germ theory, and thereby brought about a revolutionary change in the way that infectious diseases were perceived. The idea that germs are the root cause of what we now call infectious diseases created a scientific paradigm that eventually ushered in an age in which the causes, and eventually cures, of distinct infectious diseases could be systematically discovered and developed.

Infectious disease remains a complex entity, but the germ theory provides a simple framework for understanding how these diseases arise and how they might be catagorized and treated. A broadly diverse group of germs infect the various tissues of the body and respond to different classes of therapeutic compounds. Individuals vary in their susceptibility to different germs, and different diseases within the broader spectrum have distinct risk factors. Nonetheless, the germ theory that explains the underlying disease process provides a clear path to the understanding of any infectious disease.

The revolution in infectious disease research foreshadowed a similar breakthrough in cancer research that occurred a century later. The discovery of the molecular essence of the gene by James Watson, Francis Crick and their collaborators and the subsequent cracking of the genetic code ignited the explosive growth of molecular biological research in the latter part of the twentieth century. This intensive and productive effort has yielded the precise identification of genetic alterations that directly drive *tumorigenesis*, the process by which cancers arise, progressively grow, and spread. Screening and therapeutic measures based upon the cancer gene theory are predicted to significantly reduce the overall burden of cancer on future generations.

The scientific pioneers who formulated the germ theory showed that despite the complexity and diversity of infectious diseases, the underlying etiology of these diseases could be conceptually simplified. Simple concepts can be extremely powerful. Indeed, the germ theory forms the foundation for all modern attempts to classify, diagnose and treat the myriad diseases that are caused by infectious agents. A direct analogy between infectious disease and cancer is bound to be imperfect, and yet the similarity of the essential concepts is illustrative. As germs cause infections, cancer genes drive cells to form tumors.

Cancers Are Invasive Tumors

A *neoplasm* (literally 'a new growth') is any abnormal proliferative population of cells, whereas a *tumor* is a neoplasm that is associated with a disease state. Tumors are diseases in which a population of genetically related cells has acquired the ability to proliferate abnormally. The term 'cancer' simply defines those tumors which have acquired the ability to invade surrounding tissues composed of normal cells. The distinction between a *benign* and a *malignant* tumor is solely based on this invasive capacity. Cancers, then, are invasive tumors. If an invading malignant tumor reaches a blood or lymphatic vessel, a cancer can *metastasize* and grow in distant tissues. The ability of cancers to disrupt other tissues and thereby spread is what makes them lethal.

As will be described in the following sections, most tumors are thought to initially arise from a single, genetically altered cell. The growth of a tumor composed of the progeny of this one cell occurs by a process known as *tumorigenesis*. As tumors grow from small, benign lesions to malignant and then metastatic cancers, the cells that compose these tumors change genetically and thereby acquire new properties. The accumulation over time of cancer genes underlies the process of tumorigenesis.

Cancer Is a Unique Type of Genetic Disease

The classical genetic diseases are typically *monogenic* in nature; they are caused by a single faulty gene. In some cases, the inheritance of a defective gene is both necessary and sufficient to cause disease, and the incidence is exactly as predicted by the Mendelian laws of inheritance.

Sickle cell anemia is an example of such a classical genetic disease. All manifestations of this illness are directly caused by a single alteration in the gene, *HBB*, that encodes beta globin, a subunit of hemoglobin. The protein encoded by this heritable disease gene is relatively insoluble and can come out of solution under conditions of low oxygen tension, causing red blood cells to adopt the shape of a sickle and become nonfunctional. Anemia and vascular blockage are caused by the altered properties of the sickled red blood cells. There is an environmental component to acute illness, as a period of local oxygen deprivation is required to initiate the pathological process. However, the underlying cause is the disease gene. The pattern of inheritance of sickle cell anemia, like that of all monogenic diseases with high penetrance, is simple and can be predicted by the principles established by Gregor Mendel in the nineteenth century.

Like sickle cell anemia, cancer can be inherited as a monogenic trait. Large, extended families have been identified in which individuals in multiple generations develop etiologically related types of cancer at a high rate. Such families have been used to define cancer syndromes and to isolate the genes that underlie cancer susceptibility. While inherited cancer syndromes have provided a wealth of information as to the relationships between specific genes and cancer, they are relatively rare.

Cancer predisposition syndromes vividly demonstrate the genetic basis of cancer. But are all cancers genetic in origin? Clearly, the majority of cancers that affect the human population cannot be predicted by the simple principles of Mendelian inheritance. The genes that cause tumors to grow are not most often inherited, but rather are spontaneously acquired. Cancer is unique among genetic diseases in this regard. While genes that cause the classic genetic diseases are passed from generation to generation in a predictable way, cancer genes are most commonly acquired over the course of a lifetime.

What Are Cancer Genes and How Are They Acquired?

A cancer gene can be defined as a genetic variant that increases cancer risk when present in normal cells, or promotes the development of cancer as neoplasia grow. Cancer genes are distinct *alleles* of normal genes that arise as a result of mutation.

From a genetic perspective, there are two types of cells in the human body. *Germ cells* are the cells of the reproductive system that produce sperm in males and oocytes in females. *Somatic cells*, derived from the Greek work for body, *soma*, are all other cells exclusive of the germ cells. Cancer genes that arise in the germ cells are said to be in the *germline*. Individuals who inherit germline cancer genes will harbor a cancer gene in every cell, somatic cells and germ cells alike. Such individuals, known as *carriers*, are at increased risk of contracting cancer and can transmit that risk to their children. In contrast, cancer genes that arise in somatic cells are not passed on to subsequent generations.

Germline cancer genes cause a small but significant fraction of human cancers; 5–10 % of all cancers result from a heritable predisposition. Several important cancer genes that run in the germline of cancer-prone families greatly elevate the risk of cancer for individuals that inherit them. The likelihood that an allele carrier will develop cancer defines the *penetrance* of that allele. In some cases the penetrance of an inherited allele is so high that the development of cancer is virtually a certainty, and preemptive surgical treatment is indicated. Other germline cancer genes have lesser impact on overall cancer risk.

In the majority of common cancers, the cancer genes that underlie tumorigenesis arise spontaneously by *somatic mutation*. Somatic mutation is a term that describes both a process, the spontaneous acquisition of a mutation in a non-germ cell, and a product, which is the genetic alteration.[1] Somatic cells that spontaneously acquire cancer gene mutations are the precursors of cancers.

Both germline mutations and somatic mutations alter a normal gene and create a new, mutant version of that gene. As will be more extensively discussed in subsequent sections, not all mutant genes acquired via the germline contribute to cancer risk, nor do all somatic mutations cause cancer. Indeed, the majority of genes and gene mutations do not appear to be functionally related to the growth of tumor cells.

A third way that a normal cell can acquire a cancer gene is by viral infection. This is a less common mode of cancer gene acquisition overall, but one that is very important in several cancer types. As will be illustrated in sections that follow,

---

[1] The process referred to as the 'cancer gene theory' in this book is sometimes called the 'somatic mutation theory', to emphasize the predominant role of somatically acquired mutations in the development of most cancers. The term 'cancer gene theory' reflects the theoretical relatedness of somatic and germline cancer genes.

viruses play a varied role in cancer. A few cancers can be considered to be infectious diseases. But for most types of cancer, the contributory viruses do not actually carry or transmit cancer genes but instead alter the tissue environment in which cancer genes are propagated.

Mutations Alter the Human Genome

There are a number of different types of mutations that can alter the DNA sequences that define the structure and function of a gene. When such a change occurs, a new variant, or *allele* of that gene is created. Small mutations that affect a relatively short region of DNA are typically detected by DNA sequencing, while mutations that involve large regions of chromosomes can be visualized by microscopy (Fig. 1.1).

Mutations are typically categorized by the extent to which the DNA sequence is changed. *Single base pair substitutions*, often referred to as *point mutations*, simply change one base pair (bp) to another. More extensive mutations cause loss of DNA sequences or insertions of new DNA sequences. Deletions and insertions of 20 bp and fewer are typically called *micro-deletions* or *micro-insertions*, respectively, while larger losses are termed *gross deletions* or *gross insertions*. This latter type of

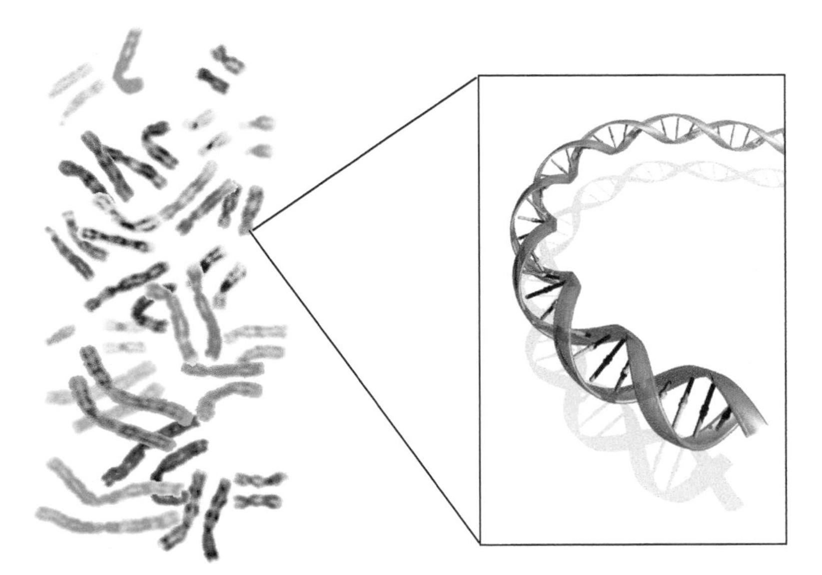

Fig. 1.1 Genetic alterations, great and small. The genetic alterations that underlie cancer can affect whole chromosomes (*left*), and therefore be detectable by cytogenetic methods. Small genetic alterations that affect individual DNA bases (*right*) are detected by molecular methods, including DNA sequencing. Images courtesy of the National Human Genome Research Institute

alteration can span many thousands of bp and be visually apparent upon microscopic examination of stained chromosomes.

Changes in chromosome structure in the microscopic size range are known as cytogenetic abnormalities. DNA breaks can give rise to chromosomal translocations in which chromosome fragments are joined with pieces of different chromosomes, as well as large deletions and inversions (Fig. 1.2). Most cytogenetic abnormalities arise somatically. However, large deletions are clearly heritable. For example the heritable form of the ocular tumor retinoblastoma, described in Chap. 3, is caused by a large deletion that is cytogenetically apparent. Germline cytogenetic alterations are present in every cell in the body, and are said to be *constitutional* in nature.

The genomic DNA sequences of tumor cells can be altered by mutations in virtually every imaginable way. Poorly characterized DNA repair processes can result in a DNA sequence inversion or a more complex type of rearrangement that combines an insertion and a deletion. Short repetitive sequences can expand in tandem arrays. Long tracts of mononucleotide sequence (eg. a lengthy, uninterrupted tract of A residues) or simple repeats can expand and contract. Recent studies have revealed clustered cytogenetic rearrangements that appear to be the end product of a catastrophic event involving chromosome breakage and random reassembly. The underlying process that causes these chromosomal rearrangements is known as *chromothripsis*, a neologism derived from the Greek word *thripsis*, which means 'shattered into pieces'.

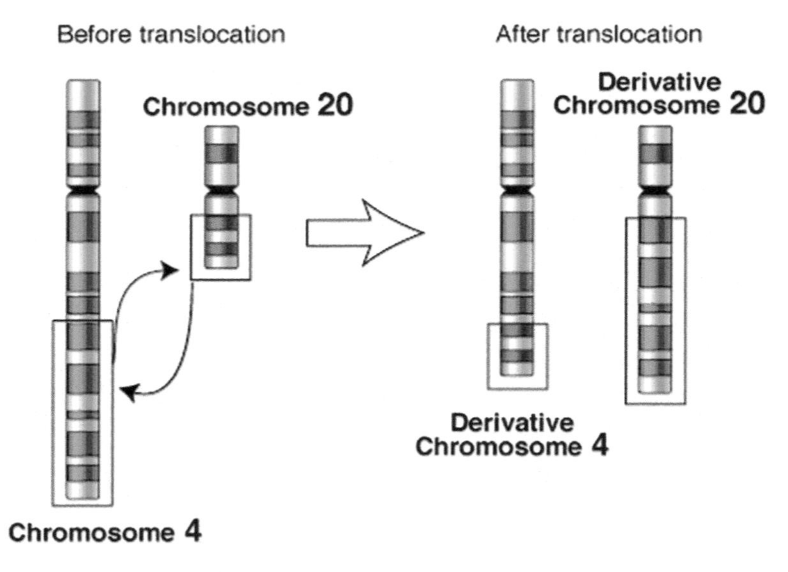

Fig. 1.2 Chromosomal translocation. The exchange of large regions of DNA between nonhomologous chromosomes is known as a translocation. A balanced exchange between two chromosomes, as depicted in this example showing a translocation between chromosome 20 and chromosome 4, is known as a *reciprocal translocation*. Translocations result in derivative chromosomes. Illustration form the National Human Genome Research Institute

Understanding how mutations occur and how these mutations affect the biology of the cell are critical to understanding the process of *tumorigenesis*, the initiation and growth of a cancer. The origins of some mutations are mechanistically clear. For example, a significant fraction of all single base pair substitutions arise as a result of a complex chemical reaction that involves the covalent addition of a methyl group to cytosine nucleotides, and the change of these bases upon the subsequent removal of this modification. Alterations occurring in mononucleotide tracts (repetitive elements that consist of a single nucleotide) can often be attributed to defects in the processes by which genomic DNA is replicated, proofread and repaired. These specific mechanisms will be described more extensively in later sections.

Much has been learned about the basic mechanisms of mutagenesis. However, the origin of many mutations, particularly of those that are structurally complex, remains incompletely understood. In the case of gross changes that result in large deletions, insertions and chromosomal rearrangements, a possible mechanistic clue is the repetitive DNA sequences that flank many characterized deletion breakpoints. A substantial portion of the human genome is composed of repetitive elements. The most abundant of these is the *Alu* repeat, an element that is about 300 bp in length. The core sequence of Alu repeats is similar to bacterial sequences that stimulate recombination by promoting DNA strand exchange between sequences that have a high degree of similarity, a property known as homology. Such evidence suggests that *Alu* repeats may represent hotspots for *homologous recombination*, a process by which separate DNA sequences are joined in a linear assembly on the basis of their similarity or identity.

Alterations in genomic DNA convert normal genes to cancer genes. But it is important to understand that not all genomic alterations contribute to cancer. In fact, only a very small number of mutational events actually promote the growth of tumors. The extent to which a mutation will promote tumor growth depends on the identity of the gene that is mutated, the precise nature of the mutation, and on the overall replicative potential of the cell in which the mutation occurs.

Genes and Mutations

How do mutations convert normal genes into cancer genes? To appreciate the fundamental cause of cancer, it is necessary to first understand the basic elements of gene structure and function.

The gene defines a functional unit of heredity. The physical location of a gene on the chromosome is known as its *locus*. A genetic locus can encompass a chromosomal region that spans from fewer than 10^3 to greater than 10^6 bp, with a mean size of approximately 5×10^4 bp. The information content of a gene lies in the sequence of the four DNA bases: the purines adenine (**A**) and guanine (**G**), and the pyrimidines cytosine (**C**) and thymidine (**T**). The *expression* of a gene is defined as the extent to which the DNA at that locus is transcribed into RNA, which in turn is processed and translated into a functional protein. Not all genes encode proteins, but most, if not all, cancer-causing mutations affect the functions of genes that encode proteins.

Protein-coding genes are composed of several basic elements (Fig. 1.3). The region of a gene that defines the protein that is ultimately expressed is the *open reading frame* (ORF). The ORF is a stretch of triplet DNA base pairs, or *codons*, that encode the distinct amino acid sequence of the expressed protein. ORFs are most often spread among multiple expressed regions of the gene, or *exons*. Intervening sequences, aptly known as introns, are removed during processing of the initially transcribed RNA, and the exons are spliced together. Further processing usually involves the capping of the 5′ end of the transcript and 3′ polyadenylation, and results a mature messenger RNA (mRNA).

Upon cursory examination of the overall structure of a typical protein-coding gene, one might intuitively predict that alterations occurring in different regions would have very different consequences. The ORF contains the sequence information that defines the primary structure of the encoded protein. Accordingly, mutations in these regions are more likely to be of functional consequence. In contrast, because introns are spliced out of RNA transcripts during processing, mutations within these regions are less likely to make a significant impact on gene expression or on the function of the encoded protein.

Mutations within exons can alter gene function and ultimately affect protein structure (Fig. 1.4). The most obvious way in which a mutation can directly alter

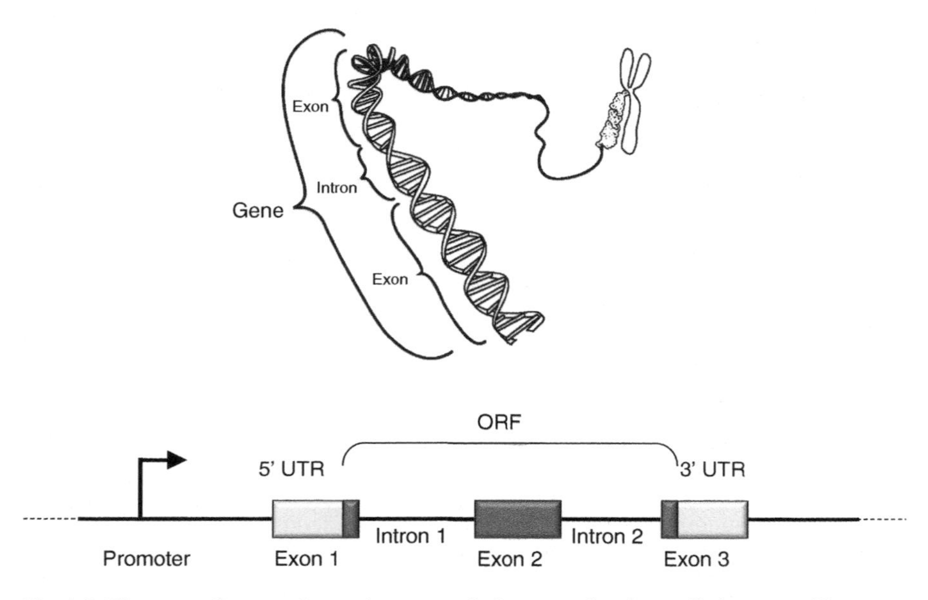

Fig. 1.3 Elements of a gene. A gene is composed of expressed regions called exons and intervening sequences called introns. In the chromosome, these elements are spatially condensed and extensively packaged (*top panel*). Most characterized genes encode proteins. As shown in a linear representation (*lower panel*), exons contain a protein-coding region known as an open reading frame (ORF). Flanking the ORF are the 5′ and 3′ untranslated sequences (UTRs). Expression of the gene requires the activity of a cis-acting promoter

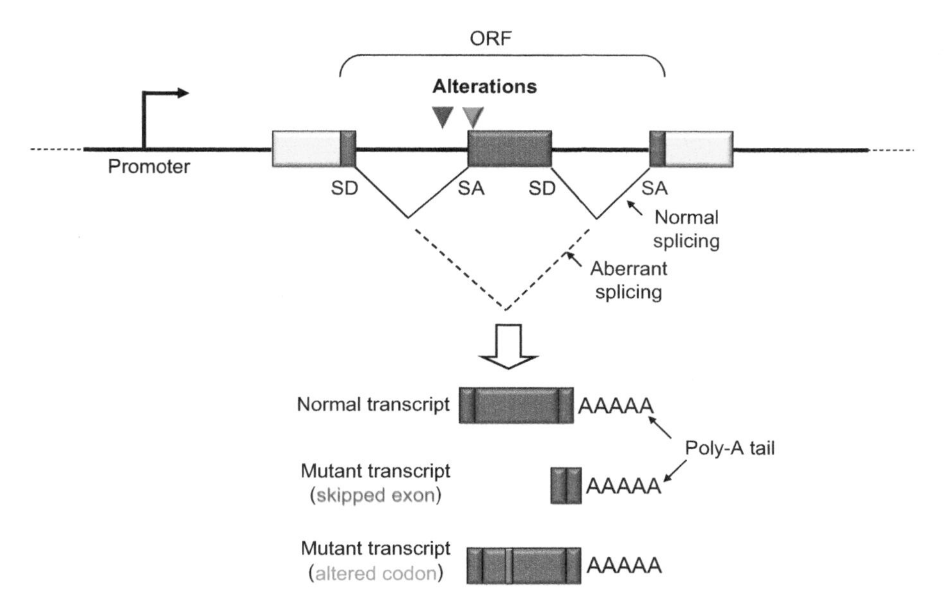

Fig. 1.4 Mutations can alter gene transcripts. The large majority of mutations that create cancer genes alter individual codons within exons (*red arrow*). Fewer than 2 % of the mutations that cause cancer interfere with RNA processing by disrupting the splice donor (SD) or splice acceptor (SA) consensus sequences. Such mutations (*blue arrow*) cause aberrant RNA splicing that can result in exon skipping

gene function is by changing one or more codons, and thereby changing the amino acid sequence of the encoded protein. Mutations can also alter the way that RNA is spliced. Correct RNA splicing is dependent on the presence of short *splice donor*, *splice acceptor*, and *branch point* consensus sequences. Mutations within these splice sites can result in exon skipping or otherwise aberrantly-spliced RNA species. Such mutations in cancers are relatively rare.

While most cancer genes arise from mutations in exons, some unusual mutations in introns have been shown to affect gene function. In rare instances, mutations within introns activate *cryptic splice sites*, essentially generating new splice sites that then lead to the production of aberrant RNA species. Other intron mutations have been shown to alter gene expression or splicing efficiency. In general, the overall contribution of mutations in regions other than exons to tumorigenesis remains poorly defined, but appears to be relatively small. This topic is discussed in more detail in Chap. 6.

A mutation in a coding sequence is much more likely to result in a change in gene function than a similar sequence change in a non-coding exon. Among the mutations that occur within coding exons, some have much larger effects than others. Some mutations result in no phenotypic effect while other changes can profoundly affect gene function and significantly increase disease risk.

Many single base pair substitutions do not result any change to the encoded protein. The reason lies in the inherent degeneracy of the genetic code; many amino acids have several codons that are synonymous. Leucine, for example, is encoded by six DNA triplets: CTT, CTC, CTA, CTG, TTA and TTG. A C→T change that results in a mutation of CTC to CTT would have no effect on the structure or function of the encoded protein. In this case, one leucine codon is simply converted to another. Such mutations are known as *silent* or *synonymous mutations*, and are the most benign type of mutation in terms of disease risk. Mutations in the third codon position, also known as the *wobble* position, are least likely to result in an amino acid change.

A single base pair substitution that causes a codon change is known as a *missense* mutation. A C→A mutation would change CTT, the codon for leucine into ATT, which encodes isoleucine (Table 1.1). In this case, a single base change results in a single amino acid change. A single base pair substitution can also change a codon that represents an amino acid into one of the termination, or STOP, codons, encoded in the DNA sequence by TAG, TAA, and TGA. Terminating mutations, also known as *nonsense* mutations, result in truncation of the open reading frame.

Missense mutations have a wide range of phenotypic effects. The effect of a missense mutation depends on both the chemical characteristics of the original and mutated amino acids and the position of the change within the structure of the encoded protein. In our previous example, leucine and isoleucine are chemically very similar and have the same molecular weight. A missense mutation that changes leucine to isoleucine might therefore be predicted to have a minimal effect on

Table 1.1 The standard genetic code

First codon position	Second codon position			
	T	**C**	**A**	**G**
T	TTT Phe (F)	TCT Ser (S)	TAT Tyr (Y)	TGT Cys (C)
	TTC	TCC	TAC	TGC
	TTA Leu (L)	TCA	TAA **STOP**	TGA **STOP**
	TTG	TCG	TAG **STOP**	TGG Trp (W)
C	CTT Leu (L)	CCT Pro (P)	CAT His (H)	CGT Arg (R)
	CTC	CCC	CAC	CGC
	CTA	CCA	CAA Gln (Q)	CGA
	CTG	CCG	CAG	CGG
A	ATT Ile (I)	ACT Thr (T)	AAT Asn (N)	AGT Ser (S)
	ATC	ACC	AAC	AGC
	ATA	ACA	AAA Lys (K)	AGA Arg (R)
	ATG Met (M)	ACG	AAG	AGG
G	GTT Val (V)	GCT Ala (A)	GAT Asp (D)	GGT Gly (G)
	GTC	GCC	GAC	GGC
	GTA	GCA	GAA Glu (E)	GGA
	GTG	GCG	GAG	GGG

The DNA codons are grouped with their corresponding amino acids (the single-letter amino acid designations are in parentheses). The degeneracy of the genetic code reduces the impact of many single nucleotide substitutions protein structure and function. In contrast, the mutation of the sequence GAG, which encodes glutamic acid, to a GTG codon for valine results is a change from a highly acidic to a hydrophobic amino acid. A single base change thereby causes the amino acid substitution that is the basis for the gross structural and functional changes in β-globin that underlie sickle cell anemia.

The position of an amino acid substitution within an encoded protein is also a key determinant of the extent to which a mutation can impact gene function. Protein structure is progressively defined by amino acid sequence (*primary structure*), by interactions between neighboring amino acids (*secondary structure*), by three-dimensional interactions between more distant peptide motifs (*tertiary structure*) and finally, by interactions between subunits of multiprotein complexes (*quaternary structure*). By definition, all missense mutations alter the primary structure. Some, but not all, missense mutations can also change the higher order structure of a protein or a protein complex. Mutations that change amino acids that directly contribute to disulfide bonds, hydrophobic interactions and hydrogen bonds affect both secondary and tertiary protein structure and often result in dramatic functional changes. For proteins that function as catalytic enzymes, mutations near the substrate or cofactor binding domains can profoundly influence enzymatic activity. Structural proteins, in contrast, are typically sensitive to mutation in regions involved in the critical protein-protein interactions that define their quaternary structure. In general, amino acid residues that are present in similar positions in homologous proteins from other species, and are therefore *evolutionarily conserved*, are more likely to have a functional impact when mutated.

Because an open reading frame is defined by a continuous array of triplet codons, any numerical alteration to this invariant pattern will have significant effects. Thus, even small deletions and insertions can completely disrupt an open reading frame. If a deletion or insertion within an open reading frame involves any number of bp not divisible by 3, that alteration will result in a shift in the reading frame. *Frameshift mutations* result in a new set of codons that encode an entirely unrelated series of amino acids in the 3′ direction (downstream) from the location of the mutation. Because the human genome is rich in the A:T bp that are present in stop codons, probability dictates that any given alternate reading frame resulting from a frameshift will have a termination codon within a short distance (Fig. 1.5). Small insertions and deletions therefore thus result in a new coding sequence that encodes both random amino acids and a truncated protein product. A mutation that occurs at the beginning of an open reading frame, which encodes the amino terminus of a predicted protein, would most often have a greater effect than a mutation at the very end of the open reading frame that preserves most of the codons.

Synonymous or nonsynonymous mutations that affect the correct splicing of exons can often lead to aberrations such as *exon skipping* and activation of cryptic splice sites. Such alterations will usually lead to a shift in the reading frame, with the same consequences as other types of frameshift mutations. In the case in which the skipped exon contains a multiple of 3 bp, the spliced mRNA product will maintain the original reading frame, with the only consequence of the mutation being the loss of the amino acid positions encoded by the skipped exon.

5′-aat agt aaa aag acg ttg Cga gaa gtt gga agt gtg-3′
N S K K T L R E V G S V
Nonsense mutation
5′-aat agt aaa aag acg ttg Tga gaa gtt gga agt gtg-3′
N S K K T L STOP
5′-gaa ata aaa gaa AAg att gga act agg tca-3′
E I K E K I G T R S
2 bp deletion, frameshift
5′-gaa ata aaa gaa gat tgg aac tag gtc a-3′
E I K E D W N STOP

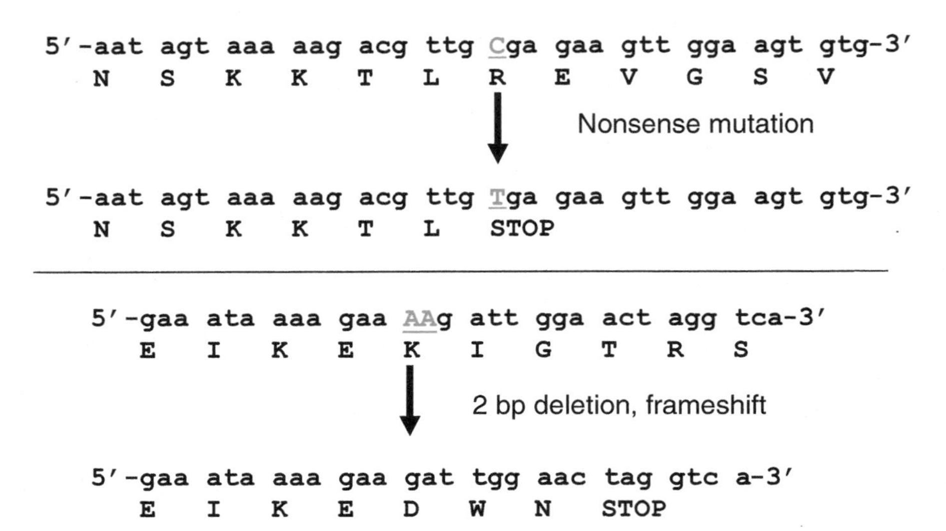

Fig. 1.5 Truncating mutations. Nonsense mutations generate STOP codons (*upper panel*). In this example, a C → T mutation (indicated in *red*) introduces a premature STOP. Insertions or deletions create frameshifts. Premature STOP triplets in occur in the new reading frame (*lower panel*). In this example, the deletion of AA (indicated in *red*) results in a frameshift and the appearance of a premature STOP several codons downstream

Premature stop codons caused by nonsense or truncating mutations do not typically result in the expression of truncated protein because mRNA transcripts that contain nonsense codons are systematically and rapidly degraded. The multistep pathway that performs this surveillance function is known as *nonsense-mediated mRNA decay*. This process can distinguish normal and premature stop codons. Nonsense-mediated mRNA decay is an evolutionarily conserved process that is thought to be a mechanism to eliminate mRNAs that encode potentially deleterious protein fragments. It has been estimated that up to one quarter of all cancer mutations are of the type that trigger nonsense-mediated decay.

In summary, nonsense mutations, insertions and deletions can significantly impact the genes that encode regulatory proteins. The phenotypic effects of such mutations can include altered protein functionality and altered levels of protein expression. In many cases, mutations result in the total inactivation of a gene. An allele that expresses no detectable protein product is known as a *null allele*. Less common genetic alterations can also cause null alleles. For example, a cytogenetically apparent deletion that eliminates an entire open reading frame would in effect create a null allele.

While many cancer-causing mutations cause the generation of null alleles, many other seemingly minor genetic alterations can also change normal genes into cancer genes. In fact, the most common cancer-causing mutations involve subtle but functionally impactful changes to the DNA sequence of the key regulators of cell growth and survival. As will become apparent in the chapters to come, small genetic changes can have large biological consequences.

Single Nucleotide Substitutions

The most common type of DNA mutation is the substitution of one single nucleotide for another. Such mutations are often referred to as a *point mutations*. (Although both base pairs are affected by a single nucleotide substitution, the base that is on the coding DNA strand is the alteration noted.)

A *transition* is a base change from one purine to the other or from one pyrimidine to the other (C → T or G → A). A *transversion* is a change from a purine to a pyrimidine or vice versa (A → T or C → G). There are four bases, so a total of 12 different types of base substitutions are possible (Fig. 1.6).

While each base can be mutated and replaced by any other base, some substitutions occur more frequently than others. The most commonly observed substitutions are C → T and G → A, which together account for nearly 50 % of all single base substitutions. These rates are much higher than would be expected by random chance. One reason for the unexpected overrepresentation of C → T and G → A base changes is the inherent mutability of the CG dinucleotide (usually written as CpG to emphasize the phosphate group that defines the 5′ → 3′ orientation of the sequence).

CpG sites are frequently the target of a chemical modification known as *DNA methylation* (Fig. 1.7). The covalent modification of the cytosine ring by a family of enzymes called *DNA methyltransferases* converts cytosine in the CpG context to

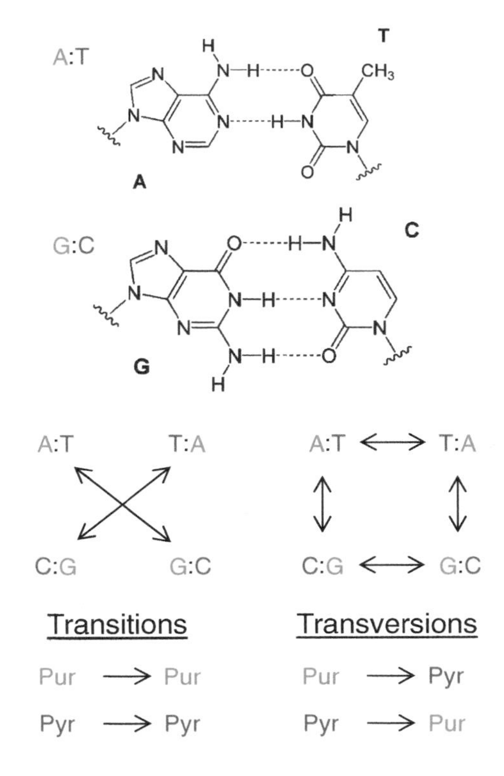

Fig. 1.6 Transitions and transversions. DNA is composed of A:T and G:C base pairs in a linear sequence. A total of 12 distinct base changes are possible

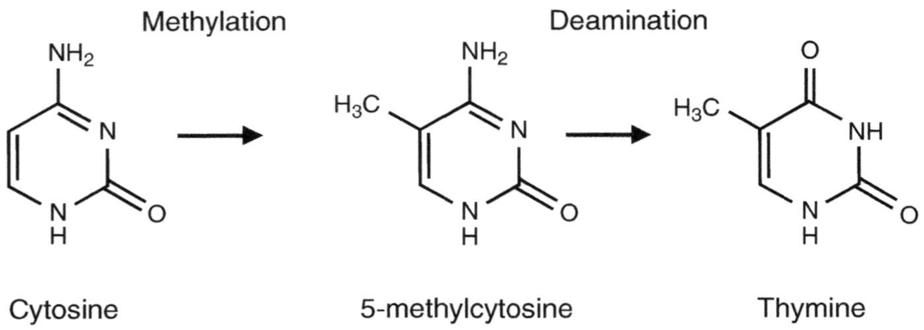

Fig. 1.7 Endogenous methylation causes a C → T transition. DNA methyltransferases convert C to 5-methylcytosine (5mC). This reaction occurs preferentially at CpG dinucleotides. The ring containing 5mC is converted to a T by loss of the NH_2-group, a chemical reaction known as deamination

5-methylcytosine (5mC). 5mC has a propensity to undergo *deamination* to become uracil, which in turn is converted to a thymidine residue during the next round of DNA replication if the deaminated base has not been repaired. (The resulting C → T transition is mirrored by a corresponding G → A transition on the complementary DNA strand.) C → T transitions arise at CpG sites at a rate that is approximately 15 times greater than at the other dinucleotide sites: CpA, CpC and CpT.

The entire human genome is comprised of 42 % G–C base pairs. Based on this number, the CpG sequence would be expected to occur at 4.41 % (0.21 C × 0.21 G = 0.041 CpG) of all dinucleotide positions. However, CpG sites occur at a much lower frequency than would be expected by chance. As a result of methylation and subsequent deamination, CpG dinuceotide sequences have been progressively lost from the human genome over the course of many generations. Thus, the inherent hypermutability of CpG sequences has led to a relative paucity of CpG sites in the human genome.

The stochastic transitions caused by CpG mutation are a source of significant genetic variation. CpG mutations in germ cells that give rise to sperm and oocytes can result in new germline mutations, often termed *de novo* mutations. Somatic mutations can also occur via this process. The inherent hypermutability of CpG dinucleotides illustrates one chemical reaction that causes spontaneous single nucleotide substitutions during DNA replication. The very process of DNA replication is in fact the greatest source of both germline and somatic mutations.

DNA replication occurs with a remarkably high degree of fidelity, as billions of nucleotides are covalently joined in precise sequence order prior to every mitotic cell division. The rate of germline base substitution mutations measured from each generation to the next is on the order of 10^{-8} per site. As the growth and development of the human embryo involves roughly 10^2 cell divisions, the overall rate of single base substitution mutations can be inferred to be approximately 10^{-10} per site for each cell division. Put another way, there is a one in 10^{10} chance that a given nucleotide pair in the human genome will be spontaneously altered during any single cell division cycle. This is the lowest per-cell division mutation rate among all organisms that have been reliably analyzed. Despite this high level of fidelity, the rare mutations that arise during normal DNA replication account for the majority of human cancers.

Mutations can arise in a proliferating cell lineage by mechanisms that include:

Slipped Mispairing in Mononucleotide Tracts Runs of identical bases can adversely impact DNA replication fidelity. At the replication fork, discontinuous synthesis of the lagging strand is mediated by the iterative extension of primers. One mechanism of mutagenesis is thought to arise from transient misalignment of the primer-template that results from the transient looping out of a base on the template strand (Fig. 1.8). A base is thus misincorporated into the primer strand, resulting in a mismatch. If the mismatch is repaired in favor of the strand with the misincorporation a mutation results. Known as the Slipped Mispairing Model, originally proposed by Thomas Kunkel, this mechanistic explanation for some replication-associated mutations is supported by an observed bias in the identity of the mutated base to a flanking base within open reading frames. In principle, slipped mispairing could also generate a 1-base insertion or deletion, depending on the primer-template misalignment and repair of the mismatch.

Limiting Availability of DNA Building Blocks Efficient DNA synthesis depends on the availability of the four deoxyribonucleotides (dATP, dCTP, dGTP and TTP, collectively referred to as dNTPs). The mobilization of dNTPs during DNA replication or DNA repair is highly regulated. Concentrations of dNTP pools are thus tightly controlled. The fidelity with which DNA polymerases replicate a template DNA strand is highly sensitive to dNTP levels. The probability of misincorporation of a base will depend partly on the ratio of the correct dNTP to the three incorrect dNTPs available to the DNA polymerase. After a misincorporation has occurred, the efficiency with which a mispaired base is excised before additional synthesis proceeds depends partly on the concentration of the next correct dNTP to be incorporated. A proportionally high concentration of the 'next' base will favor mismatch extension. By such mechanisms, perturbations in dNTP proportions or total dNTP concentration can both affect DNA replication fidelity.

Stalled Replication Forks The rate of base misincorporation can change dramatically if the progress of the replication fork is impeded. Short DNA sequences that have been identified as disproportionate targets of mutation are thought to directly cause the replication fork to stall or pause. For example, the sequences TGGA and TCGA are mutated at twice the rate that would be expected by chance alone; this sequence also resembles a site at which DNA polymerase α has been shown to transiently arrest.

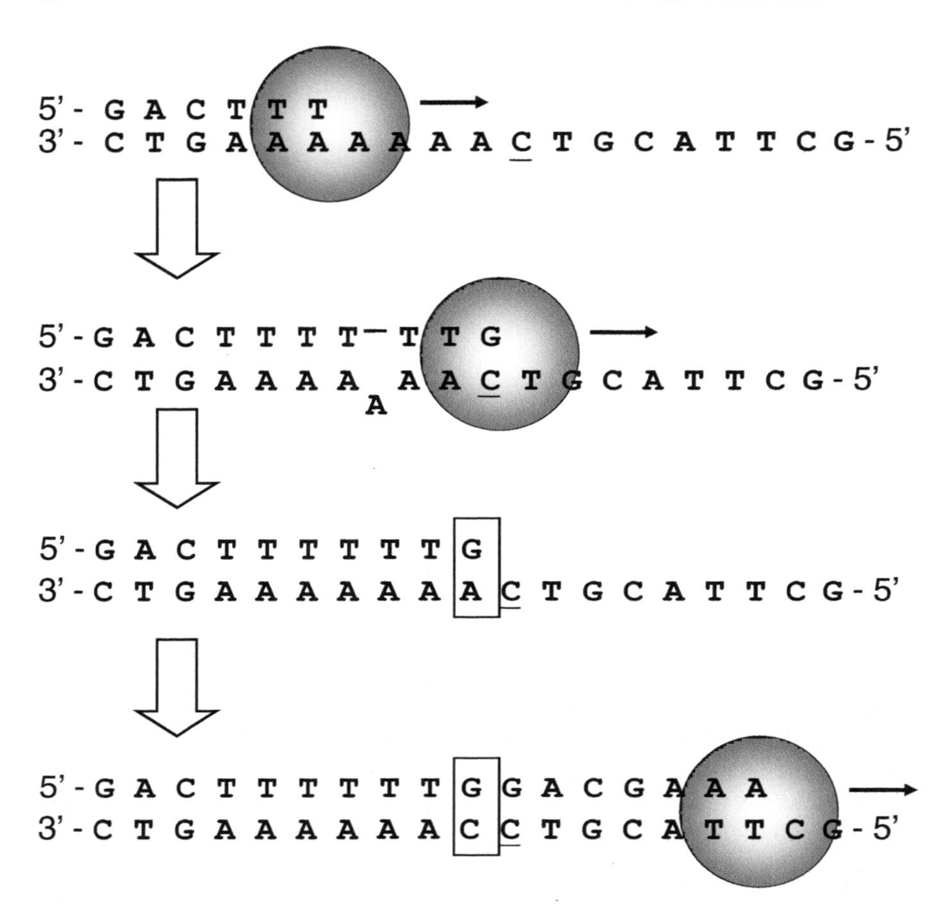

Fig. 1.8 Slipped mispairing in an A_7 tract. In this example, a DNA polymerase holoenzyme complex (shown as a sphere) encounters a tract of seven 'A' nucleotides. The looping-out of an 'A' on the template strand causes a transient misalignment of the primer and template DNAs. A 'G' is thus misincorporated into the primer strand at a position that would correctly be occupied by a 'T'. The realignment of the primer-template strand reveals a G:A mismatch. If repair fails, the replacement of the 'A' on the template strand would represent a new mutation

Gene Silencing Is Marked by Cytosine Methylation: Epigenetics

The CpG dinucleotides that are the targets of DNA methyltransferases are not distributed randomly throughout the genome. Most regions of the genome have been depleted of CpG sites by spontaneous deamination. Discrete regions known as *CpG islands* retain the number of CpG dinucleotides that would be predicted to occur randomly. CpG islands, which range in size between 0.4 and 5 kb are often associated with gene promoters.

The methylation of CpG islands near gene promoters is associated with the downregulation of gene expression, a phenomenon also known as *gene silencing.* There are striking differences in methylation patterns in normal cells and cancer cells. Globally, cancer cells have lower levels of cytosine methylation and are therefore said to be *hypomethylated.* In contrast, many promoters in cancer cells are *hypermethylated,* and their corresponding genes are transcriptionally silenced. The inheritance from one generation to the next of patterns of CpG DNA methylation is known as *imprinting.* CpG DNA methylation is thus a cause of heritable DNA base changes (C → T transitions) as well as heritable epigenetic alterations (imprinted genes).

Aberrant CpG DNA methylation and other epigenetic alterations to chromatin represent a complementary and sometimes an alternative pathway to changing the growth properties of a cell in a heritable manner. Interestingly, many known cancer genes, defined by mutations, are among the genes found to be epigenetically silenced in cancer cells. Based on such findings, epigenetic mechanisms have been proposed to account for many of the phenotypic abnormalities that arise during tumorigenesis and drive the process forward, including dysregulated cell growth, cell death and genetic instability. Some genetic mutations that have been found in cancer cells in fact appear to exert their tumorigenic effects by altering the range of epigenetic alterations. The overall contribution of purely epigenetic alterations, in the absence of accompanying mutations, to human cancer remains to be definitively determined.

Environmental Mutagens, Mutations and Cancer

It is well understood that environmental factors can significantly affect the incidence of some types of cancer. The respective contributions of tobacco smoke and sunlight to lung and skin cancers are excellent examples of this cause and effect relationship.

How do the incontrovertible relationships between cancer and the environment relate to the cancer gene theory? Part of the answer is that some environmental agents are *mutagens.* The exposure of proliferating cells to these agents increases the rate at which specific types of mutations arise. The cancer gene theory thus provides a simple explanation for why some environmental factors increase cancer incidence. Mutagens cause some of the mutations that cause cancer.

For the purposes of illustration, consider a single cancer gene, *TP53*, and the environmental factors that are known to contribute to its mutation. *TP53* is mutated in many cancers and is therefore intensively studied. Indeed, insights into how mutations in *TP53* contribute to growing cancers have fundamentally shaped the cancer gene theory. The biological effects of the *TP53* gene and the ways that *TP53* mutations contribute to cancer will be considered at length in later chapters. Here, the focus is on how environmental agents cause the mutation of *TP53* and thereby create a cancer gene. It is important to note that the mutagens discussed below alter many genes in addition to *TP53*, and that *TP53* is mutated by many additional processes that remain incompletely understood.

(The mutations indicated hereafter are described in reference to the base change that occurs on the coding, or sense, DNA strand. For example, a C → T transition on the sense strand is necessarily coincident with a complementary G → A transition on the antiparallel, antisense strand.)

Tobacco Smoke The relationship between tobacco smoke and cancer is one of the most clearly defined examples of a dose-dependent carcinogen. Smokers have a 10-fold greater risk of dying from lung cancer and this risk increases 15–25-fold for heavy smokers. Only 5–10 % of all lung cancers occur in patients that have no prior history of cigarette smoking. In addition to the well known association between smoking and lung cancer, smoking is also a significant risk factor for a number of other cancers, including head and neck cancer and bladder cancer.

Polycyclic aromatic hydrocarbons generated by the incomplete combustion of organic material during smoking are strongly implicated as the carcinogenic component of tobacco smoke. Among these, benzo[a]pyrene is by far the best studied. After ingestion, benzo[a]pyrene is metabolically altered to benzo[a]pyrene diol epoxide, or BPDE, by the P450 pathway. There are several isomers of this highly mutagenic metabolite that are formed during this process. The mucosal linings of the lungs, head and neck and the urinary bladder are all highly exposed to BPDE in smokers, further underscoring the relationship of these tissues to the cancer-causing effects of tobacco smoke.

BPDE binds directly to DNA and forms four structurally distinct covalent adducts at the N2 position of guanine (Fig. 1.9). These N2-BPDE-dG adducts constitute a significant barrier to advancing DNA replication forks in proliferating cells. The repair process that resolves such lesions results in a high proportion of G → T transversion mutations. The factors that determine whether a given N2-BPDE-dG adduct will give rise to a single base pair substitution are complex, and partially depend on the stereochemistry of the specific adduct and the sequence and methylation status of neighboring bases.

That BPDE contributes to smoking-related cancer by directly causing mutations is supported by the types of *TP53* mutations that are found in lung cancers and in heavy smokers. *TP53* mutations in lung cancers do not occur at random positions distributed across the gene, but rather are found in clusters known as *hotspots*. Hotspots are codons within a gene that are mutated at a higher frequency than would be predicted by chance alone. The base positions within the *TP53* open reading frame at which BPDE preferentially forms adducts overlap significantly with known mutation hotspots in lung cancers, strongly suggesting that BPDE directly causes the mutations that contribute to these tumors.

Ultraviolet (UV) Light Sunlight is the main cause of skin cancers. The UV-B component of sunlight, encompassing wavelengths 290–320 nm in the electromagnetic spectrum, is a mutagen that causes two types of alterations to adjacent pyrimidines: *cyclobutane dimers* and *pyrimidine (6–4) pyramidone photoproducts* (Figs. 1.10

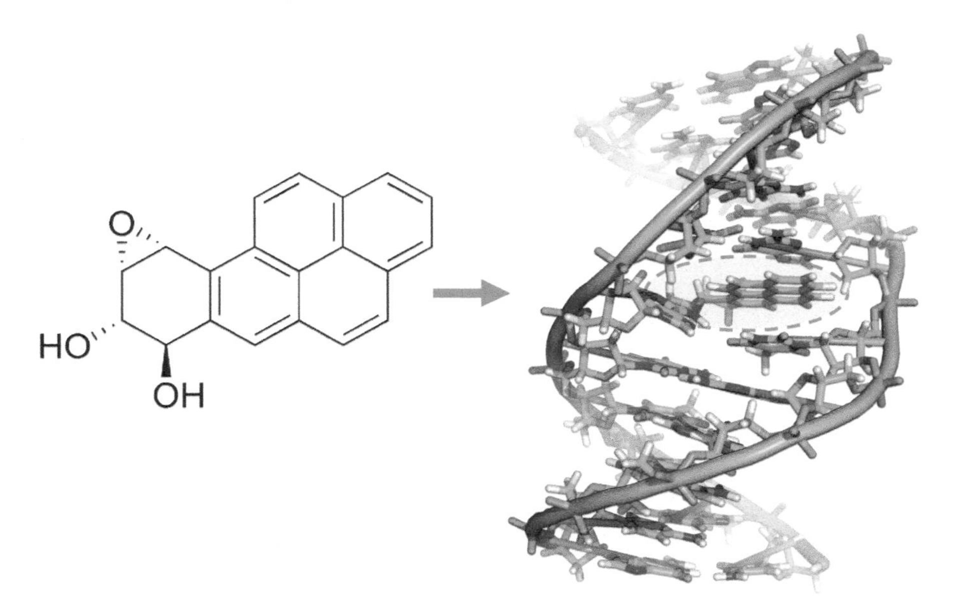

Fig. 1.9 BPDE forms a DNA adduct. The BPDE molecule (*left*) intercalates in the DNA double helix (*right*) and covalently bonds to a guanine residue at the N2 position. Illustration by Richard Wheeler. Source data from Pradhan et al. *Biochemistry* (2001) 40:5870–5881

and 1.11). Most pyrimidine photoproducts are repaired by a process known as nucleotide excision repair, a process that will be described in detail in Chap. 5. Failure of this DNA repair mechanism results in a single nucleotide substitution.

UV-B induced photoproducts largely involve pyrimidines that are adjacent to other pyrimidines. Accordingly, many of the tumor-associated mutations observed in sun-exposed skin are C → T single base transitions, with a significant number of CC → TT double base changes. In cases of the C → T single base transition, there is a significant bias towards mutation of C bases that occur in CpC dinucleotides. The CC → TT double base mutations observed occur most commonly in the context of the triplet sequence CCG. As described in earlier sections, the CpG dinucleotide is frequently methylated in the genome, suggesting that the double base changes observed probably result from the unique resolution of a photoproduct next to a methyl-cytosine (5mC) base. These base changes are unique to UV-B mediated mutagenesis, and are often referred to as the *UV signature*.

Ionizing Radiation (IR) Human tissues are intermittantly bombarded with high energy subatomic particles. Sources of ionizing radiation in the environment are both natural and anthropogenic. Depending on where they live and work, individuals encounter varying levels of radon gas that arises from the earth's crust and cosmic radiation that penetrates the atmosphere. Medical X-rays are a significant

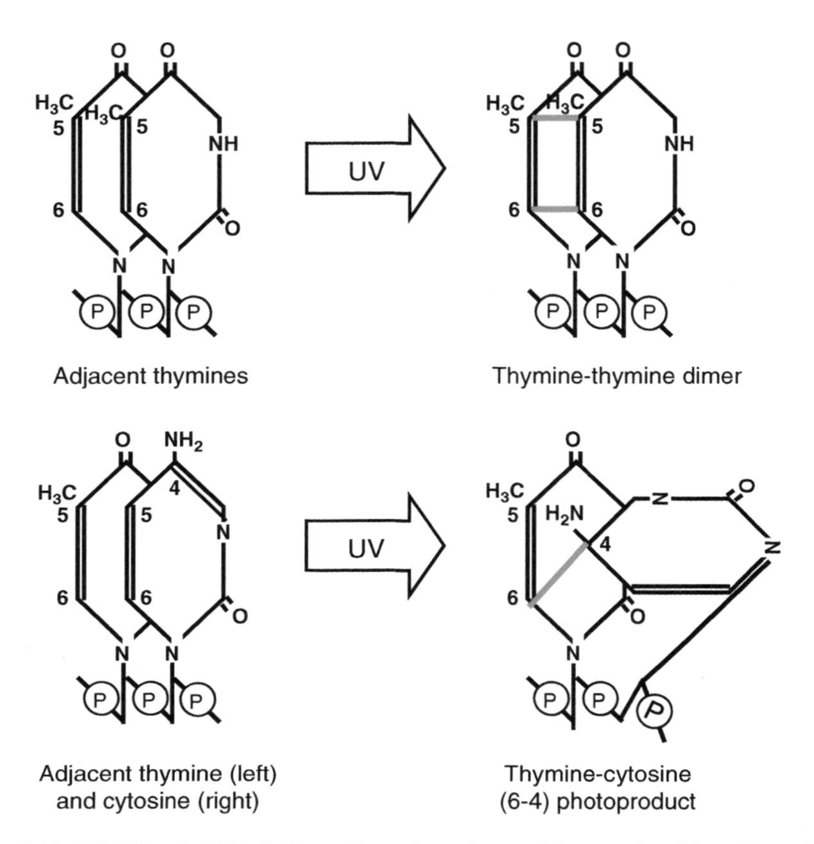

Fig. 1.10 UV-induced DNA lesions. Formation of a cyclobutane thymidine dimer (*top*). Formation of a (6–4) photoproduct between an adjacent thymidine and cytosine (*bottom*). A significant degree of distortion of the phosphodiester DNA backbone is caused by (6–4) photoproduct formation

source of exposure for some people. Radioactive fallout from nuclear weapons and nuclear accidents are problematic in more restricted areas and time periods.

When a subatomic particle of sufficient energy passes through a cell, it leaves a narrow track of ionized molecules in its wake. A large proportion of these are reactive oxygen species. These unstable and highly reactive molecules disrupt the phosphodiester bonds that form the DNA backbone and often result in a DNA break that affects both strands. Agents that create double strand DNA breaks are sometimes referred to as *clastogens*.

Ionizing radiation is a potent clastogen, but a significantly weaker mutagen. In other words, radiation causes many chromosomal breaks, but relatively few of these lesions resolve into a stable mutation that can be propagated by cell division. There are two ways in which double strand DNA breaks are repaired: *non-homologous end joining* (NHEJ), in which the two free ends of a broken chromosome are enzy-

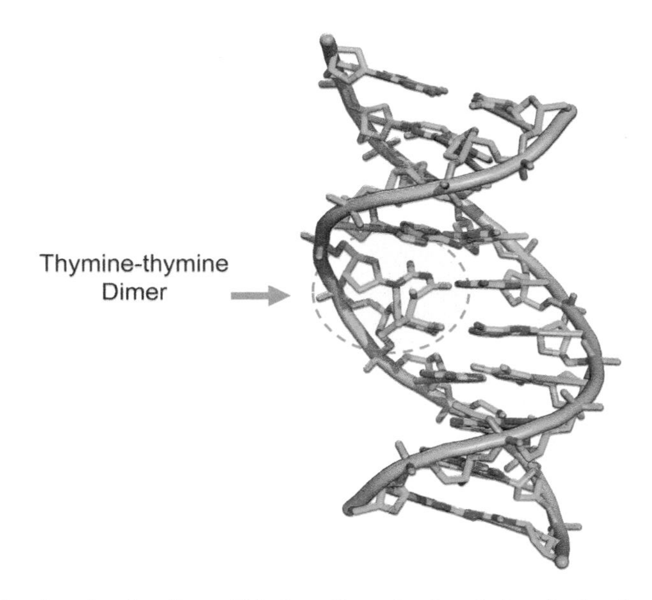

Fig. 1.11 Thymine-thymine dimer. This three-dimensional rendering of a thymine dimer reveals the local disruption of normal base-pairing. Illustration by Richard Wheeler. Source data from Park et al. *Proc Nat Acad Sci* (2002) 99:15965–15970

matically polished and then fused back together, and *homologous recombination*, a process that requires an intact sister chromatid that is used as a repair template. While homologous recombination uses extensive regions of sequence homology to align the damaged strand to the repair template, NHEJ exploits very short regions of incidental sequence similarity, termed *microhomologies*, to bring together and repair the damaged ends found at a break site. Both of these processes can reconstruct the original sequence, but NHEJ is the more error-prone of the two repair mechanisms due to erroneous pairings that occur by chance. Slippage between regions of microhomology contributes to NHEJ errors, particularly in mononucleotide repeat tracts. End processing that occurs during NHEJ also contributes to errors. Despite these sources of information loss, NHEJ has an error rate of only 1 %. The predominant mutation caused by ionizing radiation is the microdeletion, as would be expected if slippage during NHEJ was the principal mechanism of mutagenesis involved.

Single nucleotide substitutions are detected in radiation-associated cancers, although there is more limited information as to how these arise. Exposure to high doses of ionizing radiation has been shown to correlate with the appearance of several cancers, including cancer of the liver and basal cell cancer of the skin. In liver cancers associated with radiation exposure, a substantial number of single base alterations that affect the coding sequence for p53. The largest proportion of these is the $C \rightarrow T$ transition, predominantly occurring at non-CpG sites. This negative bias against the CpG dinucleotide implies that the observed transition is less likely to result from the accelerated turnover of 5mC, but rather results from the direct modification of bases by a direct effect of radiation. It is thought that direct oxidative modifications to cytosine might contribute to the later appearance of point mutations.

TP53 mutations are also found in skin cancers from individuals exposed to high levels of ionizing radiation. Long term follow-up of survivors of the atomic bomb blasts in Japan has provided valuable clues to the nature of radiation induced single base substitutions. When such individuals develop skin cancers, the etiology of the disease can be inferred from the location of the lesion. Skin cancers that occur in areas unexposed to sunlight are presumed to be associated with ionizing radiation exposure. The UV-associated basal cell cancers from these individuals contained the UV signature mutations described in the preceding section. The lesions attributable to ionizing radiation, in contrast, harbor *TP53* mutations that are C → T transitions at predominantly at non-CpG sites, similar to those observed in ionizing radiation-associated liver cancers.

Aflatoxin B1 Dietary exposure to aflatoxins is a significant risk factor for the development of liver cancer. Aflatoxins are produced by fungi, commonly found in regions of southeast Asia and sub-Saharan Africa, that grow on foods such as corn, rice and peanuts. Liver cancer is also endemic to these areas. A subtype of aflatoxin, known as aflatoxin B1 (AFB1), is a particularly potent carcinogen. Whereas the environmental agents previously discussed cause an array of different DNA base changes, exposure to AFB1 has been found to result in a single, unique alteration to the *TP53* gene. In more than 50 % of tumors that arise in areas with high levels of environmental AFB1, a G → T transversion changes codon 249 of *TP53* from AGG (encoding arginine, a basic amino acid) to AGT (encoding serine, a small nucleophilic amino acid).

Other positions in the genome are similarly mutated by AFB1. The mutagenic properties of AFB1 are acquired upon its metabolic conversion to its exo-8,9-epoxide form. The AFB1-epoxide reacts directly with guanine and forms a number of distinct adducts. These adducts are chemically reactive and promote depurination of the G and replacement with the pyrimidine T. The formation of adducts appears to be favored at the second G in GG dinucleotides, with the modification and subsequent mutation occurring at the second G. The base 3′ to the modified G also seems to confer some degree of site specificity. Overall, the known sequence biases do not fully account for all of the hotspots at which AFB1 has been shown to act, indicating that some additional structural factors remain to be discovered.

Inflammation Promotes the Propagation of Cancer Genes

As we have seen from the preceding examples, environmental carcinogens can directly convert normal genes to cancer genes by inducing mutations. In addition to their direct effects on DNA sequences, carcinogens can also promote the development of cancer by promoting the growth of cells that have acquired mutations. Many well-defined carcinogens help create localized conditions in which mutations are more likely to occur, and in which cells that harbor cancer genes can preferentially proliferate. A localized region of altered growth and cellular architecture in a tissue that is otherwise well-organized and homogeneous constitutes a tumor-promoting *microenvironment*. Cellular evidence of an inflammatory response is a central feature of such microenvironments.

Chronic inflammation is both a risk factor for initial cancer development as well as a consistent component of the microenvironment of established cancers. The relationship between inflammation and cancer was recognized as early as 1863 by Rudolf Virchow, who noted that some types of irritants could enhance cell proliferation. We now understand that inflammatory stimuli can simultaneously produce mutations and also create conditions that favor cell proliferation.

The dual effects of carcinogens in the generation of mutations and in the subsequent proliferation of mutant cells are exemplified by asbestos. Exposure to asbestos is a strong risk factor for the development of mesothelioma, a rare cancer that arises in the lining of the lungs and the pleural cavity.

Environmental asbestos exists in a number of fibrous forms. The physical properties of asbestos fibers made them a widely used component of fireproof ceramics and insulation, before the association of asbestos with lung disease was appreciated. It appears that these physical properties, combined with intrinsic chemical reactivity, make asbestos a potent carcinogen. Ingested by inhalation, asbestos fibers are engulfed by cells of the immune system by the process of phagocytosis. Longer fibers are incompletely phagocytized and are therefore inefficiently cleared from the lungs. Asbestos fibers are a chronic irritant that triggers a strong inflammatory response, clinically known as asbestosis.

The presence of asbestos in the lung leads to recruitment and activation of inflammatory cells, including pulmonary alveolar macrophages and neutrophils. The mediators of asbestos toxicity are reactive oxygen species and reactive nitrogen species that can damage DNA. Reactive oxygen species, including superoxide radicals and hydrogen peroxide, and reactive nitric oxide are released by activated inflammatory cells and irritated parenchymal cells. In addition, free radicals can be directly generated by asbestos fibers. Thus, there are two distinct sources of potentially mutagenic reactive species: the cells that are irritated by the asbestos fibers, and the fibers themselves.

Chronic inflammation is an important predisposing factor for many human cancers. It has been estimated that chronic inflammation contributes to the growth and spread of approximately one quarter of all malignancies. The best evidence that supports a role for inflammation in tumorigenesis is the clear etiologic relationship of inflammatory diseases and cancers. Diseases that have a significant inflammatory component can strongly predispose affected individuals to cancer. Some inflammatory diseases, like asbestosis, are related to an environmental exposure. Among the strongest links between chronic inflammation and carcinogenesis is the association between the inflammatory bowel diseases ulcerative colitis and Crohn's disease with the eventual development of colon cancer. Chronic inflammation has also been shown to be a significant risk factor for cancers of the esophagus, stomach, liver, prostate and urinary bladder. The underlying cause of the inflammation varies in these diseases but the relationship between chronic inflammation and the later development of cancer is similar.

Infectious agents are significant cause of chronic inflammation that promotes the growth of cancer. Accordingly, infectious agents that cause chronic inflammation have been shown to increase cancer risk. Collectively, infectious agents are thought to contribute to approximately 15–20 % of all cancers worldwide. Virus-associated cancers are particularly common and represent a significant, but theoretically tractable, public health problem.

The relationship between viruses and cancer is complex and largely beyond the scope of this text. Several carcinogenic viruses integrate into the genome and alter endogenous genes or deliver viral genes. The human papillomaviruses affect the epithelial cells of the uterine cervix and the head and neck by the transfer of genetic material (see Chap. 7). Another example is Herpesvirus 8, which integrates into the precursor cells of Kaposi sarcoma, a cancer frequently associated with acquired immune deficiency syndrome. Aside from these examples, most available evidence suggests that viruses and other infectious agents more often contribute to cancer indirectly by inducing host inflammatory responses. The Hepatitis B and C viruses, for example, cause chronic inflammation of the liver and facilitate the subsequent development of liver cancer. In parts of Asia, the combined effects of Hepatitis virus infection and exposure to the mutagen aflatoxin B1 increase cancer risk 1000-fold. Numerous infectious agents that cause chronic inflammation also significantly increase the lifetime risk of developing cancer (Table 1.2).

How does inflammation contribute to the development of cancer? The relationship between these two complex processes remains to be completely understood, but several aspects are clear. An important factor is the creation of somatic mutations by free radicals. As demonstrated by the potent carcinogen asbestos, highly reactive free radicals can be generated by both the agent and by the cellular component of the immune response. Infectious agents typically induce a strong cellular immune response, a component of which is the production of free radicals. Leukocytes and other phagocytic cells normally produce these highly reactive spe-

Table 1.2 Chronic inflammation and cancer predisposition

Infectious agent	Type	Inflammatory disease	Cancer
Hepatitis B virus	DNA virus	Hepatitis	Liver cancer
Hepatitis C virus			
Helicobacter pylori	Bacterium	Gastritis	Stomach cancer
Epstein-Barr virus	DNA virus	Mononucleosis	B-cell, non-Hodgkin's lymphoma
			Burkitts lymphoma
Human Papillomavirus	DNA virus	Cervicitis	Cervical cancer
Schistosoma haematobium	Trematode	Cystitis	Bladder cancer
Opisthorchis viverrini	Flatworm	Cholangitis	Bile duct cancer

cies to kill and denature infectious agents. Reactive oxygen and nitrogen species react to form peroxynitrite, a powerful mutagen. An elevation in the rate of mutagenesis thus appears to be a byproduct of a vigorous immune response.

The humoral component of the inflammatory response, the local production of signaling proteins known as cytokines and chemokines, also appears to be an important factor in tumorigenesis. These molecules are potent stimulators of cell division and function to recruit additional immune cells and activate local fibroblasts that will amplify the inflammatory response. Activated cells also secrete proteolytic enzymes that break down the extracellular matrix and thereby alter the tissue structure. These changes can alter cell spacing and render cells more mobile.

Importantly, the secretion of bioactive peptides promotes the outgrowth of new blood vessels, a process known as *angiogenesis*. Changes in local blood flow can expand the niches where cells can grow. The combined affects of these changes appear to provide a fertile environment for the proliferation of cells that have acquired cancer genes and the subsequent growth of tumors. The humoral component of inflammation thus transforms the microenvironment and the blood circulation in ways that favor the proliferation of cells with cancer genes.

Inflammation can play a significant role in two distinct stages of a cancer: tumor initiation and subsequent tumor growth and progression. While the majority of cancers arise in the absence of a known chronic inflammatory disease, inflammatory cells contribute to the microenvironment of most established tumors. When analyzed histologically, established tumors are commonly found to contain large numbers of infiltrating inflammatory cells (Fig. 1.12). Indeed, a significant proportion of the mass of a typical tumor is comprised of cells produced by the immune system. Viewed histologically and as gross specimens, cancers resemble wounds that do not heal.

It is not difficult to imagine how the profusion of mitogenic stimuli, the weakening of the extracellular matrix and the onset of angiogenesis that occurs in inflamed tissues might promote the continued clonal proliferation of cells that have acquired cancer genes. Obviously, the function of the immune system is not to promote cancer. On the contrary, the inflammatory response seen in many established tumors may be a futile attempt by the host immune system to eliminate those tumors. It is likely that many early tumors do in fact die off in the miasma created by the immune system, which is in many ways toxic. The growth of tumors might be best characterized as an ongoing battle between cancer cells and the immune system. This battle is gradually lost as cancer cells evade immune surveillance and acquire new phenotypes that allow them to survive and proliferate where normal, unmutated, cells would fail to thrive.

Stem Cells, Darwinian Selection and the Clonal Evolution of Cancers

In the preceding sections, we have seen how mutations arise. It this section and those that follow, we will explore how individual mutations can accumulate in a single cell lineage that gives rise to a tumor.

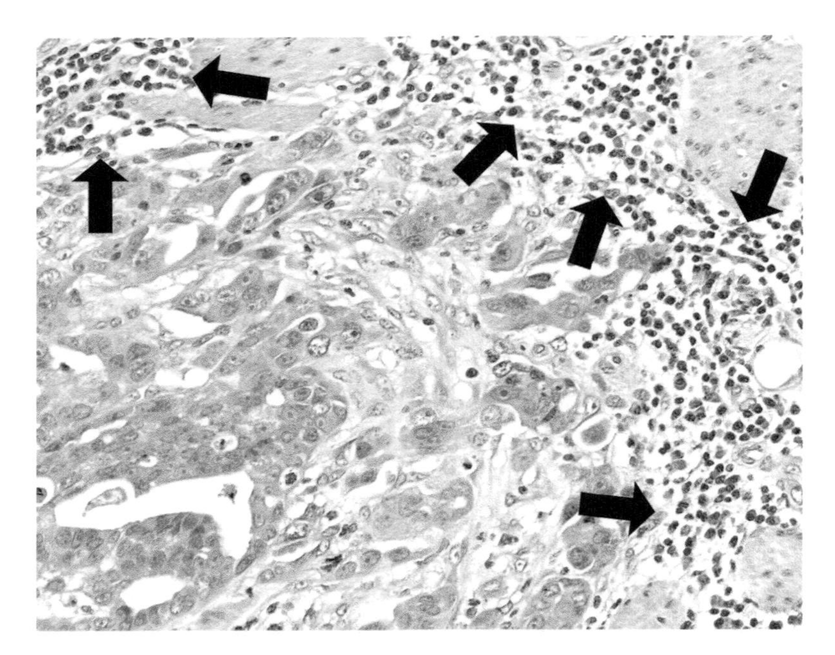

Fig. 1.12 Cancers exhibit areas of chronic inflammation. Inflammatory cells (indicated by *arrows*) are present throughout this section of a stomach adenocarcinoma. Image courtesy of Angelo De Marzo MD, PhD, The Johns Hopkins University

A useful theoretical framework for understanding how mutations drive the initiation and subsequent growth of tumors is provided by the clonal evolution model, first proposed in 1976 by Peter Nowell. According to this model, tumors arise from a single progenitor cell that has acquired a growth-changing mutation. Several lines of evidence support this idea. The pattern of X chromosome inactivation is usually uniform in cancer cell populations, an observation that is consistent with a single founder. Similarly, lymphoid neoplasms that produce immunoglobulins almost always produce a single, clonal isotype. Genetic analysis of primary tumors, from the level of DNA sequence to whole chromosomes, typically reveals phenotypically relevant mutations and structural changes that are present in all tumor cells, suggesting a unicellular origin. The preponderance of evidence indicates that the cancer cells that ultimately compose a tumor mass are vertically derived from a founder cell and therefore contain the same cancer genes. In this sense, individual tumors are clonal cell populations descended from a mutated founder.

How do such clones arise? When a somatic mutation creates a new cancer gene in a cell there exists for a time only a single copy of that newly acquired mutant allele. That mutation will only become fixed in a larger population of cells if that original cell divides and gives rise to progeny that also contain the mutant gene. The mutant clone thus expands by the process of cell proliferation. Progression of a cancer thus requires clonal expansion of cells that harbor cancer genes.

A somatic mutation that occurs in a non-dividing cell would not expand along with a growing clone and therefore could not contribute to a cancer. In fact, the majority of adult human cells do not proliferate and are said to be *terminally differentiated*, a state in which these cells are fully matured and functional. In tissues that have the capacity to regenerate, the proliferative activity that gives rise to new cells resides exclusively in a relatively small population of relatively less differentiated cells known as *somatic stem cells,* sometimes referred to as *adult stem cells.* Somatic stem cells have two defining properties: (*1*) the ability to continuously divide and generate daughter cells that remain undifferentiated (a property known as self-renewal), and (*2*) the ability to generate other daughter cells that are fated to terminally differentiate into one or more distinct cell types or lineages. Such cells replace dead or obsolete cells and thereby maintain the tissue in a steady state, known as homeostasis. Because the daughter cells that arise from a dividing stem cell can have these distinct fates, the proliferation of somatic stem cells is often referred to as *asymmetric cell division.*

As in normal tissues, the ongoing proliferative potential of some tumors exclusively resides in a stem cell-like subpopulation known as *cancer stem cells.* Like somatic stem cells, cancer stem cells have an intrinsic capacity to self-renew. But cancer stem cells do not repopulate a healthy tissue composed of a variety of differentiated cells. Instead, they add to the mass and bulk of a growing tumor, and in experimental studies, can recapitulate the tumor in a new animal. The cancer stem cell model for tumor growth does not apply to all types of cancer. Many common tumor types do not appear to rely on a distinct distinct population of cancer stem cells for their overall growth. Rather the majority of the cells that compose such tumors appear to have the capacity to proliferate indefinitely. Cancer stem cells are best described in hematologic cancers, and may not be relevant to most solid tumor types.

Why do cell clones that harbor cancer genes expand? Nowell elegantly hypothesized that cancer genes confer a selective growth advantage that allows the cells that harbor them to essentially out-compete neighboring cells. This phenomenon is in many ways analogous to speciation as explained by Charles Darwin in his theory of evolution. Natural selection occurs when an individual organism occupies a niche in which that organism's genotype confers an advantage. That advantage is selective if it promotes the production of progeny. New niches present new opportunities for individual genotypes to potentially thrive. Advantageous proliferation within a niche can eventually lead to speciation. In an illustrative analogy, tumorigenesis can be viewed as a form of cellular speciation.

Tissues represent a cellular niche. A region of tissue that encompasses a cellular niche is often called a compartment. In adults, the number of cells that occupy a self-renewing tissue compartment, such as the epithelial lining of the gastrointestinal tract or the marrow within bony trabeculae, is normally stable. Stability depends upon the delicate balance between two opposing processes: the proliferation of adult stem cells and cell death. In a stable compartment, the number of cells that arises though stem cell division is equal to the number of cells that mature into individual functionally specialized cells, stop proliferating and ultimately die. Cells thus are added to the compartment via the proliferation of stem cells, perform their

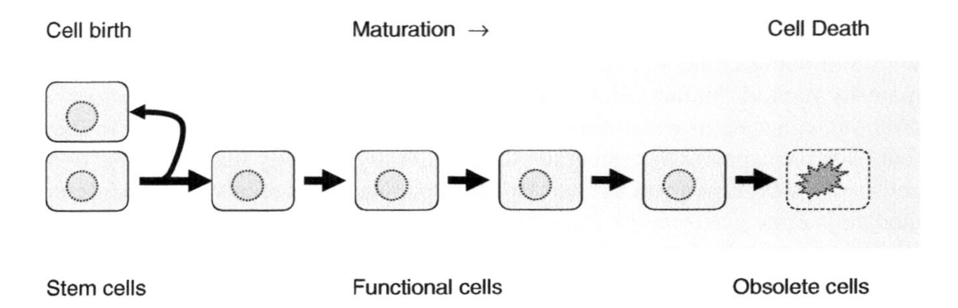

Fig. 1.13 Homeostasis within a tissue compartment. Stem cells undergo an asymmetrical division in which one daughter cell is fated to mature and the other remains an undifferentiated stem cell. Thus stem cell populations self-renew. Mature, differentiated cells carry out the various functions of the tissue, until they reach the end of their lifespans and are eliminated from the compartment. In stable compartments, the rate of cell birth is equal to the rate of cell death. Highly proliferative compartments can be completely renewed in several days

functions as mature, non-proliferating cells, and exit the compartment via cell death (Fig. 1.13). Cells that occupy highly proliferative compartments possess a large number of stem cells and typically also feature an intrinsic and highly-regulated program that actively induces cell death. This highly programmed, physiologically-activated form of cell death is known as *apoptosis*. Apoptosis is distinct from cell death that results from insult or injury in that it contributes to the stability of that tissue compartment.

The finely tuned balance between stem cell proliferation and apoptotic cell death dictates the stability of a given compartment, a property alternatively known as *tissue homeostasis*. Tissue homeostasis is disrupted when the rate of cell birth is unequal to the rate of maturation, cell death and removal.

Cancer genes cause a disruption in tissue homeostasis. If a gene confers a phenotype that increases proliferation or prevents maturation or cell death, then the cells that harbor that gene may begin to outnumber other cells in that compartment and form a neoplasm. This is the first stage of the clonal evolution of a tumor.

Selective Pressure and Adaptation: Hypoxia and Altered Metabolism

The precise growth-suppressive forces that favor the selection of cells that harbor specific cancer genes differs widely between different tissues, and in most sites remain incompletely understood. The causal relationship between inflammation and cancer provides one significant clue as to the nature of clonal selection and how the acquisition of cancer genes can facilitate adaptation, survival and proliferation.

As described previously, many cancers arise in proliferative tissues that are chronically inflamed. Inflammation creates numerous changes in the local environment (microenvironment) of a cellular compartment. The activation of free radical-producing cells, the release of humoral factors and secretion of enzymes combine to alter tissue structure and also change the microenvironmental concentrations of oxygen, glucose and hydrogen ions (as reflected in the pH). These changes produce selective pressure that favors the growth of cells that have acquired new attributes. Cells that can continue to proliferate in these conditions would be more likely to survive as a viable clone. In the terminology of Darwinian evolution, inflammation creates a new niche into which speciation can occur. A key question is: how do cancer cells adapt to new niches?

To illustrate the role of adaptation in clonal evolution, we will consider a single cellular characteristic that is known to be altered by mutation during tumorigenesis: energy metabolism. Cancer cells acquire altered metabolic states that enhance survival in adverse microenvironments.

In 1930, Otto Warburg observed that the metabolism of cancer cells differs from that of normal cells. While normal cells produce energy primarily by the aerobic process oxidative phosphorylation, the cells in tumors rely more heavily on anaerobic glycolysis, even when oxygen is available. This metabolic switch that occurs during tumorigenesis has subsequently come to be known as the *Warburg effect*.

Glycolysis is relatively inefficient. While 36–38 molecules of ATP are produced by the complete oxidation of one molecule of glucose, only 2 ATP molecules are generated by the anaerobic conversion of glucose into pyruvate.

Glycolysis

$$\text{Glucose} + 2\text{P}_i + 2\text{ADP} + 2\text{NAD}^+ \rightarrow 2\text{pyruvate} + 2\text{ATP} + 2\text{NADH} + 2\text{H}^+ + 2\text{H}_2\text{O}$$

Oxidative phosphorylation

$$\text{Glucose} + 36\,\text{ADP} + 36\text{P}_i + 36\text{H}^+ + 6\text{O}_2 \rightarrow 6\text{CO}_2 + 36\text{ATP} + 42\text{H}_2\text{O}$$

The hydrogen ions produced as a byproduct of the glycolysis reaction cause the acidification of the cellular microenvironment. Cancer cells thus appear to acquire a phenotype that is both energetically inefficient and environmentally toxic. The obvious drawbacks of this metabolic switch are apparently outweighed by at least one critical attribute: the ability to survive and proliferate under conditions of oxygen deprivation.

The structure of normal tissues is constrained by blood supply. Blood flow enhances tissue oxygenation and thus facilitates aerobic respiration. Cell proliferation is a process that requires a significant amount of energy – energy that in normal cells is generated via oxidation of glucose. Proliferation of normal cells is therefore favored in regions that are well-oxygenated. Conversely, proliferation of normal cells is limited in tissue spaces that have low oxygen tension, an environmental state known as *hypoxia*. In normal cell compartments, proliferation is spatially restricted to regions that are close to the local blood supply. Experimentally, hypoxia has been detected in tumor tissues that are more than 100 μm from the nearest blood vessel.

In areas that are relatively distant from the blood supply, hypoxia creates a niche with a distinct selective pressure. While cancer cells tend to metabolize glucose inefficiently, they also have a lower reliance on oxygen because their glycolytic pathways are upregulated. Cancer cells are thus adapted to a niche that is inhospitable to normal cells.

Multiple Somatic Mutations Punctuate Clonal Evolution

Genetic analysis of cancer samples shows that most cancer cells contain multiple cancer genes. This implies that multiple somatic mutations are required during the process of tumorigenesis. A large body of experimental evidence has shown that this is in fact the case. How does the process of clonal evolution relate to the acquisition of multiple mutations?

Somatic mutations can occur by a variety of processes, including the stochastic deamination of methylated cytosines, errors during DNA replication and repair, and chemical mutagenesis caused by environmental carcinogens and inflammatory agents. In rare instances, somatic mutations will convert a normal gene into a new allele that promotes tumorigenesis. A proliferative cell clone harboring a cancer gene will expand beyond the confines of its normal niche if that cancer gene provides a unique advantage that allows it out-compete its neighbors that do not harbor the mutation. This outgrowth of cells becomes a microscopic neoplasm.

What happens next? In most cases, nothing happens. In tissues that have been carefully studied, it appears that most neoplastic clones fail to progress and eventually die off. Most neoplasms therefore represent a dead end for that clonal lineage. In these cases, the growth advantage attained by a neoplasm is apparently not sufficient to allow sustained expansion. Perhaps the expanding cell clone encountered a new selective pressure, such as a successful immune response by the host. An expanding cell clone might also fall victim to the byproducts of its own proliferative success by contributing to a critical shortage of oxygen or overabundance of metabolically-derived acid. The barriers to tumor growth, and therefore the selective pressures that appear as a tumor grows, are many and varied.

Proliferating cell clones are neoplasms by definition, but not all neoplasms develop into cancers. Just as a very small proportion of cells that are mutated give rise to neoplasms, only a small proportion of neoplasms progress to clinically evident cancers. Again, an analogy can be made to the evolution of biological life forms. Most genetic changes are predicted to lead to either no advantage or a disadvantage. Mutations are most often a dead end. In biology as in the biological microcosm that is cancer, only the rare mutation creates a selective advantage. The neoplasms that do progress to tumors are rare products of clonal evolution.

As a neoplasm grows, the local microenvironment undergoes changes. Concomitant with cell proliferation is the local decrease in the concentrations of metabolic precursors and an increase in metabolic products. As the number of cells increase, the ratio of the cells that occupy the periphery of the neoplasm (which contact the neighboring normal cells) to the cells that are in the middle of the neoplasm (which only contact other cells of the proliferating clone) gets progressively smaller. The space occupied by the proliferating cell mass will alter the spacing between adjacent cells and one another and between all cells and the nearest blood vessel. Local oxygen, glucose and hydrogen ion concentrations will all change. Once a tumor becomes invasive, the cells at the leading edge of the invasion encounter new niches that present unique barriers. A small proportion of cells that break free of the original tumor mass and travel to distant parts of the body will survive detachment, transit through the blood or lymphatic system, and reseed to grow as a new metastatic tumor, often in a very different type of tissue.

During tumorigenesis, newly acquired genetic alterations confer new properties to the tumor cells. The rare neoplasms that progress acquire additional cancer genes by somatic mutation. In such cases, a clone containing the initiating mutation expands and eventually a single cell within that clone acquires an additional mutation. If this new mutation favors proliferation in the contemporary microenvironment, then that cell may give rise to a new clonal population that is better adapted to continued growth. The new clone may outgrow the previous clone as it continues to expand. In this manner, multiple rounds of mutation followed by waves of clonal expansion eventually give rise to a clinically apparent cancer (Fig. 1.14).

Clonal evolution is an iterative and dynamic process. The two steps of this process are somatic mutation and clonal expansion into constantly changing niches. Both steps are equally important. Somatic mutation gives rise to the phenotypes that favor improved growth and survival, while clonal expansion provides a growing number of proliferative cells that can subsequently acquire additional mutations.

Tumor Growth Leads to Cellular Heterogeneity

The clonal evolution model for cancer progression provides a theoretical framework for understanding how the lengthy process of tumorigenesis begins, and the forces that propel it forward. How well does this theory conform to the observed genetic characteristics of real tumors?

In its simplest interpretation, the clonal evolution model would predict that the majority of cells in a tumor would be genetically identical. That is, the ultimate wave of clonal expansion would have given rise to the majority of cells that compose the bulk of any identified tumor. In reality, the cells that compose many tumors, particularly late stage solid tumors, do not appear to be completely identical. Multiple biopsies of different regions of a tumor, or distinct metastases, often reveal cell populations that have unique mutations not shared by all of the other cells in the tumor. Such observations strongly suggest that multiple subclones can expand in parallel during tumorigenesis and coexist in late stage tumors.

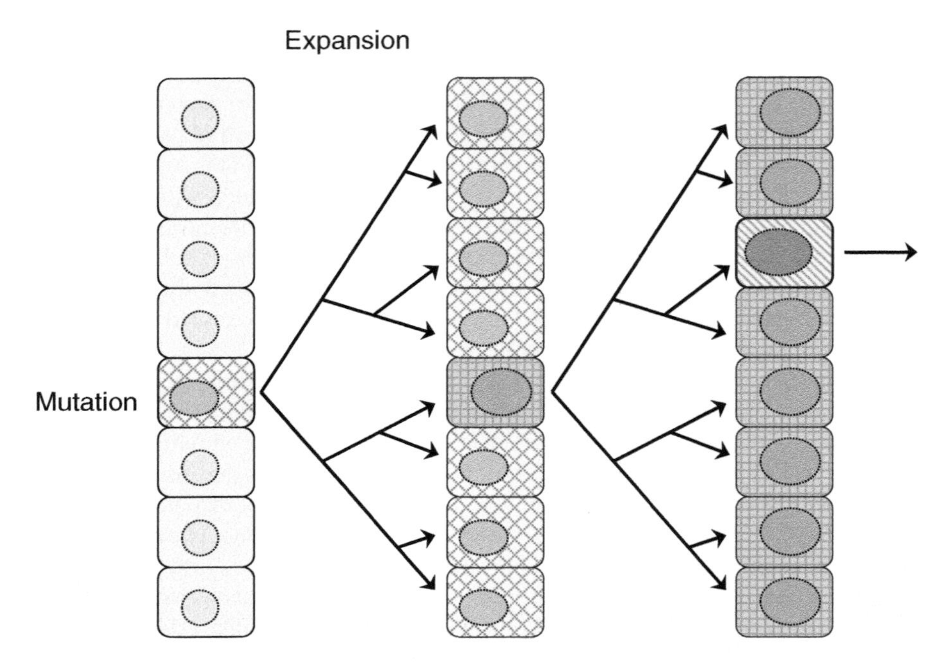

Fig. 1.14 Clonal evolution of a neoplasm. A single cell in a normal tissue acquires an alteration that confers a growth advantage. That cell divides and thus expands over time into a distinct clone. A cell within that clone acquires a second mutation that provides an additional growth advantage. A tumor results from iterative rounds of mutation and clonal expansion. Concept from *The Genetic Basis of Human* Kinzler and Vogelstein, eds., McGraw Hill (2002)

Highly penetrant cancer genes such as mutated *TP53* are typically found to be uniformly present in all cells of a given tumor in which such an alteration has been identified, suggesting that mutation of *TP53* provides a relatively strong selective advantage. It is possible that in the case of mutations that provide a weaker selective advantage, or a selective advantage that is only manifest within a distinct niche, cell clones that fail to acquire this new characteristic would nonetheless continue to expand, perhaps at a slightly lower rate or by a different route. In patients with diagnosed cancers, anti-tumor therapies can create new selective pressures that favor the outgrowth of distinct cellular subclones. Some of the mutations that occur in expanding neoplastic clones do not appear to provide any selective advantage whatsoever. Such mutations, propagated simply because they happened to arise in an already expanding clone, or were present in the original precursor cell, are known as *passenger mutations*.

The ongoing acquisition of passenger mutations contributes to tumor heterogeneity, particularly in larger tumors that are generationally farther removed from their cellular precursors. Spatial variations in the tumor microenviroment might also create unique selective pressures that unequally favor some subclones over others.

From an evolutionary perspective, genetic heterogeneity increases the adaptability of a population to new environmental challenges. Consistent with this concept, cell-to-cell intratumoral genetic heterogeneity is a characteristic that can enhance the overall viability of a tumor in the face of alterations to their microenvironment, including those induced by drugs designed to kill tumor cells or to slow their growth. Indeed, tumor heterogeneity has been reported to correlate with therapeutic resistance. These concepts will be further described in Chap. 6.

Tumors Are Distinguished by Their Spectrum of Driver Gene Mutations and Passenger Gene Mutations

Cancer-associated gene mutations fall into two general functional categories: (1) mutations that provide a selective growth advantage and are therefore are required for tumorigenesis and, (2) mutations that merely occur before or during tumorigenesis and do not directly contribute to the ongoing proliferation of cancer cell clones. These two categories of gene mutations have been referred to as *drivers* and *passengers*, respectively. Cancer genes contain driver mutations, by definition. Driver genes confer selective advantages during clonal evolution, and thus 'drive' the process forward. In contrast, passenger gene mutations do not appear in tumors as a result of evolutionary selection. Rather, a passenger gene mutation occurs by chance in a cell that harbors a driver gene mutation. As a clone that contains a cancer gene expands, the passenger mutation is propagated along with a driver gene mutation, and in that sense merely comes along for the ride. Normal, proliferative tissues that are non-cancerous often have significant numbers of mutations that have no apparent effect on cell growth or tissue morphology. Such observations provide strong evidence that many clonal passenger mutations found in established tumors were likely present in the normal precursor cells, prior to the initial round of clonal expansion.

Each cancer harbors its own distinct set of genetic alterations. There is considerable overlap in the genes that are recurrently found in tumors of the same type, and also in tumors from different sites altogether. A relatively small number of driver mutations are commonly found in many cancers (Fig. 1.15). Known as *recurrent driver mutations,* such commonly observed genetic alterations provide important insights into to the cellular processes that are typically defective in one or more cancer types. In contrast, specific passenger mutations are rarely found in multiple cancers. This is because passenger mutations arise at random, and only expand by virtue of their coincidence with driver mutations. Passenger mutations are therefore much less likely to arise independently in more than one tumor. Driver mutations arise at random as well but, because of their effect on cell growth, clones that harbor them tend to expand.

Colorectal Cancer: A Model for Understanding the Process of Tumorigenesis

Clonal evolution is an interesting hypothesis that incorporates the concepts of mutation, clonal expansion and population dynamics to explain how tumors arise in cellular compartments. But does it really describe what happens in a tumor? What is

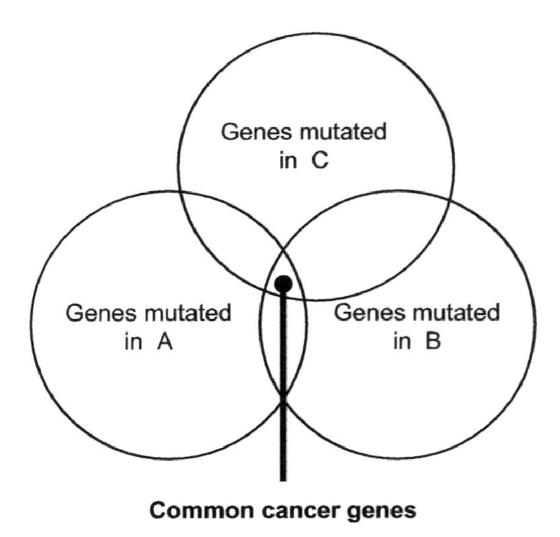

Fig. 1.15 Common and unique drivers of cancers from the same tissue. The driver mutations found in cancers are diverse and often tissue-specific. In this example, comparison of the set of genes mutated in tumors A, B and C shows that some driver mutations are unique to each tumor in which they occur, but there is also significant overlap. A small proportion of mutated genes are common to all three tumors; these represent highly prevalent cancer genes

the evidence that tumors actually arise in a step-wise manner consistent with the clonal evolution theory?

The earliest and perhaps best evidence comes from classic genetic studies of tumors in the large bowel. Tumors that arise in the epithelium of the colon and rectum are very common. Nearly one half of the US population is affected by colorectal tumors, most of which are benign. Nearly 5 % of the US population will develop colorectal cancer, the second leading cause of cancer-related death. The most common histological type is adenocarcinoma, which arises from epithelial and glandular cells.

Unlike many types of tumors, tumors of the colon and rectum are highly accessible. Through the use of endoscopy, a widely used screening technique, colorectal tumors can be directly visualized at all different stages of growth. At the time of diagnosis, tissue specimens can be readily be obtained for DNA analysis. The high prevalence and accessibility of colorectal tumors has provided a unique opportunity to study the genes that contribute to tumorigenesis at each step of the disease process. Collectively, these studies have provided a paradigm for understanding how the accumulation of cancer genes gives rise to a cancer.

The gastrointestinal system is composed of readily defined tissue compartments. Several cell types contribute to the luminal surface of the gastrointestinal tract known as the mucosa (Fig. 1.16). The normal mucosal surface of the colon is composed of invaginations known as crypts, which function to maximize the surface area of the large bowel. These crypts are lined with a single layer of epithelial cells of three different types: absorptive cells, mucus-secreting goblet cells, and neuroepithelial cells. At the base of each crypt are 4–6 adult stem cells, which give rise to the mature cells of the crypt. These proliferative cells predominantly multiply in the

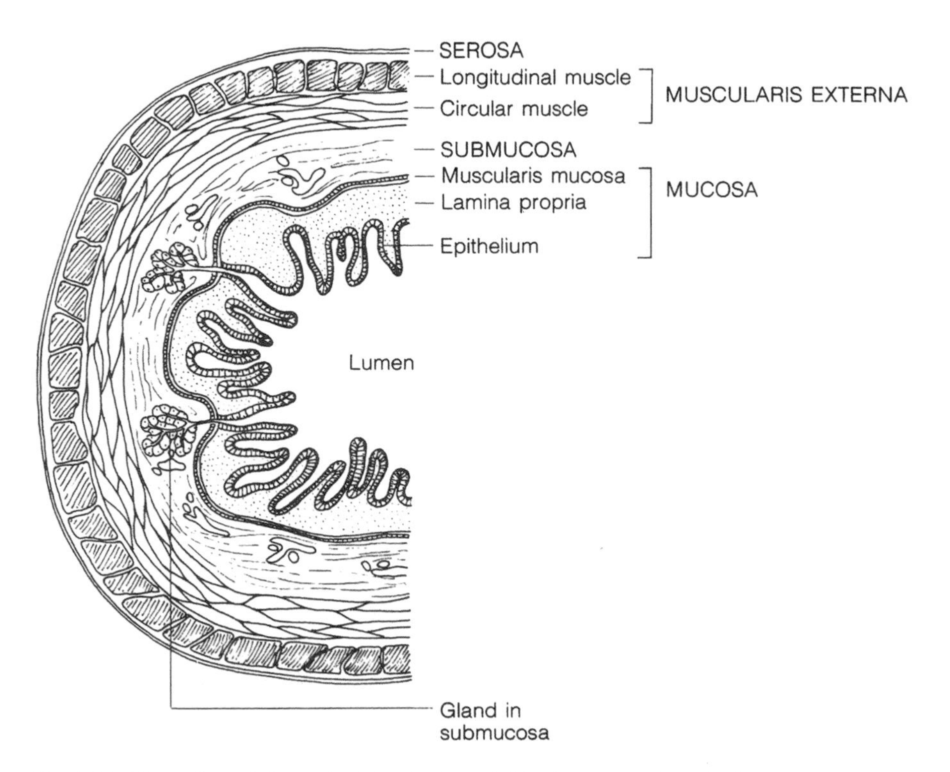

Fig. 1.16 The lining of the gastrointestinal tract. The inner-most layer is the mucosa, a membrane that forms a continuous lining of the entire gastrointestinal tract. In the large bowel, this tissue contains cells that produce mucus to lubricate and protect the smooth inner surface of the bowel wall. Connective tissue and muscle separate the muscosa from the second layer, the submucosa, which contains blood vessels, lymph vessels, nerves and mucus-producing glands. External to the submucosa is the muscularis externa, consisting of two layers of muscle fibers, one that runs lengthwise and one that encircles the bowel. The fourth layer, the serosa, is a thin membrane that produces fluid to lubricate the outer surface of the bowel so that it can slide against adjacent organs. Drawing courtesy of the National Cancer Institute

lower one third of the crypt, differentiate in the upper two thirds and are eventually extruded at the apex of the crypt and thereby lost into the lumen (Fig. 1.17). The epithelial cells of a crypt are thus a clonal population derived from a self-renewing population of stem cells at the base. Colonic crypts are a well-defined cellular compartment, where cells are born, mature, function and die in a linear space.

The smallest colorectal neoplasm that is observable within the colonic mucosa, either by microscopy or by staining with the dye methylene blue, is the aberrant crypt focus. These lesions can affect one crypt or span several adjacent crypts. An aberrant crypt focus is the earliest indication that the delicate balance between cell birth, maturation and death within a crypt has been perturbed.

The earliest grossly observable manifestation of a colorectal tumor is the polyp, a growth of cells that often extends into the bowel wall and projects into the intestinal lumen. Polyps fall into two histological classes: non-dysplastic (also called

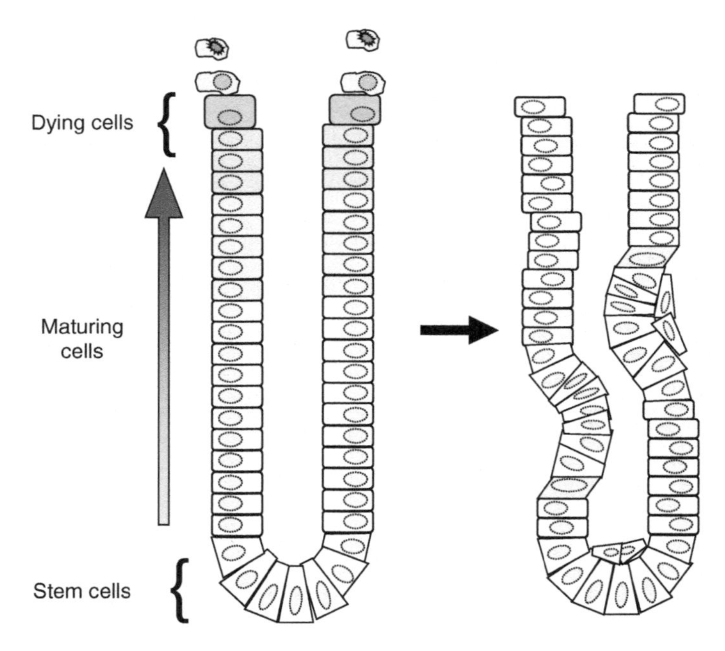

Fig. 1.17 Cell birth and death in a colon crypt. The invaginations of the colorectal epithelium form structurally-defined tissue compartments known as crypts. In this simplified representation, an increase in cell birth or decrease in cell death leads to hypercellularity and loss of tissue organization

hyperplastic) and dysplastic (also called adenomatous) polyps. Non-dysplastic polyps have an ordered epithelial structure that is similar to that of normal crypts. These tumors are benign and are thought to have a low tendency to progress. In contrast, adenomatous polyps exhibit a significant degree of dysplasia, a histologic characteristic that suggests an underlying cellular disorder. Epithelial cells can line up in multiple layers, and frequently have enlarged nuclei at atypical locations within the cell. Larger adenomas often contain projections of dysplastic crypts that confer what is known as a 'villous' morphology. Adenomas become more dysplastic as they grow larger in size. With size they also become more likely to invade surrounding tissues, at which point they are defined as malignant.

Tumor growth can be discontinuous. For example, a small polyp may remain dormant for years or even decades. But when a subsequent mutation occurs in one proliferating cell, a new wave of expansion can occur. A small but significant proportion of adenomas progress and become malignant tumors. The size of an adenoma is a reliable indicator of its malignant potential. Few adenomas that are less than 10 mm in diameter will progress to malignancy, but adenomas larger than 10 mm will have an estimated 15 % chance of becoming malignant in the subsequent 10 years. Advanced colorectal tumors can locally metastasize to the mesenteric lymph nodes or travel more distantly, typically to the peritoneum and the liver.

Benign polyps can usually be resected during colonoscopy, but malignant tumors require more extensive surgery. The probability of a cure is significantly lower if a tumor has metastasized. In such cases, surgery is combined with a form of adjuvant therapy such as chemotherapy or treatment with ionizing radiation.

In seminal studies conducted in the 1980s and 1990s, Bert Vogelstein, Kenneth Kinzler, and Eric Fearon demonstrated how specific genetic alterations underlie the stepwise progression of colorectal tumors. The illustration of the defined stages of a colorectal tumor combined with the mutations commonly associated with these transitions is often referred to as a Vogelgram (Fig. 1.18). The detailed study of colorectal neoplasia form a paradigm for understanding how cancer genes contribute to tumorigenesis.

Do Cancer Cells Divide More Rapidly Than Normal Cells?

Cancer is often described in lay terms as a disease caused by cells that are 'out of control'. This is an apt description. Cancer cells do not respond appropriately to the controls that inhibit growth, including spatial, humoral and metabolic signals that would halt the proliferation of normal cells. However, it might be inferred that 'out of control' cancer cells are dividing more rapidly and thus have a shorter doubling time than normal proliferating cells. There is little evidence that this is the case, and in fact the opposite may be true.

Malignant tumors occur disproportionately in older people. The incidence of polyps, the precursors of cancer, and advanced tumors in different age groups indicates that colorectal cancers result from several decades of clonal evolution. By the time an adenoma reaches 10 mm in diameter, and therefore has the potential to progress into a malignant cancer, it may contain roughly 10^9 cells. This number of cells could theoretically be achieved by only 30 sequential population doublings ($2^{30} = 10^9$), if all progeny were to continually proliferate. There is little evidence that growing cancer cells divide at a faster rate than do the stem cells in the base of a normal crypt. The epithelial cells in a normal crypt are replaced every 3–4 days by the proliferation of stem cells at the base of the crypt. At this rate, normal crypt epithelia turn over about 100 times every year. By this simple measure, the stem cells that give rise to normal colonic epithelia appear to be much more highly proliferative in nature than the proliferative tumor cells of colorectal cancers.

An abnormally high proliferation rate is not required to account for a typical tumor mass, given the time frame in which solid tumors are known to arise. Therefore, from a theoretical perspective, there is no reason to expect that the cells in a neoplasm will proliferate more rapidly than normal dividing cells. The idea behind the clonal evolution model is that neoplasms continue to divide, and fail to die, in changing microenvironments to which they are well-adapted. The net growth rate of an expanding neoplastic clone is the rate of cell division (or cell birth) minus the rate of cell death. Each driver mutation has been estimated to confer only a very slight increase, on the order of 0.4 %, in the net growth rate. However, the compounding effects of this small rate difference, over decades, results in the large number of cells that compose late stage, metastatic tumors.

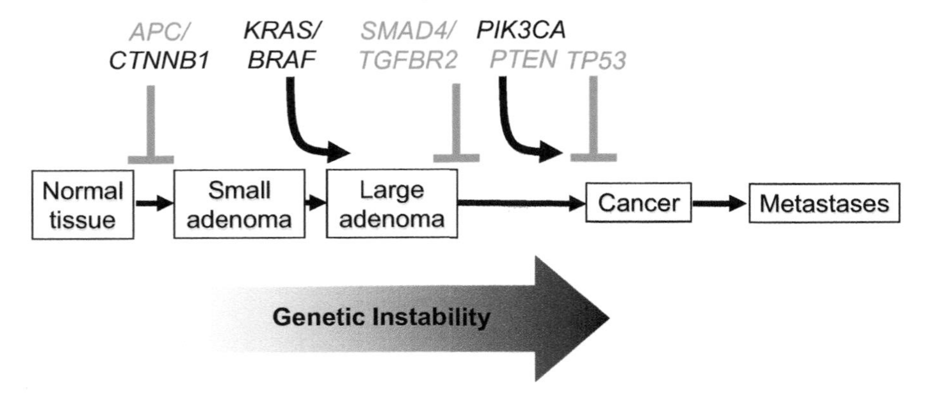

Fig. 1.18 Genetic alterations drive colorectal tumorigenesis. The Vogelgram illustrates the relationship between the histological stages of colorectal tumor development and the cancer genes that facilitate clonal expansion. Some cancer genes directly promote the growth of tumor cells (shown in *black*). Mutations in other cancer genes remove barriers to tumor growth (shown in *red*). The larger cellular pathways that are controlled by these genes can inhibit (red stops) or promote (black arrows) tumor progression when they are dysregulated by mutated cancer genes. The acquisition of successive genetic alterations is accelerated by the process of genetic instability. Concept from Fearon & Vogelstein, *Cell* (1990) 61:759

Some cancer phenotypes may in fact impede growth. In many cancers, it is clear that the process of cell division is complicated by chromosome abnormalities. As will be extensively discussed in later chapters, many cancers have abnormal numbers of chromosomes, as well as chromosomal structural abnormalities. These abnormalities are associated with defects in the cellular machinery that monitors the segregation of chromosomes during mitosis. Examination of dividing cancer cells occasionally reveals chromosomes trapped between two separating daughter cells, a phenomenon known as an anaphase bridge (Fig. 1.19). Such defects present a challenge to cell division, and could theoretically make the process of cell proliferation *less* efficient in cancer cells. The problem with cancer cells, then, is not that they divide too rapidly, but that they grow in an uncontrolled fashion that allows them to eventually perturb tissue homeostasis.

Cancer cells use an inefficient form of metabolism that allows them to adapt to adverse niches. Similarly, the basic cell division process, known as the cell cycle, appears to be defective in many cancer cells as well. Presumably, any inefficiency in cell division is outweighed by the evolutionary benefits conferred by an elevated level of genetic instability, as will be described in Chap. 4.

Germline Cancer Genes Allow Neoplasia to Bypass Steps in Clonal Evolution

To this point we have exclusively considered somatic mutations as the source of selectable genetic variation. While the majority of cancer genes that contribute to tumor progression are indeed acquired somatically, inherited cancer genes also play

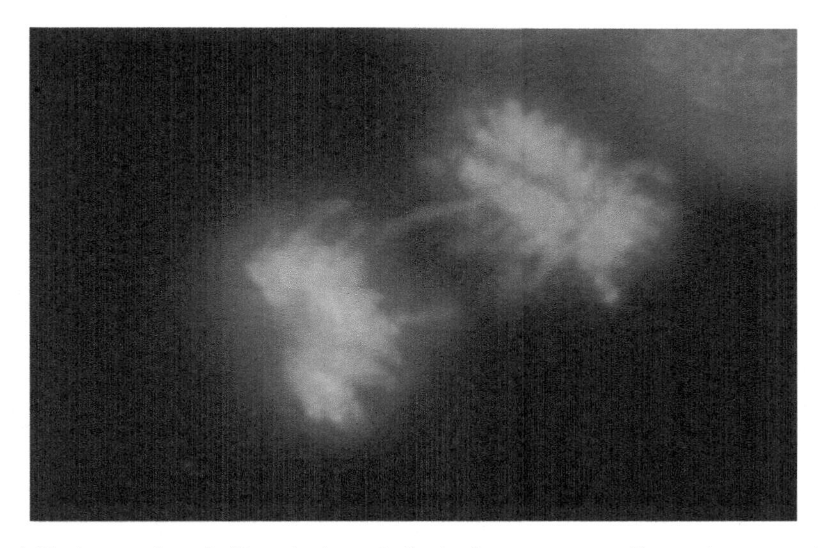

Fig. 1.19 An anaphase bridge. At the end of mitosis, two cancer cells remain connected by incompletely segregated chromosomes

an important – and highly illuminating – role in the clonal evolution of some cancers.

Inherited cancer genes can increase cancer risk. A key observation – that ultimately leads to the explanation of cancer predisposition – is that cancers with a strong familial component often occur earlier in life than similar cancers occurring in individuals with no clear family history of that disease. Clearly, inherited cancer genes must contribute in a significant way to the clonal evolution of tumors.

Well-characterized cancer genes typically exhibit an autosomal dominant pattern of inheritance. In these cases, the presence of only a single allele of a cancer gene causes the associated phenotype, an increased cancer risk. By the laws of Mendelian inheritance, one half of the offspring of an individual that carries such a cancer gene would be expected to inherit that gene and to experience a similarly elevated cancer risk (Fig. 1.20). It is important to emphasize that while cancer development is dependent on the acquisition of a finite number of distinct, somatically-acquired mutations, an increased *risk* of cancer can be transmitted from generation to generation in a Mendelian fashion.

Germline cancer genes increase the risk of cancer because such genes essentially 'short circuit' the process of clonal evolution that drives the process of tumorigenesis. A germline cancer gene is, by definition, present in every cell of an individual. Therefore, such a gene will be present in every neoplasm that might arise by chance. A cancer gene that is already in the germline does not have to be re-acquired by somatic mutation. In this case, a rate-limiting step in the process of tumorigenesis is eliminated. The presence of a germline cancer gene in an expanding cell clone essentially allows that clone to skip one iterative cycle of mutation and clonal expansion. An inherited cancer gene that circumvents a rate limiting step in tumorigenesis would thus be expected to increase the overall lifetime risk of cancer and

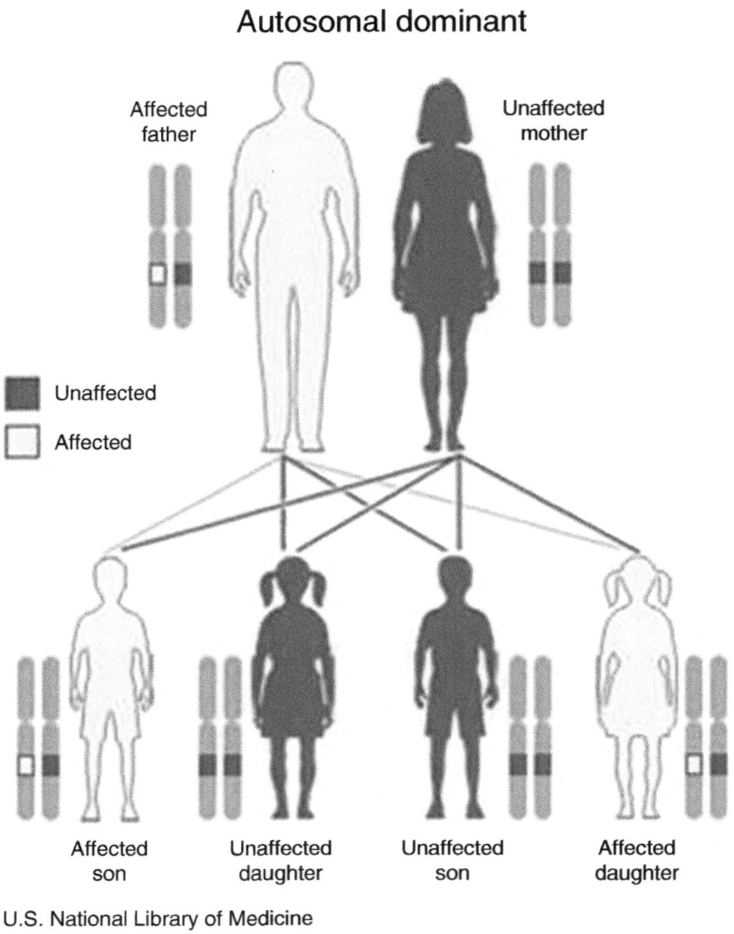

Fig. 1.20 Cancer predisposition can be inherited in autosomal dominant fashion. By this mode of inheritance, one half of the offspring will harbor a germline cancer allele from the affected (cancer-predisposed) parent. Illustration courtesy of the US National Library of Medicine

also to cause cancers to arise at a younger age. These observations are entirely consistent with – and thus serve to reinforce – the idea that clonal evolution selects for cells that harbor cancer genes.

Cancer Syndromes Reveal Rate-Limiting Steps in Tumorigenesis

Estimates of the proportion of colorectal cancers that can be attributed to the inheritance of cancer genes have ranged between 15 and 30 %. Among all cancer types, about 5–10 % have a known heritable component. Most cancers arise in the absence of significant inherited predisposition and are known as *sporadic* cancers. Nonetheless, inherited cancer syndromes have provided fundamental insights into the genetic basis of tumorigenesis.

Colorectal cancers provide a useful model for understanding how the accumulation of somatic mutations leads to the initiation and progression of sporadic tumors. Studies of heritable colorectal cancer syndromes confirm and expand this model by showing how germline cancer genes are additive with somatic mutations, and thereby accelerate the process of tumorigenesis. The contribution of germline cancer genes is exemplified by two heritable colorectal cancer syndromes: familial adenomatous polyposis (FAP) and hereditary nonpolyposis colorectal cancer (HNPCC). Each of these diseases is caused by the inheritance of a cancer gene in an autosomal dominant manner. Although both of these syndromes predispose affected individuals to colorectal cancer, the effects of these genes on colorectal epithelial cells are very different.

Patients with FAP develop large numbers of colorectal polyps at a young age. Typically, hundreds to thousands of these benign lesions will develop during the second and third decade of life. About 1 in every 10^6 colorectal epithelial stem cells gives rise to a polyp in these patients. Even in these patients, most stem cells proliferate normally, and only a small proportion go on to form a observable neoplasm. As in the case of polyps that occur sporadically, the majority of polyps in FAP patients do not progress. However, the sheer number of polyps leads to a significant risk that one or more of these tumors will progress to an invasive, malignant cancer.

The genetic defect in FAP patients is a germline mutation in the *adenomatous polyposis coli* (*APC*) gene that is present about 1 in 5000–10,000 individuals. Patients with germline mutations in *APC* have a much higher risk of developing colorectal cancer than the general population, and also often develop manifestations in other tissues including retinal, bone and skin lesions and brain tumors. The genetics of *APC* mutations will be described in Chap. 3; the roles of the APC protein in the cell will be discussed in Chap. 6.

That the inheritance of a mutant gene causes a plethora of early colorectal tumors is strong evidence that *APC* mutation affects a rate limiting step in tumor initiation. FAP patients are remarkable because of the number of colorectal tumors they develop. In contrast, the process by which these benign lesions subsequently progress appears indistinguishable from that seen in sporadic tumors. For this reason, *APC* has been described as a genetic *gatekeeper* that is required for maintaining tissue homeostasis. Gatekeepers such as *APC* function in stem cells to keep the proper balance between cell proliferation, differentiation and death. By this analogy, an *APC* mutation opens the gate to the subsequent rounds of clonal expansion and mutation that eventually lead to a cancer.

The role of *APC* in cancer is not limited to the inherited alleles that cause FAP. On the contrary, somatically acquired mutations of *APC* are present in the overwhelming majority of all colorectal neoplasms, most of which are sporadic. *APC* inactivation by mutation is therefore a nearly universal step in the initiation of colorectal tumors. Although FAP is a rare syndrome affecting fewer than 1 % of all families, the genetic analysis of FAP has provided important insights into the both inherited and sporadic forms of a very common cancer.

HNPCC, also known as Lynch syndrome, is another Mendelian disease associated with an increased risk of colorectal cancer. The genes that cause HNPCC, and the mechanisms by which mutations in these genes affect disease risk, are clearly distinct from those of the more rare syndrome FAP. The comparison of these two diseases sheds light on the rate-limiting steps of colorectal tumorigenesis.

Unlike FAP, HNPCC is not characterized by an increase in polyps. In HNPCC-affected individuals, adenomas occur at the same rate as in the general population. However, the adenomas that arise in HNPCC patients have a much greater likelihood of progressing to cancer. These tumors have several unique features. The degree of histological differentiation is often low as compared with sporadic tumors of the same size, which normally is an indicator of an aggressive lesion. Contrary to this negative prognostic factor, colorectal cancers in HNPCC patients typically have a more favorable outcome than matched sporadic cancers. This might indicate that HNPCC-associated colorectal tumors evolve somewhat differently than sporadic tumors. HNPCC also affects tissues beyond the colon and rectum, and affected individuals are at an increased risk of cancers in the endometrial lining of the uterus, small intestine, ovary, stomach, urinary tract, and brain.

While FAP is caused by different mutations within a single gene, *APC*, HNPCC is caused by several different mutant genes that are inherited through the germline of affected families. The genetic heterogeneity of this disease entity complicated epidemiological analysis and obscured the true nature of HNPCC for many years. The combination of genetic heterogeneity and the high rate of sporadic colorectal cancers in the general population have made the prevalence of HNPCC difficult to precisely quantify.

The mutated genes that cause HNPCC normally function to ensure the fidelity of DNA replication. The maintenance of DNA replication fidelity is one of the mechanisms by which the genome is stabilized during multiple rounds of cell division. Misincorporated DNA bases cause mismatches between the template strand and the newly replicated strand. DNA mismatches that escape the proofreading functions of the replicative DNA polymerases are removed and corrected by a process known as DNA mismatch repair (MMR). The genes that are required for this process are mutated and thereby functionally inactivated in HNPCC. HNPCC thus arises as a result of the failure of the MMR process. Most cases of HNPCC can be attributed to germline mutation of two genes, *MSH2* and *MLH1*, with a few cases attributable to a third MMR gene, *PMS2*. Proteins encoded by these genes function to repair single-base pair mismatches and unpaired bases, which tend to occur at high frequency at highly repetitive sequences. Long tracts of repeat sequences are known as *microsatellites*. The genetic defects that underlie HNPCC tend to cause microsatellite instability, which can be readily measured, and an overall increase in the spontaneous mutation rate. The process of MMR and the contribution of genetic instability to tumorigenesis will be discussed in greater detail in Chap. 4.

The germline cancer genes that cause HNPCC lead to genetic instability and a corresponding increase in the somatic mutation rate. However, HNPCC genes do not appear to contribute significantly to the rate of tumor initiation. HNPCC patients do not have an elevated number of polyps. The mutation of *APC* initiates the growth of tumors regardless of whether an MMR defect is present or not. The increased rate of mutation caused by the loss of mismatch repair function causes an increased rate of tumor development. HNPCC accelerates tumor progression by increasing the rate at which critical somatic mutations are acquired.

Interestingly, both FAP and HNPCC patients develop colorectal cancers at the median age of 42 years, which is 25 years earlier than the median age of patients with sporadic forms of the disease. Given that FAP is a disease of cancer initiation while HNPCC is a disease of tumor progression, the similar age of cancer onset implies that both initiation and progression are similarly rate-limiting.

The Etiologic Triad: Heredity, the Environment, and Stem Cell Division

Germline cancer genes contribute to familial cancers, but 90–95 % of all cancers arise sporadically and are solely caused by somatic mutations. Many of these sporadic cancers are associated with well-defined risk factors, such as tobacco smoke, sunlight or viral infections. Such agents can greatly increase the rate of somatic mutation, and thereby increase the incidence of cancers that occur in mutagen-exposed tissues. However, mutations would arise even in an idealized environment devoid of mutagens. The replication of human DNA is a highly coordinated and closely monitored process that copies the information content of the genome with high fidelity, but the error rate is not zero. Mutations spontaneously arise at a low but measurable rate. The chance that a mutation will occur in a proliferating cell population increases with every round of DNA replication that accompanies each cell division. Rare mutations that arise as a result of stochastic replication errors are sometimes referred to as *replicative mutations*. What proportion of cancers can be attributed to replicative mutations?

It is useful and interesting to examine the incidence of cancers at different sites. Common cancers tend to occur in tissues that are highly proliferative. To quantify this association, Cristian Tomasetti and Bert Vogelstein analyzed the relationship between the cumulative amount of normal cell proliferation and the incidence of cancer in different tissues. Using compiled data on cancer incidence in the US, and extracting quantitative assessments of stem cell numbers and division rates from various tissues from the literature, they were able to plot cancer incidence in 31 different tissues against the respective amount of cell proliferation in each of those tissues (Fig. 1.21). The results were unexpectedly striking. Across all the tissues that could be reliably assessed, there was a highly positive correlation between the total number of stem cell divisions and the lifetime risk of cancer. Tissues that are inherently more proliferative, such as the lung, liver and colon, give rise to cancers at much higher rates than tissues with low numbers of proliferative cells, such as bones, brain and thyroid. The linearity of this correlation was found to be robust even with the most commonly increased cancers arising from heredity (heritable forms of colorectal cancer), environmental chemicals (lung cancer in smokers) and infectious agents (liver cancer in individuals infected with hepatitis C virus, head and neck cancer in individuals infected with human papillomavirus) included in the analysis.

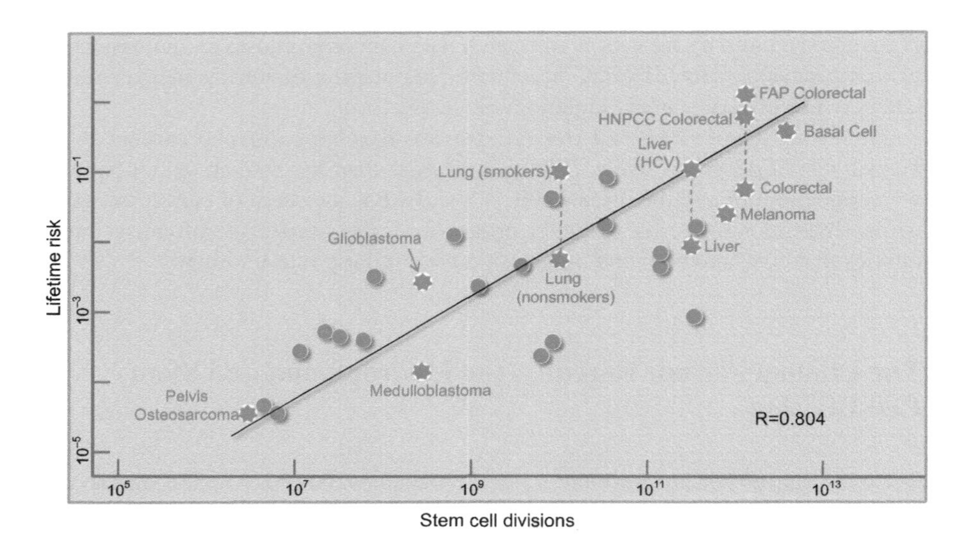

Fig. 1.21 Cancers arise more frequently in tissues that are highly proliferative. The lifetime risk of cancer in any given tissue is positively correlated with the total number of stem cell divisions that occur in that tissue. The linearity of this relationship (R close to 1) supports a large role for replicative mutations in human cancers. This study examined 31 types of cancer, from diverse tissues. Common tumors of the breast and prostate were excluded from this analysis because of uncertainty in the absolute number of stem cells in these tissues. Data from Tomasetti & Vogelstein, *Science* 347, 78 (2015)

The quantification of stem cell proliferation performed in this study allowed an estimation of the total contribution of replicative mutations to all cancers. If replicative mutations were the only contributing factor in the development of cancer in all the tissues assessed, the plot of total stem cell divisions on the X-axis versus the lifetime risk of cancer would form a perfectly straight line, and the two variables would have a linear correlation (a value designated R) of exactly 1. The actual data points derived by Tomasetti and Vogelstein were determined to have an R = 0.804. In statistical analysis of linear regression, the coefficient of determination (defined as R^2) indicates how well the observed data fit a linear model. The R^2 calculated by Tomasetti and Vogelstein was 0.804*0.804 = 0.646. Therefore, this straightforward analysis suggested that about 65 % of the variation in cancer incidence across different tissues is attributable to replicative mutations. Hereditary and environmental factors added together accounted for only about one third of the overall variation in cancer risk. Other studies, including one from Yusuf Hannun and Song Wu, have attempted to refine and extend this type of analysis by differentiating between the intrinsic and extrinsic factors that contribute to replication-associated mutation. The results obtained via this modified approach suggest a lower, but still substantial, contribution by unavoidable mutations to the overall incidence of cancer.

Mutations that arise as a random result of DNA replication have a surprisingly large effect on cancer incidence. One important implication of this finding is that every human being is at risk of developing cancer. The risk of cancer can be dramatically elevated by our lifestyle choices, diet and occupational exposures, and accordingly reduced by preventive measures. Some cancers are clearly preventable. Public health efforts that encourage smoking cessation, promote the use of sunscreens, reduce the incidence of viral infections and minimize exposure to toxic chemicals and radiation can each significantly reduce the incidence of some types of cancer. But recent mathematical approaches to understanding the sources of cancer gene mutations strongly suggest that many cancers are the result of stochastic events that are beyond anyone's control.

Understanding Cancer Genetics

This chapter outlines the essential elements of the cancer gene theory. Cancer genes can be inherited, or they can arise in somatic cells via interactions with environmental mutagens or by chance errors of DNA replication. Mutations occur at a significant rate, but most mutations do not contribute to tumorigenesis, and most neoplasia do not develop into invasive cancers. Proliferative cells that acquire cancer genes can occasionally expand in an iterative, clonal fashion, eventually becoming large, invasive, genetically heterogeneous tumors. The upcoming chapters will delve into the specific genes that cause cancer and how they give rise to the cellular phenotypes that lead to malignancy.

The Vogelgram illustrates several features of the cancer gene theory that explain how sequential genotypic changes cause the evolving phenotypes of growing cancers. These key concepts will be expanded in the upcoming chapters:

There are two types of cancer genes. Tumorigenesis is driven by mutations that result in the activation of oncogenes (Chap. 2) and the loss of function of tumor suppressor genes (Chap. 3).

Cancers exhibit genetic instability. The rate at which mutations and complex genetic rearrangements occur is not constant during the process of tumorigenesis, but rather is increased in most expanding clones as compared to normal cells (Chap. 4).

Cancer genomes reflect the underlying processes of tumorigenesis. The unique genome of a cancer cell results from the accumulation of driver gene mutations and passenger gene mutations (Chap. 5).

Cancer genes populate intracellular pathways. Cancer genes encode proteins that are components of complex molecular circuits, known as pathways. The pathways altered in cancers increase survival, alter cell fate or impact the ability of the cell to repair its DNA (Chap. 6).

Different types of cancers harbor a variety of cancer genes. Tumors of a given type have recurrent genetic defects (Chap. 7).

Cancer genes can mark the early stages of a cancer, or define potential targets for new forms of therapy. The genes that are altered during tumorigenesis can be detected in the germline of cancer-predisposed individuals, or in the bodily fluids of individuals with established cancers. These genes also represent molecular targets for new modes of clinical intervention (Chap. 8).

Further Reading

Antonarakis SE, Krawczak M, Cooper DN (2000) Disease-causing mutations in the human genome. Eur J Pediatr 159(Suppl 3):S173–S178
Coussens LM, Werb Z (2002) Inflammation and cancer. Nature 420:860–867
De Marzo AM et al (2007) Inflammation in prostate carcinogenesis. Nat Rev Cancer 7:256–269
Fearnhead NS, Wilding JL, Bodmer WF (2002) Genetics of colorectal cancer: hereditary aspects and overview of colorectal tumorigenesis. Br Med Bull 64:27–43
Fearon ER (1997) Human cancer syndromes: clues to the origin and nature of cancer. Science 278:1043–1050
Fearon ER, Vogelstein B (1990) A genetic model for colorectal tumorigenesis. Cell 61:759–767
Gatenby RA, Vincent TL (2003) An evolutionary model of carcinogenesis. Cancer Res 63:6212–6220
Haber DA, Settleman J (2007) Cancer: drivers and passengers. Nature 446:145–146
Hollstein M et al (1999) New approaches to understanding p53 gene tumor mutation spectra. Mutat Res 431:199–209
Kamp DW, Weitzman SA (1999) The molecular basis of asbestos induced lung injury. Thorax 54:638–652
Kelly PN, Dakic A, Adams JM, Nutt SL, Strasser A (2007) Tumor growth need not be driven by rare cancer stem cells. Science 317:337
Klein CA (2006) Random mutations, selected mutations: a PIN opens the door to new genetic landscapes. Proc Natl Acad Sci U S A 103:18033–18034
Lynch M (2010) Rate, molecular spectrum, and consequences of human mutation. Proc Natl Acad Sci U S A 107:961–968
Merlo LM, Pepper JW, Reid BJ, Maley CC (2006) Cancer as an evolutionary and ecological process. Nat Rev Cancer 6:924–935
Modica-Napolitano JS, Kulawiec M, Singh KK (2007) Mitochondria and human cancer. Curr Mol Med 7:121–131
Nowell PC, Rowley JD, Knudson AG Jr (1998) Cancer genetics, cytogenetics--defining the enemy within. Nat Med 4:1107–1111
Salk JJ, Fox EJ, Loeb LA (2010) Mutational heterogeneity in human cancers: origin and consequences. Annu Rev Pathol 5:51–75
Scadden DT (2004) Cancer stem cells refined. Nat Immunol 5:701–703
Smallbone K, Gatenby RA, Gillies RJ, Maini PK, Gavaghan DJ (2007) Metabolic changes during carcinogenesis: potential impact on invasiveness. J Theor Biol 244:703–713
Smela ME, Currier SS, Bailey EA, Essigmann JM (2001) The chemistry and biology of aflatoxin B(1): from mutational spectrometry to carcinogenesis. Carcinogenesis 22:535–545
Spencer SL et al (2006) Modeling somatic evolution in tumorigenesis. PLoS Comput Biol 2:e108
Stein LD (2004) Human genome: end of the beginning. Nature 431:915–916
Tomasetti C, Vogelstein B (2015) Variation in cancer risk among tissues can be explained by the number of stem cell divisions. Science 347:78–81
Vaux DL (2011) In defense of the somatic mutation theory of cancer. Bioessays 33:341–343
Weinberg RA (1996) How cancer arises. Sci Am 275:62–70
Wu S, Powers S, Zhu W, Hannun YA (2016) Substantial contribution of extrinsic risk factors to cancer development. Nature 529:43–47

Chapter 2
Oncogenes

What Is An Oncogene?

An oncogene is a mutated form of a normal cellular gene – called a *proto-oncogene* – that contributes to the development of a cancer. Proto-oncogenes typically regulate basic processes that direct cell growth and cell differentiation. Most proto-oncogenes are highly conserved in evolutionarily diverse species, underscoring the fact that genes of this class play central roles in fundamental cellular processes. Mutations of proto-oncogenes that cause their conversion to oncogenes cause many of the perturbations in cell growth and differentiation that are commonly seen in cancer cells.

An oncogene is a type of cancer gene. While all cancer genes are created by mutation, oncogenes are unique in that they are caused by mutations that alter, but do not eliminate, the functions of the proteins they encode. Proteins encoded by oncogenes typically show an increased level of biochemical function as compared with the protein products of the corresponding, non-mutated proto-oncogene.

Most proto-oncogenes encode enzymes. The oncogenic forms of these enzymes have a higher level of activity, either because of an altered affinity for substrate or a loss of regulation. To reflect these gains of function, the mutations that convert proto-oncogenes to oncogenic alleles are known as *activating mutations*.

The Discovery of Transmissible Cancer Genes

The first cancer genes to be discovered were oncogenes. Indeed, the oncogene concept was the first redaction of what would eventually become the cancer gene theory.

Oncogenes were initially discovered as intrinsic components of viruses that cause cancer. Present-day molecular oncologists can trace their scientific lineage to the pioneering virologists of the early twentieth century. This group of technologically advanced and elite scientists established many of the laboratory methods and

F. Bunz, *Principles of Cancer Genetics*, DOI 10.1007/978-94-017-7484-0_2

reagents that are essential to modern cancer research. The early virologists created a scientific infrastructure that would facilitate studies of cells and genes. In a tangible way, the revolution triggered by the germ theory begat a successive revolution in cancer research.

By the early twentieth century, the germ theory was firmly established, as were scientific methods for the systematic study of infectious agents. It was both technically feasible and intellectually compelling to explore whether cancer, like many other common diseases, might have an infectious etiology. Particularly interesting at that time were viruses, which were a new and largely mysterious entity. Viruses were largely uncharacterized, and defined simply as submicroscopic infectious agents present in tissue extracts that would pass through fine filters.

Early experimental observations that laid the foundation for the discovery of oncogenes predated the era of molecular biology. In 1908, Vilhelm Ellerman and Oluf Bang demonstrated that a filtered extract devoid of cells and bacteria could transmit leukemia between chickens. Leukemia was not yet recognized as a form of cancer at that time, so this work initially had little impact. Two years later, Peyton Rous discovered that chicken sarcomas could be serially transmitted from animal to animal by cell-free tumor extracts (Fig. 2.1). The causative agent in the cell filtrates, the Rous sarcoma virus (RSV), was among the first animal viruses to be isolated. The discovery of oncogenic viruses like RSV for the first time led a cancer-causing agent to be studied from a genetic perspective.

The idea that infectious agents cause cancer has a long and tortuous history. The contagious nature of cancer was promulgated in classical times by the widespread

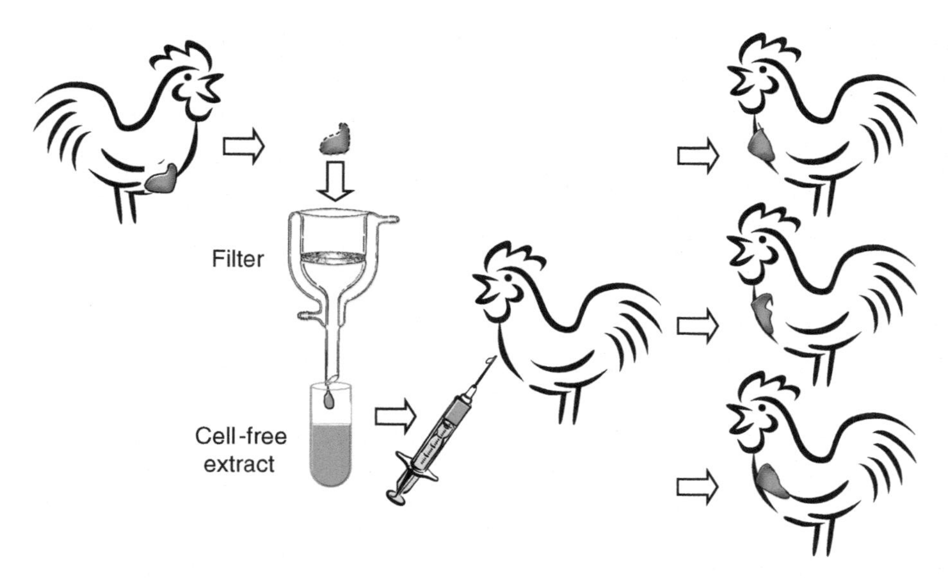

Fig. 2.1 The Rous experiment. Chicken sarcomas can be horizontally transferred between animals via injection of a cell-free filtrate. This experiment demonstrated the infectious nature of this avian cancer

belief that cancer was commonly transmitted between individuals by intimate contact, particularly between spouses, from mothers to children and from patients to caregivers. Such thinking persisted well into the nineteenth century, when they were gradually disproven by rigorous epidemiologic analysis.

A resurgence of interest in infectious agents as common causes of cancer was prompted by the formulation of the germ theory at the end of the nineteenth century. Various bacteria, yeasts, fungi, protozoa, spirochetes and coccidia were, at times, briefly implicated as potential agents that could transmit cancer, but subsequent studies failed to support a positive association. As negative results accumulated, the idea that cancer has an infectious etiology fell out of favor once again.

The initial reports by Rous were therefore met with a considerable amount of skepticism. It was suggested that his cell-free filtrates contained active cell fragments or even submicroscopic cells. The prevailing climate of antipathy towards an infectious cause of cancer substantially delayed full acceptance of Rous' work. The idea that viruses could cause cancer was dogmatically rejected as late as the 1950s, despite intermittent reports showing that other cell-free solutions could induce diverse cancers, including breast cancer, in experimental animals. Eventually, the preponderance of evidence grew too large to discount. Peyton Rous was awarded the Nobel prize in 1966, 55 years after his pioneering work was first published.

Interest in viruses as a cause of human cancer reached a new peak with the discovery of DNA tumor viruses in the 1960s. As the name of this category of viruses suggests, these common viruses – which include the papilloma-, parvo-, and polyoma-viruses – can cause tumors in animals and induce cancer-like characteristics in cultured cells. These findings led to the resurgence of the idea that viruses might be involved in the etiology of human cancer. The contemporary discovery of the DNA tumor virus simian virus 40 (SV40) as a contaminant in polio vaccine stocks that had been previously administered to millions of people was, in this context, troubling. However, as was the case with other infectious agents that had generated interest decades earlier, large follow up studies failed to establish a causal relationship between the DNA tumor viruses and common human cancers. Despite the fact that most of the viruses in this class are not a significant cause of cancer (with the very notable exception of the papillomaviruses), DNA tumor viruses have nonetheless been very useful tools for cancer research. The most widely mutated gene in human cancer, *TP53*, was initially discovered by virtue of its physical association with an SV40 viral protein in cultured cells (see Chap. 3).

As discussed in Chap. 1, most of the viruses that impact the incidence of human cancer stimulate a chronic inflammatory response. Inflammation, in turn, creates a microenvironment that promotes the acquisition, by mutation, of cancer genes and the proliferation of cells that harbor cancer genes. The DNA tumor viruses are different in that they inactivate specific host proteins, and thus create a proliferative advantage for both the cell and the infecting virus.

There is no known virus that causes cancer in humans in the dramatic way that RSV causes cancers in chickens. Nonetheless, the use of RSV to induce chicken tumors provided an invaluable model system that showed how a simple genetic element could cause cells to acquire cancer phenotypes. Prior to the complete sequencing of the human genome, much of the information contained in the genome was unavailable or inaccessible. Cancer-associated viruses presented researchers with relatively short, well-defined regions of DNA sequence that were known to directly relate to cancer development. Viral genes could be fully sequenced and experimentally manipulated with recombinant DNA technology that was developed in the 1970s and the 1980s. The unraveling of the complex relationship between the genes of cancer-associated viruses and human genes was a pivotal step in the elucidation of the cancer gene theory.

Viral Oncogenes Are Derived from the Host Genome

The sarcoma virus isolated by Rous is one of the most potent carcinogens known. Inoculation of chickens with RSV results in the appearance of tumors within several weeks. This acute onset is in stark contrast to the development of most human tumors, which take decades to develop. Clearly, viruses like RSV have evolved a unique mechanism to trigger the cellular changes that cause cancer.

RSV belongs to a category of viruses now known as the *retroviruses*. Retrovirus particles contain genomes that are in the form of ribonucleic acid (RNA). After infection with RSV, the retroviral RNA genome is copied into DNA by the virus-encoded enzyme *reverse transcriptase*. The viral DNA then integrates into the host genome, and thus becomes a *provirus*. The provirus is replicated along with the host genome by the host DNA replication machinery, and is also transcribed by host RNA polymerase complexes. The proviral RNA transcripts are packaged into new virions, completing the virus life cycle (Fig. 2.2).

Retroviruses can cause cancer in two different ways. Depending upon where they integrate, proviruses can disrupt the functions of host genes, usually by altering their transcriptional regulation. In effect, a proto-oncogene can be changed into an oncogene upon integration of a provirus. Typically, cancers caused by the disruption of a host gene by a provirus have a long latent period and take a long time to develop. The viruses that cause such tumors are accordingly known as *slowly transforming retroviruses*. In contrast, acutely transforming retroviruses such as RSV carry their own cancer genes.

RSV contains a cancer gene known as *SRC* (pronounced "sark"). The protein encoded by *SRC* is an enzyme that localizes near the cell membrane and covalently modifies proteins in response to growth signals (Fig. 2.3). Specifically, *SRC* encodes a protein tyrosine kinase, a class of enzymes that catalyzes the addition of a phosphate group onto the tyrosine residues of multiple protein substrates, thereby altering their function. Each covalent modification catalyzed by the *SRC*-encoded protein is one of a series of enzymatically controlled events that collectively function to mediate signals that promote cell growth and division. In short, the *SRC*-encoded protein signals the cell to grow. The biochemical modes by which the enzymes encoded by cancer genes act as cellular messengers will be discussed in detail in Chap. 5.

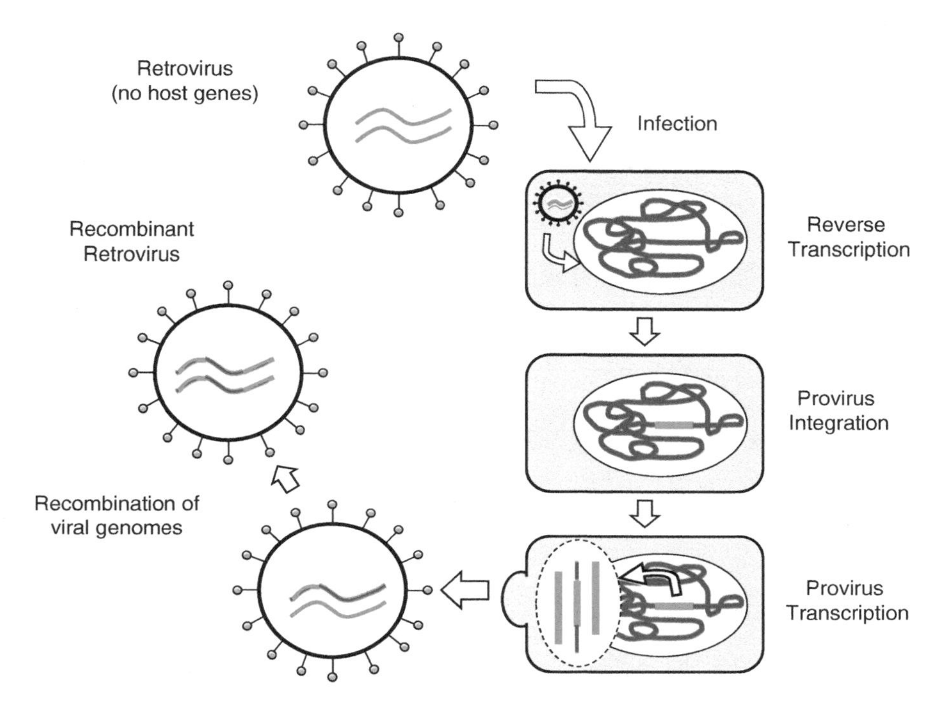

Fig. 2.2 The acquisition of oncogenes by retroviruses. The retrovirus capsule contains 2 copies of the viral RNA genome. After infection, the viral genome is copied into DNA by reverse transcriptase and integrates into the cellular genome as a provirus. If the provirus is integrated in close proximity to exon sequences, proviral transcripts can be spliced with host cell exons. These hybrid transcripts are packaged into a virion, resulting in a heterozygous viral genome. The viral genome undergoes recombination during a second round of infection. The resulting recombinant virus contains coding genetic elements that originated in the host cell

In a landmark study published in 1976, J. Michael Bishop, Harold Varmus and their colleagues demonstrated that the retroviral genes that rapidly trigger the growth of avian cancers are actually variants of genes that are already present in the host genome. There are in effect two related *SRC* genes. The cellular form of the *SRC* gene is a proto-oncogene that encodes a protein containing a tyrosine residue in the carboxy-terminus. This residue is a substrate of an enzyme that regulates growth in concert with the SRC protein (see Chap. 6). When phosphorylated at this tyrosine residue, the *SRC*-encoded protein is rendered functionally inactive and does not transduce growth signals. In contrast, the *SRC* gene carried by RSV, *V-SRC*, encodes a protein that has a truncated carboxy-terminus, and therefore does not contain the tyrosine residue that is the target of the inhibitory signal (Fig. 2.2). The *V-SRC* encoded protein thus is missing a regulatory feature present in the *SRC* encoded protein. The role of SRC and protein phosphorylation in cancer is described in detail in Chap. 6.

How did a host gene come to reside in a retrovirus? The answer lies in the retrovirus life cycle (Fig. 2.2), during which retroviruses shuttle in and out of the host genome. It appears that retroviruses acquire cellular genetic material over the course

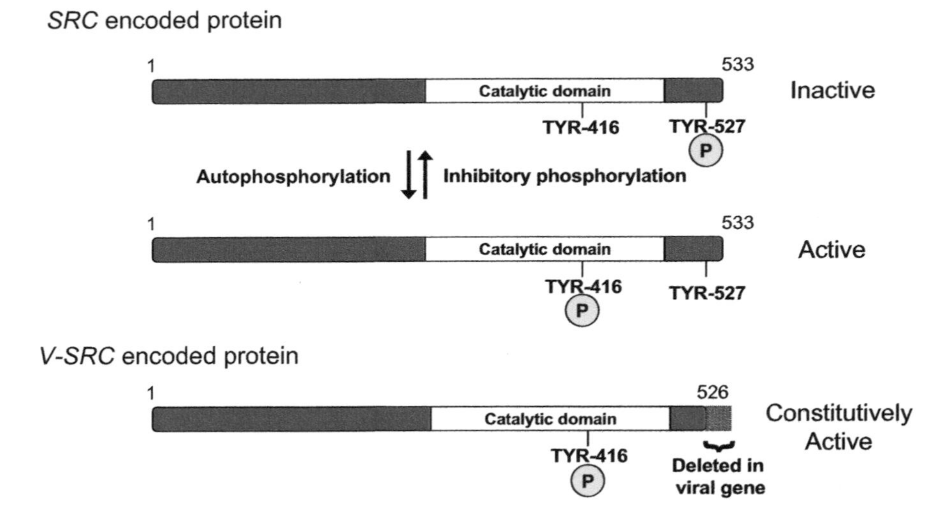

Fig. 2.3 Viral and cellular *SRC* genes. Cellular *SRC* (formerly designated *C-SRC*) is a protein tyrosine kinase that consists of 533 amino acids. Tyrosine autophosphorylation at residue 416 within the kinase domain causes a conformational change and results in the activation of kinase activity. Phosphorylation at tyrosine 527 by upstream inhibitory kinases prevents *SRC* – encoded protein activation. The viral oncogene *V-SRC* does not encode the c-terminal 7 amino acids, and therefore does not contain the negative regulatory element

of these cycles by recombination of the viral DNA with cellular DNA, and incorporate these genes into their own genomes. Evolutionary forces would favor proviruses that can most effectively propagate. Once integrated, the fate of a provirus becomes linked to the fate of the host cell genome. Proviruses that contain genes such as *V-SRC* trigger DNA replication and cell proliferation and thereby promote their own production.

The discovery that cancer-causing retroviruses contain altered forms of host genes fundamentally changed the focus of cancer research. This critical finding showed that the key to understanding cancer lies in the genome of the cancer cell itself. For the first time it was clear that altered cellular genes could cause cancer.

The Search for Activated Oncogenes: The RAS Gene Family

The oncogenes that most often contribute to the development of human cancers are not transmitted by viruses, but rather are acquired by the somatic mutation of proto-oncogenes. The horizontal transfer of cancer by RSV-containing cell extracts does not reflect the means by which human cells acquire oncogenes. Nonetheless, viruses such as RSV did provide important insight as to what oncogenes look like and to how they might induce cellular changes.

The idea that oncogenes could be transmitted by some viruses fostered creative strategies to isolate additional genes that might have oncogenic potential. Genetic material can be efficiently transferred to cultured cells by chemical techniques that were developed during the 1970s. When introduced into primary cells growing in culture dishes, oncogenes can cause observable changes in growth properties. In a process known as *in vitro* transformation, cells that are experimentally forced to express many types of oncogene undergo changes in morphology, lose contact inhibition and begin to grow in piles known as foci (Fig. 2.4). These quantifiable changes formed the basis of numerous experiments that led to the discovery of several widely mutated oncogenes.

Potent oncogenes were found to be carried by two retroviral strains, the murine Harvey and Kirsten sarcoma viruses. These retrovirus-associated DNA sequences (or RAS genes) were designated *HRAS* and, *KRAS* respectively. The Harvey and Kirsten retroviruses were not naturally occurring pathogens, but had been experimentally derived by repeated passage of murine leukemia viruses through laboratory strains of rats. During the creation of these new, highly carcinogenic viruses, *HRAS* and *KRAS* had been acquired in altered, oncogenic form from the host genome. Using DNA transfer schemes, the laboratories of Robert Weinberg and Geoffrey Cooper, and Mariano Barbacid and Stuart Aaronson independently isolated variants of the RAS gene family directly from human cancer cells.

That retroviral oncogenes are related to the oncogenes created by the somatic mutation of proto-oncogenes was underscored by the discovery of the RAS genes. Activated RAS alleles were the first cancer genes to be found in cells derived from naturally-occurring human cancers. It was shown that the RAS genes isolated from human bladder and lung carcinoma cells were homologous to the RAS genes harbored by the Harvey and Kirsten retroviruses. Soon thereafter, Michael Wigler and colleagues isolated a third RAS gene family member that had no known viral homolog, from a neuroblastoma. The third RAS gene was accordingly designated *NRAS*. These three genes are encoded by distinct loci but are highly related, both structurally and functionally.

The wild type RAS proto-oncogenes do not induce focus formation in the *in vitro* transformation assay. The gain of function that leads to the acquisition of this property is conferred by an activating point mutation. The bladder carcinoma from which the cellular *HRAS* gene was first isolated was found to have a single base substitution that changed codon 12 from GGC (glycine) → GTC (valine). Subsequent DNA sequence analysis of large numbers of human tumors has revealed a high frequency of RAS gene mutations in several common tumor types. The majority of these cancer-associated mutations involve just three codons: 12, 13 and 61. Different tumor types differ greatly in the overall frequency of RAS gene mutations, and also in the RAS family member that is predominantly mutated (Table 2.1).

Interestingly, the first oncogenes discovered were not representative of naturally-occurring activated oncogenes. Although activated *HRAS* was among the first oncogenes to be discovered in a tumor, mutations in this RAS family member are

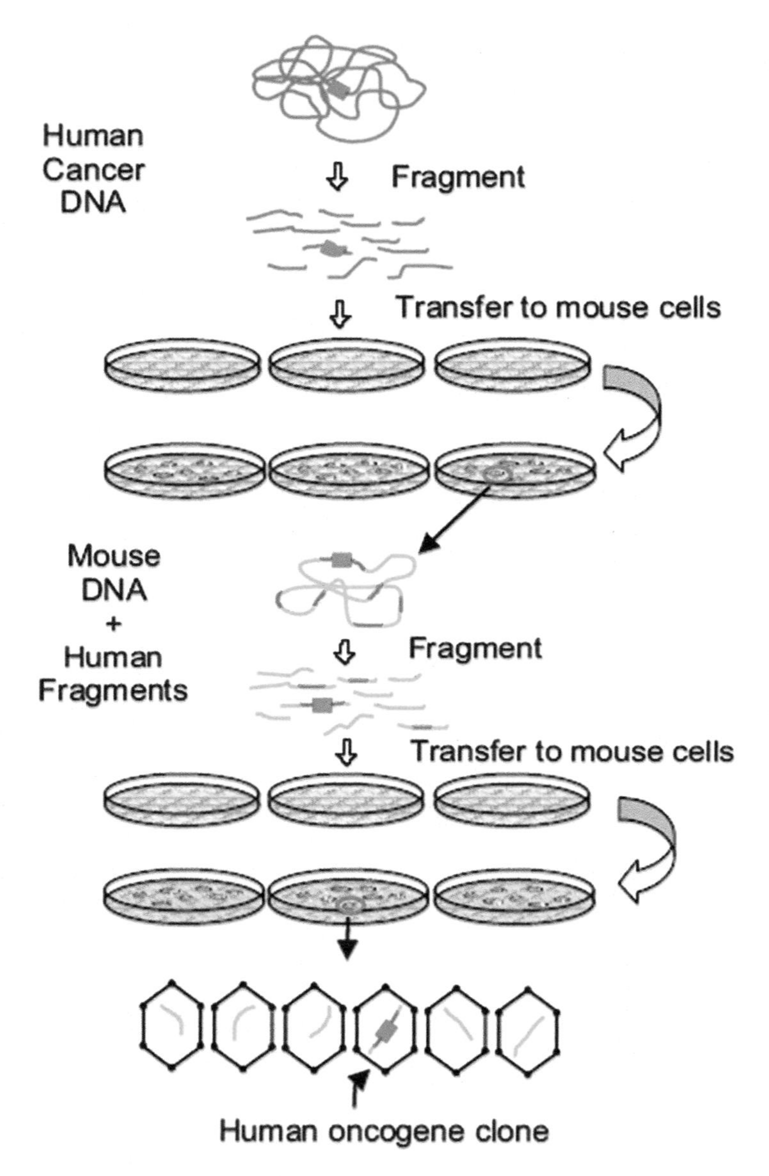

Fig. 2.4 Oncogene discovery by *in vitro* transformation. Genes transferred from human genomic DNA (*blue*) can alter the growth properties of mouse fibroblasts. Genomic DNA is sheared into small fragments, which are introduced into mouse cells grown in monolayer cultures. Appearing after a period of growth, discrete foci represent clones of mouse cells that have altered growth and cell-cell interactions. Genomic DNA from these clones (*yellow*) can contain multiple integrated fragments of human DNA. A second round of transfer allows the isolation of individual human fragments. DNA from the second clone is packaged into a bacteriophage library, which is then screened with a probe corresponding to human genomic DNA-specific repeat elements. Assays of this type were relatively non-specific. Foci can be caused by actual oncogenes that are activated in cancer cells, but also by proto-oncogenes activated by the gene transfer process and growth regulatory genes that are not found to be mutated in cancers

Table 2.1 Mutations in the *RAS* gene family

Cancer type	Mutation frequency (%)	RAS family member
Pancreatic carcinoma	95	*KRAS*
Colorectal carcinoma	50	*KRAS*
Lung carcinoma	40	*KRAS*
Acute Myelogenous Leukemia	25	*NRAS*
Melanoma	15–30	*NRAS*

not widespread in cancers. Similarly, *NRAS* was first isolated from a neuroblastoma, yet subsequent studies have failed to detect *NRAS* mutations in a significant proportion of these tumors. It remains a possibility that the mutated RAS genes identified by *in vitro* transformation arose during the maintenance of tumor-derived cell lines in culture (*in vitro*), rather than by somatic mutation that occurred during tumorigenesis. Nonetheless, the initial identification of the RAS family of oncogenes was an important achievement that paved the way for the systematic analysis of common cancer mutations. Mutations in *RAS* family members are involved in a significant proportion of a number of common malignancies.

RAS genes are ubiquitously expressed and presumably have the same function in all cells. Why then is mutation of *KRAS* a dominant feature of pancreatic tumors and present at much lower frequencies other malignancies? Why are *NRAS* mutations but not other RAS family mutations prevalent in acute myelogenous leukemias? The basis for the tissue specificity of RAS mutations, and indeed of cancer gene mutations in general, remains largely unknown. One might assume that tissue-specific gene alterations arise in cancers at a detectable frequency because they provide a selective advantage under the unique micro-environmental conditions of given cellular compartment.

The cellular role of the RAS-encoded proteins involves the coupling of signals that arise at cell membrane receptors with downstream intracellular signaling molecules. The mutation of conserved codons in the RAS family members affects the regulation of the enzymatic activity of RAS proteins. The nature of RAS protein activity and the cellular functions of the RAS gene family will be discussed in detail in Chap. 6.

Complex Genomic Rearrangements: The MYC Gene Family

The MYC gene family first emerged as a viral gene, *V-MYC*, harbored in the genomes of four independent isolates of avian leukemia virus. Among the tumors caused by these oncogenic retroviruses is myelocytomatosis, a tumor composed mainly of myelocytes, a type of white blood cell. It is from this rare tumor that the name of a commonly activated oncogene family was derived. The cellular homolog of *V-MYC* is the proto-oncogene *C-MYC*, now simply known as *MYC*. There exist two structurally and functionally related genes that were discovered subsequently, originally designated *N-MYC* and *L-MYC* and now known as *MYCN* and *MYCL*. The latter two genes were isolated as oncogenes from a neuroblastoma and a lung carcinoma, respectively.

In contrast to the genes in the *RAS* family, which are activated by single nucleotide substitutions, *MYC* and related genes are typically activated by larger and more complex genomic rearrangements. The encoded protein product is most often not structurally altered by *MYC* gene activation, but increased in quantity. The consequence of *MYC* activation is an increase in gene expression. Even modest increases in *MYC* expression caused by activating mutations are thought to significantly contribute to tumorigenesis in some tissues.

The *MYC* genes encode transcription factors that directly affect the expression of genes involved in diverse aspects of cell growth and death. The *MYC* genes are sometimes referred to as nuclear proto-oncogenes, reflecting their role in controlling the transcription of genes in the cell nucleus. The function of the *MYC* genes in the alteration of gene expression in cancer cells will be discussed in Chap. 6.

The three *MYC* genes share a common genomic structure that consists of three exons. Including intronic regions, each spans approximately 5 kb. This compact genetic unit has been found to be rearranged in a number of ways that result in the aberrantly high expression of MYC proteins. Studies of *MYC* genes in cancers have revealed several general mechanisms by which proto-oncogenes can be activated.

All of the activating mutations that convert *MYC* genes to their oncogenic forms increase the protein levels. There are several mechanisms by which this occurs. The number of functional *MYC* genes can increase as a result of the amplification of the genomic region containing a *MYC* gene. Alternatively, the level at which a MYC gene is expressed can be altered if that gene is repositioned in proximity to a highly active promoter element, usually as a result of a chromosomal translocation. These genetic changes are types of somatic mutations that are stably propagated by cancer cell clones during their evolution.

Proto-oncogene Activation by Gene Amplification

In normal cells, proto-oncogenes exist as single copy genes. That is, a single genomic locus contains one copy of each exon, intron and regulatory element. Due to the diploid nature of the human genome, a total of two alleles of each gene will be present in each cell.

The copy number of a gene can increase as a result of the amplification of a subchromosomal region of DNA. The increase in gene copy number leads, in turn, to a corresponding increase in the overall expression levels of that gene. The process by which genomic amplification occurs remains incompletely understood, but is thought to involve repeated rounds of DNA replication that occur during a single cell cycle.

The unit of genomic DNA that is amplified is known as the *amplicon*. Amplicons vary in size, but typically range in size between 10^5 and 10^6 base pairs. The number of amplicons found within a region of amplification also varies broadly. An amplicon can contain varying numbers of genes depending on the size and location of the genomic region contained within the amplicon. Overall genomic structure is typically preserved within amplified regions, with amplicons ordered in repetitive arrays in head-to-tail orientation (Fig. 2.5).

If the copy number is high or if an amplicon is particularly large, the amplified region may be directly observable by cytogenetic methods. Amplified regions of the genome can exist in extrachromosomal bodies known as *double minutes*, which are small structures that resemble chromosomes but do not contain centromeres. Double minutes can integrate into a chromosome. The region of integration can often be distinguished cytogenetically as a region that stains homogenously with dyes used to reveal chromosome banding patterns. The integration of double minutes is thought to be reversible. Accordingly, the integrated and extrachromosomal forms of amplified genomic DNA are interchangeable. Double minutes and homogeneous

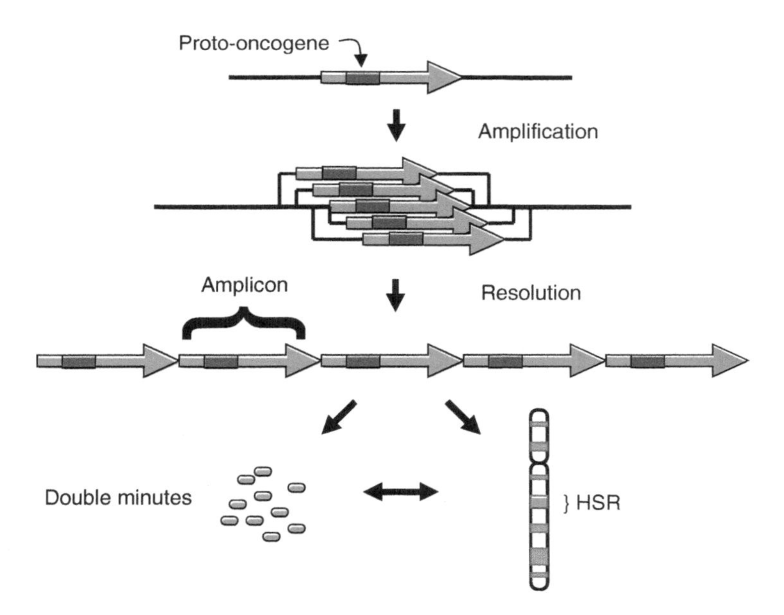

Fig. 2.5 Oncogene activation by gene amplification. A genomic region (*red arrow*) containing a proto-oncogene is amplified as a result of multiple rounds of DNA replication during a single cell cycle. Resolution of the over-replicated region results in a tandem array of amplicons in a head-to-tail orientation. The amplified region can alternatively be maintained as double minutes, or integrated into a chromosome to form a heterogenous staining region (*HSR*). It is believed that these two configurations are interchangeable

staining regions are not seen in cytogenetic analysis of normal cells, but are observed in a significant number of tumor cells.

Upon amplification of a MYC locus, *MYC* is converted from a proto-oncogene to an oncogene. The most notable role for *MYCN* amplification is in the growth of neuroblastomas, tumors that arise from immature nerve cells. These tumors almost exclusively affect young children. Amplification of the genomic region on chromosome 2p24 containing *MYCN* can be detected in about 25 % of neuroblastomas. The degree of amplification of *MYCN* in neuroblastomas can be extensive; as many as 250 copies have been found in some of these cancers. The extent of *MYCN* amplification has been found to correlate with both the stage of the disease, and independently with the rate of disease progression and outcome. These findings provide evidence that *MYCN* amplification directly contributes to neuroblastoma progression.

Amplified *MYC* genes are commonly found in a number of tumors in addition to neuroblastomas. The first example of *MYC* amplification was observed in a myelocytic leukemia, and the gene was named accordingly. Small-cell cancers of the lung have been found to variously contain amplification of one of the three MYC genes, *MYC*, *MYCN* and *MYCL*. *MYC* amplification is found in approximately 20–30 % of breast carcinomas and appears to be correlated with a poor clinical outcome.

Another gene that is commonly amplified in a broad spectrum of cancers is *ERBB2*, previously referred to as *HER2/neu*. *ERBB2* amplification has been found in a significant proportion of breast and ovarian cancers and also in adenocarcinomas arising in the stomach, kidneys and salivary glands.

The *ERBB2* gene was first identified as the cellular homolog of an oncogene, *VERBB2*, carried by the avian erythroblastic leukemia virus, a retrovirus. At around the same time, an oncogene termed *NEU* was isolated from a rat neuroblastoma cell line by *in vitro* transformation, while a gene known as *HER2* was discovered by virtue of its similarity to a previously discovered gene that encodes a cell surface signaling protein called human epidermal growth factor receptor. Efforts to determine the chromosomal locations of these genes suggested – and DNA sequencing subsequently proved – that *HER2/neu* and *ERBB2* are in fact the same gene.

Genetic alterations that activate *ERBB2* are among the most common somatic mutations found in breast cancer, occurring in about 15 % of tumors analyzed. Most of these alterations are gene amplifications that result in increased *ERBB2* expression. The amplicons that include the entire *ERBB2* locus vary between cancers but span a common region of about 280 kb in length. This core amplicon includes several loci in addition to *ERBB2*, but genetic analysis strongly suggests that it is the enhanced expression of *ERBB2* that confers clonal selectivity. Amplified regions typically contain about 20 copies of the *ERBB2* amplicon, but have been found to contain as many as 500 copies. Analysis of the *ERBB2* coding regions has revealed relatively few alterations that affect the open reading frame, confirming that the increase in gene dosage is the primary mode of activation.

ERBB2 encodes a protein that functions as a receptor on the cell surface that transduces growth signals. The activation, by amplification, of this proto-oncogene results in the overexpression of the ERBB2 receptor and a resulting hypersensitivity to growth factors. The *ERRB2*-encoded protein is a prototype of an important class of oncogene-encoded proteins that will be described further in Chap. 5.

Amplification of *ERBB2* in breast cancers is a useful prognostic marker. While amplification of *ERBB2* does not appear to correlate with disease characteristics such as tumor size, there is a significant correlation with the spread of cancer cells to local lymph nodes, which is independently a negative prognostic sign. Breast tumors that harbor *ERBB2* amplification tend grow more aggressively. Statistically, patients with *ERBB2* positive cancers exhibit a significantly shorter time to relapse following standard therapy and reduced long-term survival. The recent development of specific therapy that targets *ERBB2* function makes the identification of patients with *ERBB2* overexpressing tumors a priority. The molecular basis for targeted therapies is discussed in Chap. 8.

Oncogenes activated by gene amplification contribute to many common types of cancer (see Table 2.2).

Table 2.2 Oncogenes frequently amplified in human cancers

Oncogene	Cellular function	Type of cancer	%
MYC	Transcription factor	Breast ca	20
		Ovarian ca.	30–40
		Prostate ca.	15
		Pancreatic ca.	15
CCND1	Cell cycle regulator	Esophageal ca.	35
		Head and Neck ca.	25
		Breast ca	15
		Bladder ca.	10–15
CCNE1	Cell cycle regulator	Uterine serous cell ca.	45
		Ovarian ca.	20
CDK4	Cell cycle regulator	Sarcoma	20
		Glioblastoma	20
EGFR	Growth factor receptor	Glioblastoma	30–50
ERBB2	Growth factor receptor	Breast ca	20–35
		Gastric ca	10
MDM2	Regulation of tumor suppressor protein	Sarcoma	20–25
		Glioblastoma	10–15
MET	Protein tyrosine kinase	Breast ca.	20
PIK3CA	Lipid kinase	Lung squamous cell ca.	40
		Ovarian ca	30
		Esophageal ca	20

Proto-oncogenes Can Be Activated by Chromosomal Translocation

A chromosomal break presents a unique challenge to a growing cell. Cells that contain broken chromosomes cannot continue to grow and divide; proliferation can only continue once a chromosomal break is repaired. The resolution of such breaks is critical to cell survival, but the process of repair frequently results in mutations. One such mutation is the chromosomal translocation.

A translocation is the transfer of a chromosome segment to a new position, often on a nonhomologous chromosome. In some cases the repair process results in the exchange of pieces between nonhomologous chromosomes; such an exchange is termed a reciprocal translocation (see Chap. 1).

Gross structural rearrangements like translocations can juxtapose proto-oncogenes with genetic elements that normally would be unrelated. Proto-oncogenes can be activated by translocations in two ways, depending on the location of the breakpoint. A translocation can put the exons of two separate genes under the control of a single promoter element. The splicing together of previously unrelated exons can then result in the expression of a single hybrid protein that contains elements of each of the two genes involved. Alternatively, a translocation can preserve a complete open reading frame but place it under the control of a more active promoter.

An example of a proto-oncogene that can be activated by chromosomal translocation is *MYC*. The expression of *MYC* is normally tightly regulated. This tight transcriptional control is altered in some lymphomas and leukemia in which the *MYC* gene is repositioned, via translocation, into the vicinity of a highly active promoter. The repositioning of *MYC* into the vicinity of these strong promoters is sufficient to activate *MYC*, and thereby convert it into a functional oncogene.

Chromosomal Translocations in Liquid Tumors

Somatically acquired chromosomal translocations are frequently found in the liquid tumors: the leukemias and lymphomas. Although translocated chromosomes have been found in many solid tumors, translocations are highly prevalent in liquid tumors and are in some cases pathognomonic. Translocations that convert proto-oncogenes to oncogenes have been found in over 50 % of leukemias and in a significant proportion of lymphomas.

Some common genetic alterations are repeatedly observed in cancers of a single type from many different patients. Such alterations are said to be *recurrent*. Many of the recurrent translocations found in liquid tumors are structurally conserved and defined by common breakpoints. These breakpoints often occur in closely spaced clusters. The location of the breakpoints or breakpoint clusters that define translocations is highly disease-specific. In other words, cancers that arise in a particular type of cell will typically harbor similar translocations.

Recurrent translocations, like other genetic alterations, are cell lineage-dependent. The recurrent translocations involving *MYC* indicate why this is the case. The chromosomal translocation resulting in the juxtaposition of *MYC* and highly expressed immunoglobulin genes is a common feature of both B-cell leukemia and Burkitt lymphomas, particularly those arising in children. These cancers arise from a common stem cell, the lymphoid progenitor, in which immunoglobulin gene expression is highly activated. In contrast, *MYC* is activated in T-cell leukemias by translocation and juxtaposition with highly expressed T-cell receptor genes. In these distinct cancers, both the oncogene and the mode by which is it activated are recurrent. Based on these patterns of activation, one can infer that increased expression of *MYC* confers a particularly strong survival advantage in these distinct tissue compartments.

Chronic Myeloid Leukemia and the Philadelphia Chromosome

The activation of a proto-oncogene by a recurrent translocation is best illustrated by the example of chronic myeloid leukemia (CML). In 95 % of CML patients, the cancer cells contain a unique derivative chromosome named after the city in which it was discovered, the Philadelphia chromosome (Fig. 2.6). The Philadelphia chromosome was originally identified in 1960 by Peter Nowell and David Hungerford and upon detailed cytogenetic analysis in 1973 by Janet Rowley, was found to result

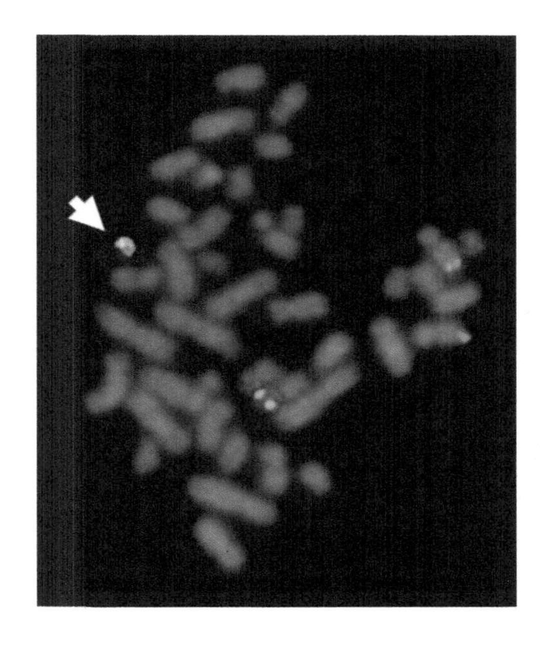

Fig. 2.6 The Philadelphia chromosome. The Philadelphia chromosome (indicated by *arrow*) stained in a mitotic spread. Fluorescence *in situ* hybridization probes are derived from *BCR* (*green*) and *ABL* (*red*). The spots in other chromosomes represent the untranslocated *BCR* and *ABL* genes

from a reciprocal translocation involving chromosomes 9 and 22. The small proportion of CML patients that do not exhibit a typical Philadelphia chromosome have translocations that are structurally more complex, but still ultimately involve the same chromosomal regions. Subsequent to its discovery in CML patients, the Philadelphia chromosome was also found to be present in 3–5 % of children and 30–40 % of adults with acute lympohcytic leukemia (ALL).

CML is a cancer that arises in blood cell progenitors and spreads throughout peripheral blood and bone marrow. CML affects all age groups, but is most common in older adults. The natural history of CML unfolds in clinically defined stages. Within 3–5 years after its detection, CML typically progresses from a relatively benign chronic disease to an acute illness known as blast crisis, which is life-threatening. While the CML cells found during the chronic stage are mature, those found during blast crisis are relatively undifferentiated and resemble those found in patients with acute leukemias.

Interestingly, the only environmental factor known to increase the risk of CML is exposure to high-dose ionizing radiation. It appears that the double strand DNA breaks caused by ionizing radiation can facilitate the translocation that creates the Philadelphia chromosome. In most cases, no predisposing factors are identified and the initiating translocation thus appears to result from a stochastic process. Regardless of the mechanism by which they arise, the rare cells containing the Philadelphia chromosome are then clonally selected and expanded by the process of clonal evolution. The recurrence of a single translocation in CML suggests that this genetic alteration must provide the cancer precursor cells with a unique and essential survival advantage.

At the molecular level, the consequence of the translocation involving chromosomes 9 and 22, denoted t(9;22), is the unique juxtaposition of two genes, *BCR* and *ABL*. *ABL* is a proto-oncogene homologous to an oncogene originally found in the retroviral genome of the Ableson leukemia virus. In the absence of translocation, the expression of the *ABL* proto-oncogene is tightly regulated. The *BCR* gene, in contrast, was so named because of its location within the breakpoint cluster region on chromosome 22. *BCR* expression is driven by a strong, constitutively active promoter. Strictly speaking, *BCR* is not considered a proto-oncogene, and in fact its normal cellular role is unknown. The *BCR* promoter functions to transcribe *ABL* exons when the two genes are fused by translocation (Fig. 2.7).

The t(9;22) reciprocal translocation results in the creation of two separate fusions between the *BCR* and *ABL* genes. The *BCR-ABL* gene is created on the derivative of chromosome 22, the Philadelphia chromosome, while a corresponding *ABL-BCR* fusion gene is created on the derivative chromosome 9. Numerous experiments have demonstrated that it is the product of the *BCR-ABL* gene that is oncogenic. Like a substantial number of proto-oncogenes, the *ABL* gene encodes a protein tyrosine kinase. The fusion gene encodes the catalytic domain of this enzyme, while the expression of this domain is controlled by the *BCR* promoter. It appears that the BCR peptide mediates oligomerization of the BCR-ABL fusion protein, causing constitutive activation of the protein tyrosine kinase domain in the ABL peptide.

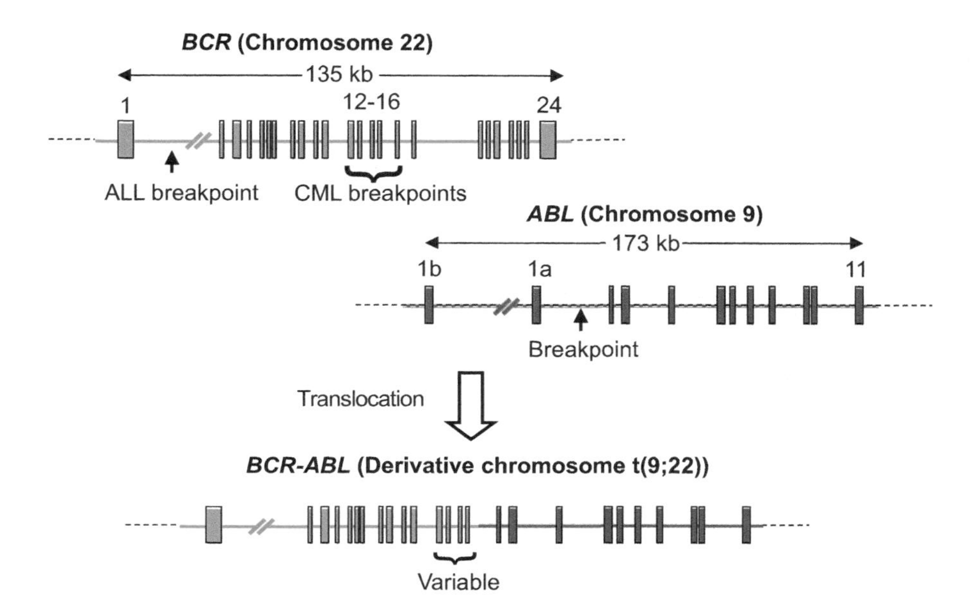

Fig. 2.7 The creation of *BCR-ABL* by translocation. The BCR locus on chromosome 22 spans roughly 135 kilobases (kb) and is composed of 24 exons. Within this gene is a recurring breakpoint, found in acute lymphocytic leukemia-associated translocations, and also a cluster of breakpoints found in chronic myeloid leukemias. The ABL locus on chromosome 9 spans 173 kb and has 11 exons. Two first exons are alternatively utilized. A single recurrent breakpoint occurs upstream of exon 2. In the t(9;22) derivative, the *BCR* and *ABL* genes are fused, and together form a single open reading frame. The different CML-associated breakpoints in *BCR* result in the variable inclusion of *BCR* exons 12–15 in different allelic forms of *BCR-ABL*

The mutational activation of tyrosine kinases and their roles in the cell are discussed in detail in Chap. 6.

The precise junction between chromosome 9 and chromosome 22 sequences varies between different groups of CML patients. While there is a single breakpoint on chromosome 9, the breakpoint on chromosome 22 is actually of cluster of distinct breakpoints variably found in different groups of patients. Accordingly, the portion of *BCR-ABL* that is composed of *ABL* sequence is invariant. However, the existence of multiple breakpoints within the *BCR* locus results in the creation of distinct in-frame fusions. The chimeric proteins encoded by these different gene fusions differ at their N-termini and can be distinguished by their molecular weight (Fig. 2.8). CML is monoclonal in nature, and so only one *BCR-ABL* encoded protein is detectable in each patient. Depending on the site of the break point in the *BCR* gene, the fusion protein can vary in size from 185 to 230 kDa.

The different *BCR-ABL* fusion proteins can be correlated with different clinical outcomes. Most CML patients express the 210 kDa form of the fusion protein. A subgroup of CML patients has been identified that express a 230 kDa BCR-ABL

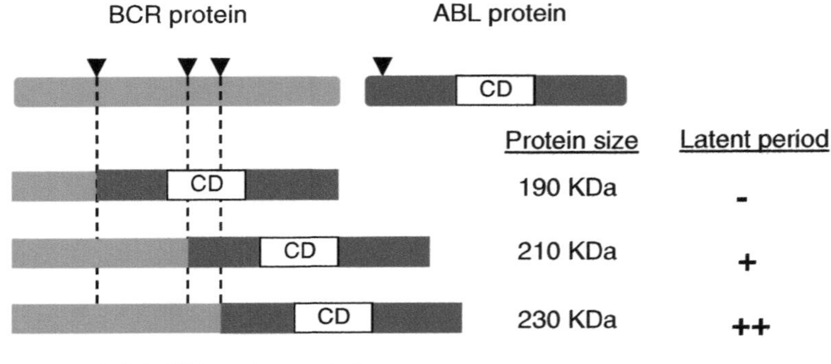

Fig. 2.8 BCR-ABL-encoded proteins. The primary structures of the native BCR and ABL proteins are shown. *Arrowheads* indicate the regions of defined by the recurrent breakpoints. The various breakpoints in *BCR* lead to the appearance of distinct fusion proteins with molecular weights of 190, 210 and 230 kilodaltons (kDa). The 190 kDa protein is restricted to ALL, an acute disease that is not characterized by a latent period. The 210 kDa is the most prevalent CML associated version, while the 230 kDa protein is found in a subset of CML patients that typically exhibit an extended period of disease latency

encoded protein. These patients have a distinct disease course that is typified by decreased numbers of white cells in the peripheral blood and delayed progression to blast crisis. Patients with highly-aggressive ALL express either the 210 kDa form or a unique 190 kDa protein. The 190 kDa protein has been shown to be a more active tyrosine kinase than the 210 kDa protein, suggesting that different levels of activity affect the clinical course of these diseases.

Because the presence of the various gene fusion products correlates with both the type and course of disease, these molecules are useful markers for diagnosis and prognosis. The presence of a chimeric RNA species transcribed from a fusion gene is readily detectable by commonly employed RNA/DNA amplification techniques. Thus, the expression of these unique oncogenes provides a convenient and highly informative marker than can be directly used in the clinic.

The catalytic activity of the *BCR-ABL* encoded tyrosine kinases can be directly inhibited by drugs. Therapy based on this approach has been highly successful at delaying blast crisis and has significantly improved the overall outlook for patients with CML. The fact that specific therapy directed at the *BCR-ABL* gene product is highly effective demonstrates conclusively the central role of the *BCR-ABL* oncogene in CML pathogenesis. The effects of tyrosine kinase activation on cancer cell proliferation will be discussed in Chap. 6; novel therapeutic approaches to specifically target these enzymes will be described in Chap. 8.

Oncogenic Activation of Transcription Factors in Prostate Cancer and Ewing's Sarcoma

Cytogenetic analysis is considerably more difficult in solid tumor samples, and so the role of translocations was first appreciated in the liquid tumors. But recurrent translocations activate oncogenes in solid tumors as well.

Prostate cancers are often caused by driver gene mutations that alter the cells' normal responses to male sex hormones, known as *androgens*. The most frequently detected oncogene in prostate cancers is a fusion gene that is created by a translocation involving two loci on chromosome 21. The translocation creates a novel fusion gene that contains the 5' untranslated region of *TMPRSS2*, an androgen-regulated transmembrane receptor protein and the proto-oncogene *ERG*. ERG encodes a transcriptional regulator that is one of a large family of evolutionarily conserved proteins that mediate several basic cellular functions, including cell division, differentiation and migration, which are normally active during embryonic development. The products of the *ERG* gene had previously been observed to be expressed at high levels in many prostate cancers. The discovery of the *TMPRSS2-ERG* fusion gene in 2005 provided a mechanistic explanation for this androgen-dependent upregulation.

The founding member of the transcription factor family that includes *ERG* is an oncogene that was found to be transduced by the leukemia virus E26, or ETS. A second ETS-family member designated *ETV1* has also been found to be activated by fusion to upstream elements of *TMPRSS2* in a smaller number of prostate cancers. The encoded proteins of the ETS family of genes contain a common protein domain that is important for the protein interactions that facilitate sequence-specific DNA binding.

Ewing's sarcoma is a rare tumor of bone or soft tissue that occurs in children and young adults, most frequently in male teenagers. These highly aggressive tumors can occur in various anatomic sites, but most often are found in the bones of the pelvis, femur, humerus, ribs and clavicle. The cells that compose Ewing's sarcomas are morphologically similar to those found in diverse types of pediatric solid tumors, making accurate diagnosis difficult. This challenge prompted focused investigation into cytogenetic changes that could potentially provide a diagnostically useful marker. A distinguishing characteristic of Ewing's the majority of sarcoma cells was found to be the presence of a reciprocal translocation between chromosomes 11 and 22, abbreviated t(11;22).

Molecular analysis revealed that t(11;22) consistently juxtaposes the *FLI1* gene on chromosome 11 and the *EWS* gene on chromosome 22 (Fig. 2.9). *FLI1* is a proto-oncogene that was originally identified in mice as the integration site common to two retroviruses that cause leukemias and sarcomas, including the Friend leukemia virus for which the locus was named. Like *ERG*, *FLI1* is a gene in the ETS family and shares many of the basic functional attributes of these genes. The *EWS* gene, named for its discovery as the locus at the Ewing sarcoma breakpoint, is the proximal component of the *EWS-FLI* oncogene. The proto-oncogene *EWS* encodes a

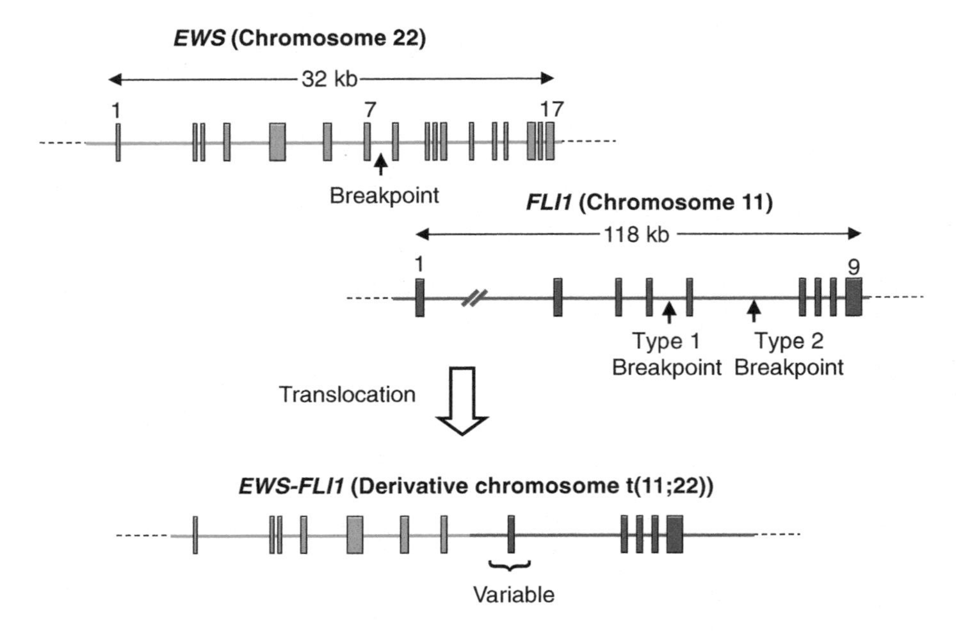

Fig. 2.9 The creation of *EWS-FLI1* by translocation. The *EWS* locus on chromosome 22 spans roughly 32 kb and is composed of 17 exons. In patients with Ewing's sarcoma, a recurring breakpoint is found the 7th intron. The *FLI1* locus on chromosome 11 spans 118 kb and has 9 exons. Within this gene are two recurrent disease-associated breakpoints. In the t(9;22) derivative, the *EWS* and *FLI1* genes are fused, and contain a single open reading frame. The Type 1 and Type 2 fusions result in two distinct *EWS-FLI1* genes that differ in the inclusion of one *FLI1*-derived exon

multifunctional RNA binding protein that is involved in gene expression, cell signaling and RNA processing and transport.

In the Ewing's sarcoma translocation, the chromosomal breakpoints occur within the introns of *FLI1* and *EWS*, and result in the in-frame fusion of the promoter and upstream elements of *EWS* and the downstream elements of *FLI1*. The precise locations of the breakpoints vary from tumor to tumor. The most frequent junction, occurring in 60 % of cases, joins exon 7 of EWS to exon 6 of *FLI1* in what is termed a Type 1 fusion. Approximately 25 % of cases are associated with a so-called Type 2 fusion, which includes exon 5 of *FLI1*. As was seen to be the case in CML, the fusion variants correlate with distinct clinical outcomes. In particular, the Type 1 fusion is associated with a significantly better prognosis than the other fusion types.

In all t(11;22) breakpoints, the RNA-binding domain encoded by *EWS* is replaced with the DNA-binding domain encoded by *FLI1*. The *EWS-FLI1*-encoded fusion protein is thus a chimera. Though the target sequences recognized by the DNA-binding domain of the *EWS/FLI1* gene product are indistinguishable from those recognized by native *FLT1*, the chimeric protein is more active and is found to transactivate 5–10 times more transcription than native *FLI1*. Of direct clinical relevance are functional differences between the alternative forms of *EWS-FLI1*. The protein product of the Type 1 fusion was found to be a less effective transcriptional transactivator than the other fusion gene products. This difference in activity correlates closely with the more benign clinical course associated with this alteration.

The *EWS-FLI1* fusion is the most common gene product of chromosomal translocation in Ewing's sarcoma, occurring in about 90 % of cases. These alterations are also found in rare tumors that are similar to Ewing's sarcoma. The *EWS* gene has also been found to be fused with several other members of the ETS family of transcription factors in both Ewing's sarcoma and in related disorders. About 10 % of Ewing's sarcomas exhibit fusion of *EWS* with *ERG*, the same gene that is activated in prostate cancers harboring the *TMPRSS2-ERG* fusion.

The discovery of these molecular similarities has led to the reclassification of a group of molecularly and clinically related diseases, which is now referred to as the Ewing's sarcoma-related family of tumors. Cumulatively, these molecular data suggest that the dysregulation of ETS-mediated transcription by *EWS* fusion is a critical step in the clonal evolution of the Ewing's sarcoma family from their stem cell progenitors.

Oncogene Discovery in the Genomic Era: Mutations in *PIK3CA*

The identification of the majority of known oncogenes predated the sequencing of the human genome. The prototypical oncogenes described in previous sections were isolated on the basis of their homology to genes carried by oncogenic retroviruses or on their ability to induce colony formation in an *in vitro* transformation assay. These early oncogenes were not discovered because they were necessarily involved in large numbers of cancers. Rather, they emerged as a consequence of idiosyncratic properties that facilitated their discovery by the tools available at the time. While these groundbreaking discoveries provided a paradigm for understanding how genes cause cancer, the actual genes that emerged were not necessarily those that contributed to the greatest number of cancers. For example, studies of *SRC* provided the first critical link between tumorigenic retroviruses and the activation of host cell genes. While the SRC protein is active in many tumors, the mutational activation *SRC* is not a predominant feature of human cancer.

The complete sequencing of the human genome by 2000 facilitated a shift from the functional approaches to gene discovery that had dominated the field of cancer genetics, to the more direct approach of scanning cancer cell genomes in search of mutations. Cancer gene discovery came to rely less on cellular experimentation and more on informatics, the study and processing of large and complex datasets. In the genomic era, new oncogenes are discovered not on the basis of an idiosyncrasy or serendipity, but on the basis of their frequency of mutation in cancers.

An example of an oncogene identified by high throughput DNA sequencing is *PIK3CA*. *PIK3CA* is a member of a family of genes that encode a class of enzymes known as *phosphatidylinositol 3'-kinases* (PI3Ks). The PI3K enzymes first became a focus of interest to cancer researchers in the 1980s, when it was found that PI3K activity was linked to the protein products of viral oncogenes, such as SRC. PI3K enzymes function in the signaling pathways involved in tissue homeostasis, including cell proliferation, cell death, and cell motility. The organization of these signaling pathways and the role of PI3Ks in cancer phenotypes will be described in detail in Chap. 6.

The known roles of the lipid kinases in cancer-associated cellular processes and the association of these enzymes with known viral oncogenes formed the rationale for the large scale analysis of all genes in this family. As part of an early attempt to scour the genome for cancer genes, a group at Johns Hopkins University used informatics to identify eight members of the PI3K family, on the basis of similarities in their coding sequences. Each of the PI3K genes identified contained a putative kinase domain at its C-terminus. The research team proceeded to sequence the 117 exons that, in total, encoded the kinase domains of each of the PI3K-family members in a panel of colorectal tumors. Recurrent mutations were found in a single family member, *PIK3CA*. Expanding their analysis to include all *PIK3CA* coding exons in nearly 200 tumor samples, the Johns Hopkins group established that *PIK3CA* is mutated in more than 30 % of colorectal cancers.

The majority of mutations that occur in *PIK3CA* during colorectal tumorigenesis are single nucleotide substitutions that result in missense mutations. These mutations do not occur at random points along the *PIK3CA* open reading frame, but rather occur in clusters known as *hot spots*. Most frequently mutated was a helical domain that largely defines the three dimensional structure of the encoded protein. The C-terminus portion of the lipid kinase domain was also mutated in many cancers. The amino acid residues that are affected by hot spot mutations are highly conserved among evolutionarily-related proteins. Functional studies of *PIK3CA* mutants have shown that hot spot mutations cause an increase in the enzymatic activity of the encoded protein.

Subsequent sequencing studies revealed hot spot mutations of *PIK3CA* in brain tumors, and breast, lung, endometrial, urinary bladder and gastric cancers. *PIK3CA* is amplified in significant numbers of ovarian, esophageal and prostate cancers (Table 2.3 and Fig. 2.10). Overall, the mutated and amplified alleles of *PIK3CA* are among the most prevalent of all cancer genes.

Table 2.3 Activating mutations in *PIK3CA*

Cancer type	Mutation frequency (%)
Breast ca.	30–35
Endometrial (uterine) ca.	35
Colorectal ca.	15–30
Gastric ca.	25
Ovarian ca.	<5
Glioma	10
Lung ca.	5–20

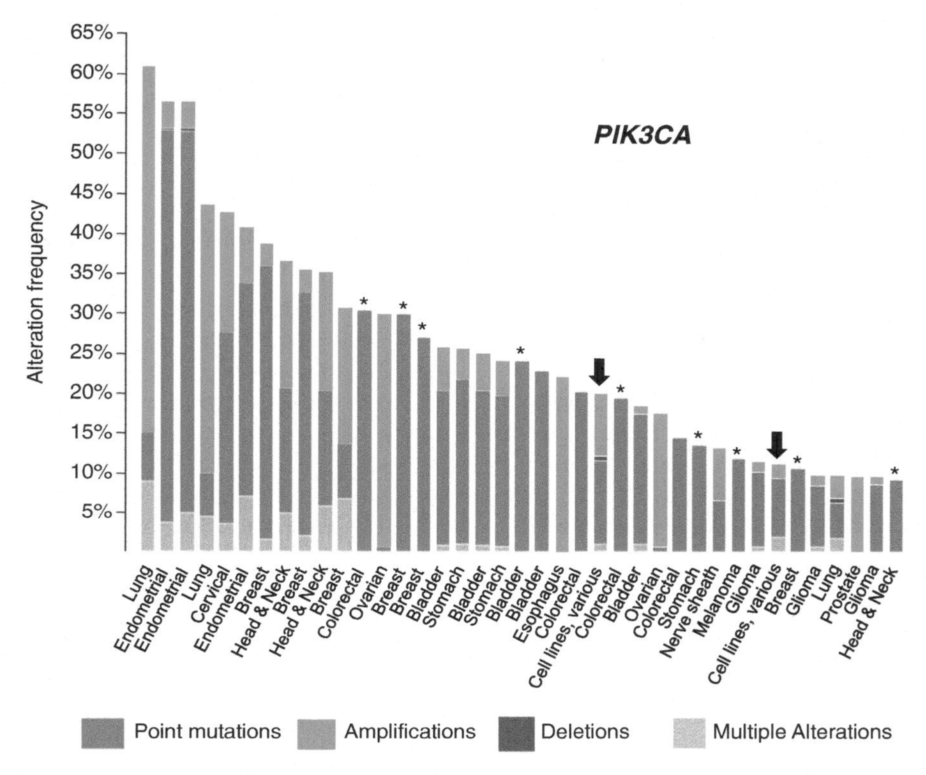

Fig. 2.10 A meta-analysis of *PIK3CA* across tumor types reveals a high frequency of point mutations and amplification. Since its identification as an oncogene in colorectal cancers, *PIK3CA* has been examined in many tumor types. Relatively minor discrepancies between studies can in some cases be attributed to different methodologies and distinct patient populations. However, the frequency of *PIK3CA* mutation in tumors of a given type is largely consistent. Mutations are more prevalent than amplifications. The rare deletions that have been observed are probably incidental or artifactual. * denotes a study in which amplifications were not assessed. ↓ denotes a study of cell line collections that were derived from various tumor types. The results shown here are in whole or part based upon data generated by the TCGA Research Network: http://cancergenome.nih.gov/

Selection of Tumor-Associated Mutations

Mutations identified via high throughput approaches are not identified on the basis of their function, but on the basis of their sequence. With a high degree of sensitivity and specificity, genomic DNA sequencing can reveal all base changes, passenger mutations and driver mutations alike. The evaluation of the *PIK3CA* mutations found in cancers provides an example of the features that practically distinguish passengers and drivers.

What is the evidence that *PIK3CA* is a cancer gene and not simply a target of passenger mutations? The first and strongest piece of evidence is the high frequency of *PIK3CA* mutations in tumors. Passenger mutations are clonally expanded by chance and thus occur at random, non-recurrent positions. The observed mutations in *PIK3CA* hot spots were found to occur at a rate that was over 100-fold above the background rate of nonfunctional alterations that had previously been observed in colorectal cancer cells. In contrast, analysis of other genes, such as the other members of the PI3K family, has revealed non-recurrent base changes that are consistent with passenger mutations.

A second piece of evidence is the proportion of silent mutations to missense mutations observed. Silent mutations, otherwise known as *synonymous mutations*, should confer no selective advantage because by definition such mutations do not result in changes to the encoded protein. Missense mutations, or *nonsynoymous mutations*, potentially confer a selectable advantage. Among mutations that are propagated by chance alone, nonsynonymous mutations would be expected to occur at a rate that is about two-fold greater than the rate of synonymous mutations. This is simply a function of the numbers of potential bases changes that can occur at random within an open reading frame. The nonsynonymous mutations found in the *PIK3CA* gene occur at a frequency 30 times higher than synonymous mutations in the same gene. This overrepresentation of nonsynonymous mutations suggests that they conferred a selective advantage, and thus contributed to tumorigenesis.

The clustering of *PIK3CA* mutations in evolutionarily conserved hot spots also suggests that these mutations are significant. As described in Chap. 1, evolutionarily-conserved protein elements tend to be fundamental to protein function. Therefore, the frequency of mutation at these key codons provides another convincing piece of evidence that the mutations observed in colorectal tumors are highly likely to confer functional phenotypic changes that, in turn, promote cancer cell growth.

Multiple Modes of Proto-oncogene Activation

There are several ways in which changes to the genome can result in the activation of proto-oncogenes. Whether a mutation results from a small sequence alteration such as a single base substitution, gene amplification, a chromosomal translocation or another more complex gross chromosomal rearrangement, the contribution of an oncogene to tumorigenesis is qualitatively the same. Somatic mutations that activate proto-oncogenes increase the activity of the encoded protein.

Increased protein activity can result from increased levels of gene expression, as we have seen in the examples of the commonly amplified *MYC* and *ERBB2* oncogenes and in the cases in which *MYC* is relocated to a position upstream of a highly active promoter. Alternatively, somatic mutations can result in the expression of a mutant protein. In the case of the *RAS* gene family, activating point mutations cause a loss of regulation and result in constitutive enzymatic activity. In the case of the more complex *BCR-ABL* and *EWS-FLI1* oncogenes, the fusion of unrelated genes results in both a change in transcriptional activation and in some cases a change in protein structure. Both of these factors can contribute to increased activity of oncogenic proteins.

Another general theme that emerges from a survey of frequently activated oncogenes is that the same oncogene can be activated by different kinds of mutations in different cancers. *MYC* is activated by amplification in a significant proportion of breast and ovarian cancers, but activated by rearrangements in Burkitt lymphoma, and in B-cell and T-cell leukemias. The mechanism of activation in a single cancer type is not always exclusive. While *ERBB2* is most frequently activated by amplification in breast cancers, non-synonymous single base substitutions are found in lower levels in breast, ovarian, gastric, and colorectal cancers. Similarly, *PIK3CA* is activated by single base substitutions in a wide range of carcinomas. While single base substitutions within *PIK3CA* mutations are occasionally found in high grade ovarian carcinomas, a greater proportion of such tumors harbor amplifications of this locus.

In some cases, the causal relationship between a cancer cell lineage and a specific mechanism of proto-oncogene activation is fairly obvious. In the cellular precursors of many leukemias and lymphomas, for example, immune response genes are normally transcriptionally much more active than in any other cell type. It is easy to imagine that a translocation event that results in the juxtaposition of a growth promoting gene such as *MYC* with a transcriptionally active gene would result in a strong selectable advantage, and the outgrowth of that clone.

In most types of cancers, the reason for an apparent bias towards the activation of a proto-oncogene by one mechanism over another is unclear. One important factor, to be discussed in more detail in Chap. 4, is that different types of cancer cells appear to be inherently prone to different kinds of genomic alterations. Some cancers are characterized by gross numerical and/or structural chromosomal abnormalities, while others exhibit a preponderance of changes that occur at the nucleotide level. The acquisition of different forms of genetic instability during tumorigenesis is an important factor in determining the spectrum of somatic mutations present in an advanced cancer.

Oncogenes Are Dominant Cancer Genes

A single nucleotide substitution at a critical position is sufficient to activate a proto-oncogene and convert it to an oncogene. The activating mutation results in a growth advantage, in spite of the continued presence of a normal, unmutated allele in every cell. Because the phenotype conferred by an oncogenic mutation is not influenced by the presence of the remaining wild type allele, oncogenes are, by definition, dominant alleles.

The oncogenic mutations found in a tumor sample are almost never present in the normal cells of that same individual. (The few known exceptions to this pattern are described in the following section.) Generally, activated oncogenes do not run in the germlines of cancer-prone families. Extensive examination of proto-oncogenes and oncogenes in normal tissues and in cancers has revealed that the mutations that convert proto-oncogenes to oncogenes are almost always acquired by somatic mutation.

Cancer genes can be acquired by somatic mutation or by inheritance. Cancer predisposition is an inherited trait, and therefore the genes that confer this trait must be present in the germline. Oncogenes are not commonly found in the germline and therefore are not a major factor in cancer predisposition. Clearly, this is true for oncogenes that are highly *penetrant*, those that exert strong phenotypic effects regardless of environment or genetic background. Heritable predispositions to cancer development are attributable to different type of cancer gene: the tumor suppressor gene. The nature of these important cancer genes will be described in Chap. 3.

Germline Mutations in *RET* and *MET* Confer Cancer Predisposition

All of the oncogenes described thus far are activated by somatic mutations that occur during tumorigenesis. An interesting exception to this general pattern is the *RET* oncogene, which is somatically mutated in cancers, but is also found in the germline of individuals that are predisposed to inherited cancers of the endocrine system.

Multiple endocrine neoplasia type 2 (MEN2) is a rare, autosomal dominant cancer syndrome. There are several clinically distinct subtypes of this inherited disorder, designated MEN2A, MEN2B and familial medullary thyroid carcinoma (FMTC). Affected individuals most commonly develop an atypical form of thyroid carcinoma which is derived from a population of cells that have an origin in the neural crest. Other endocrine cancers, benign lesions and developmental abnormalities are variably seen in the different MEN2 subtypes.

MEN2-related cancers are caused by germline mutations in the *RET* proto-oncogene. The *RET* proto-oncogene is located on chromosome 10 and contains 21 exons that encode a membrane-bound tyrosine kinase. Like many other oncogenes, *RET* was first discovered during *in vitro* transformation assays using genomic DNA from lymphomas and gastric tumors. The first isolates of this gene were chimeras that had formed during the transfection process, and so the gene was accordingly designated by the acronym for 'rearranged during transfection'. The oncogenic forms of *RET* that have been found in sporadic cancers are similarly rearrangements. These somatic rearrangements vary in different cancers, but commonly put the tyrosine kinase domain in-frame with highly expressed genes, thereby resulting in its constitutive activation. These types of mutations are different from those that cause MEN2.

In contrast to the *RET* mutations found in sporadic cancers, the mutations harbored by individuals affected with MEN2 are usually single nucleotide substitutions. Activating point mutations that convert *RET* into an oncogene typically affect the extracellular domain of the *RET*-encoded protein and lead to ligand-independent activation of the kinase and constitutive activation of downstream mitogenic pathways. (These pathways and the manner in which they related to cancer cell phenotypes will be described in Chap. 5.) Most commonly, mutations in *RET* affect exons 8 and exons 10–16. The precise location of the mutations appears to confer distinct disease phenotypes.

RET is one of a small number of oncogenes that causes an inherited predisposition to cancer. Another oncogene known as *MET* is carried in families affected by hereditary renal cell carcinoma. Like the MEN2 syndomes, hereditary renal cell carcinoma is rare, but highly illustrative of the role that oncogenes can play in some inherited forms of cancer.

The role of the oncogenic forms of *RET* and *MET* in heritable cancers is highly unusual. Activated oncogenes are dominant alleles. As will be extensively described in Chap. 3, the cancer genes that contribute to hereditary forms of cancer are typically recessive alleles that are unmasked during the process of tumorigenesis. Highly penetrant, dominant cancer genes would confer a growth advantage onto every proliferative cell in the body, a phenotype that would presumably compromise the viability of carriers. The role of oncogenes in inherited cancer predisposition is therefore limited.

Proto-oncogene Activation and Tumorigenesis

How do oncogenes fit into the sequence of genetic alterations that underlie tumorigenesis? Activated oncogenes can be found in nearly all colorectal cancers. The oncogenes that commonly contribute to colorectal tumorigenesis are associated with discrete clinico-pathological stages of the disease (Fig. 2.11).

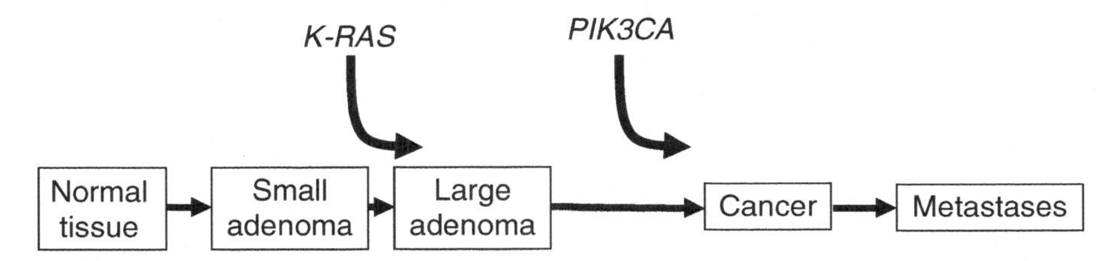

Fig. 2.11 Oncogenes and colorectal cancer progression. Oncogenic mutations in *KRAS* and *PIK3CA* contribute to the later stages of tumor progression. While *KRAS* mutations are occasionally found in very small aberrant crypt foci (ACF), the lesions that harbor these mutations do not appear to progress. In contrast, *KRAS* activation plays an important role in the transition from small to large adenomas, which have significant potential to become malignant. *PIK3CA* mutations are largely found in invasive cancers

The first cancer genes to be firmly associated with colorectal cancers were activated members of the RAS family. Single base substitutions within *KRAS* or less often in *NRAS* are found in approximately 50 % of all colorectal cancers. Among the precancerous lesions, adenomas greater than 1 cm in size exhibit a frequency of *RAS* mutations that is similar to that seen in invasive cancers. In contrast, smaller adenomas (<1 cm) rarely exhibit *RAS* mutations. This finding suggests that *RAS* mutations are acquired during adenoma progression. In support of this hypothesis, dissection of adenomas has revealed small subpopulations in which *RAS* mutations has occurred. Presumably, these subpopulations represent clones that are beginning to progress and that have the potential to give rise to more invasive clones.

Interestingly, *RAS* mutations can be found in some very early lesions arising in the colorectal mucosae. In a distinct histological subset of the earliest lesions, the aberrant crypt foci, *RAS* mutations are found at a high rate. However, such lesions are self-limited and appear to have little, if any, potential for progression. This is a very illuminating finding that underscores a basic principle of tumorigenesis. Clearly, *RAS* mutations can occur in any cell population, but they alone are not sufficient to promote the continued growth of a neoplasm. Rather, the stepwise expansion of tumor cell clones requires a defined sequence of events. While *RAS* mutations appear to be of primary importance in the progression of adenomas to more advanced tumors, this effect is stage-specific and requires prior genetic alterations.

Mutational activation of *PIK3CA* also occurs frequently in colorectal cancers. Like *RAS* mutations, *PIK3CA* mutations are not often found in early stage tumors. Rather, *PIK3CA* mutations most often arise late in the process of tumorigenesis, when a tumor begins to invade surrounding normal tissues. One can infer that the increased activity of the *PIK3CA*-encoded protein provides a survival advantage to cancer cells as they penetrate the barriers that physically separate tissue compartments.

Further Reading

Bishop JM (1981) Enemies within: the genesis of retrovirus oncogenes. Cell 23:5–6

Epstein MA (2001) Historical background. Philos Trans R Soc Lond B Biol Sci 356:413–420

Garraway LA, Sellers WR (2006) Lineage dependency and lineage-survival oncogenes in human cancer. Nat Rev Cancer 6:593–602

Martin GS (2004) The road to Src. Oncogene 23:7910–7917

Mitelman F, Johansson B, Mertens F (2007) The impact of translocations and gene fusions on cancer causation. Nat Rev Cancer 7:233–245

Rowley JD (2001) Chromosome translocations: dangerous liaisons revisited. Nat Rev Cancer 1:245–250

Sawyers CL (1999) Chronic myeloid leukemia. N Engl J Med 340:1330–1340

Schwab M (1999) Oncogene amplification in solid tumors. Semin Cancer Biol 9:319–325

Thomas RK et al (2007) High-throughput oncogene mutation profiling in human cancer. Nat Genet 39:347–351

Vogt PK (2010) Retroviral oncogenes: a historical primer. Nat Rev Cancer 12:639–664

Weinberg RA (1997) The cat and mouse games that genes, viruses, and cells play. Cell 88:573–575

Chapter 3
Tumor Suppressor Genes

What Is a Tumor Suppressor Gene?

A *tumor suppressor gene* is a type of cancer gene that is created by a loss-of-function mutation. In contrast to the activating mutations that generate oncogenic alleles from proto-oncogene precursors, tumor suppressor genes and the proteins they encode are functionally *in*activated by mutations.

Tumor suppressor genes typically control processes that are fundamental to the maintenance of stable tissue compartments. Such cellular processes include the maintenance of genetic integrity, the regulated progression of the cell cycle, differentiation, growth inhibitory cell-cell interactions, and a form of programmed cell death known as *apoptosis*. Mutational inactivation of tumor suppressor genes contributes to the loss of tissue homeostasis – the hallmark of a developing neoplasm.

As described in Chap. 2, the mutations that convert proto-oncogenes to oncogenes are single nucleotide substitutions, amplifications, or chromosomal rearrangements that increase the activity or abundance of proto-oncogene-encoded proteins. Nonsense, frameshift and splice site mutations do not in most cases lead to proto-oncogene activation. In contrast, tumor suppressor genes are inactivated by mutations; a distinct spectrum of mutations has this inactivating effect. The open reading frames of tumor suppressor genes are commonly truncated by nonsense mutations or altered by small insertions, deletions, and splice site mutations. Larger deletions can eliminate exons or even entire genes. Tumor suppressor genes can also be inactivated by single base substitutions that alter functional sites in the encoded protein.

F. Bunz, *Principles of Cancer Genetics*, DOI 10.1007/978-94-017-7484-0_3

The Discovery of Recessive Cancer Phenotypes

The first cancer genes to be discovered were oncogenes. For a time it was accordingly believed that the cancer phenotype resulted primarily from activating mutations that led to gains of function. An early piece of evidence that other types of genetic alteration might also be important in cancer was provided by Henry Harris and his colleagues.

In a 1969 study, Harris adopted a novel approach to study the genetic factors that were involved in cancer cell phenotypes (Fig. 3.1). Previously, it had been established

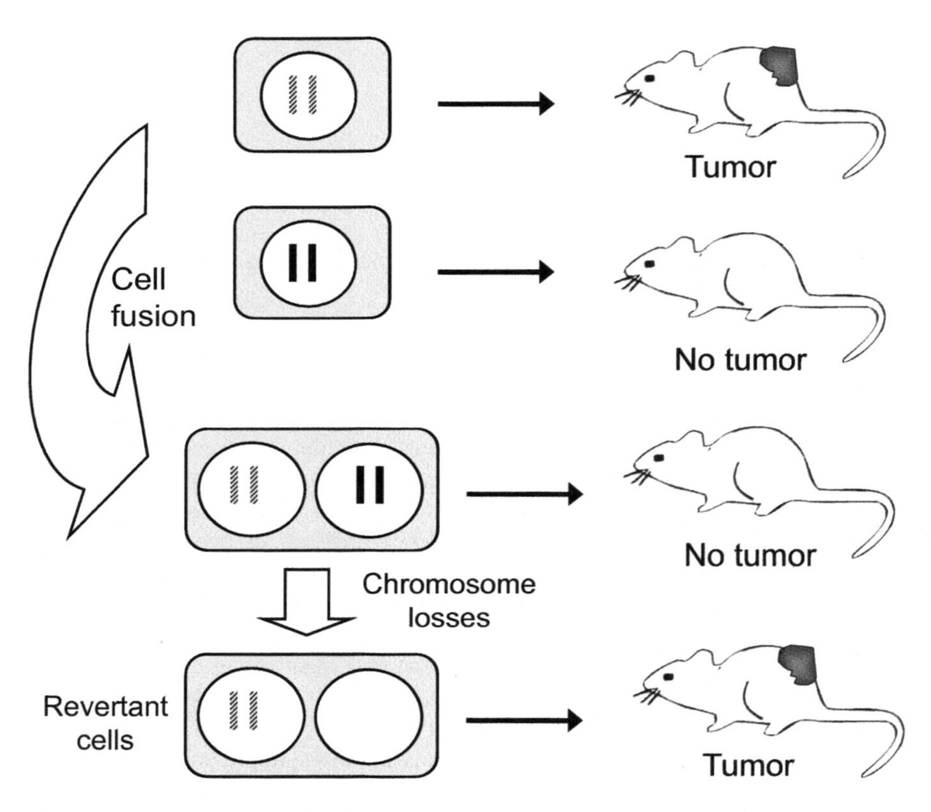

Fig. 3.1 Tumor suppression is a dominant phenotype. Two distinct types of cultured cells can be distinguished upon their introduction into mice: tumorigenic cells (which form tumors when experimentally introduced just below the skin of mice) and non-tumorigenic cells. Fusion of these two types of cells allows them to share their genetic material. Cells containing both sets of chromosomes are not tumorigenic, demonstrating that the alleles that cause tumor formation (carried on the hatched chromosomes, in the illustration below) are recessive. Because the chromosome complement of the fused cells are unstable, over time cells appear that have lost wild type alleles (carried on the solid chromosomes) contributed by the non-tumorigenic cells. These rare cells revert to a tumorigenic phenotype. In this simplified illustration, only the relevant pair of homologous chromosomes is shown in each cell

that cells of different types could be experimentally fused, and thereby made to share their genes. Among the phenotypes that many cultured cancer cells share is an ability to grow into tumors when implanted into mice, a property is known as tumorigenicity. Tumorigenicity is an experimental trait that is believed to be reflective of the malignant nature of the tumor from which cultured cancer cell was derived. Harris found that when tumorigenic cells derived from a murine tumor were fused with non-tumorigenic cells, the resulting hybrid cells were non-tumorigenic. The genome of the non-tumorigenic cells therefore suppressed tumorigenicity of the cancer cells in a dominant manner.

Continued observation of the fused hybrids revealed the basis for this effect. When the non-tumorigenic hybrid cells were cultured for extensive periods, newly tumorigenic subpopulations began to appear. Cytogenetic analysis revealed chromosomal losses in these subclones, also known as revertants. Subsequent studies with human cells demonstrated that the suppression of tumorigenicity was sustained as long as both sets of parental chromosomes were retained. The transfer of individual chromosomes was found to similarly suppress the tumorigenicity of human cancer cells, even if an activated oncogene, such as a mutant *RAS* gene, was expressed in the hybrids. Thus, it was apparent that the underlying cause of reversion to the tumorigenic phenotype was not chromosomal losses in general, but rather the loss of specific chromosomes that could actively suppress tumor growth. The investigators concluded that tumorigenicity was a recessive trait that could be suppressed by the transfer of a specific chromosome, and perhaps even by the transfer of a single dominant gene.

Somatic cell genetic studies such as these supported the idea that at least some aspects of the malignant cancer cell phenotype are recessive traits that arise through genetic losses. It is important to understand that the primary assay used in these studies, the generation of tumors upon introduction of cells into a mouse, does not recapitulate the many selective pressures faced during the evolution of a naturally occurring tumor. Thus, the chromosomal additions in the fused hybrids and subsequent losses by the revertants presumably affected only a subset of cancer-associated phenotypes. Indeed, other cancer cell phenotypes such as immortality and anchorage-independent growth were found to be retained in the non-tumorigenic somatic cell hybrids. These results are consistent with the idea that cancer cells arise by the accumulation of multiple genetic alterations that cause complex phenotypic traits. The genetic alterations that promote the progressive process of tumorigenesis cause the conversion of proto-oncogenes to oncogenes and the loss of tumor suppressor genes.

Retinoblastoma and Knudson's Two-Hit Hypothesis

Retinoblastoma is a tumor of the eye that arises from immature cells within the retina (Fig. 3.2). Though retinoblastoma is a relatively rare tumor, occurring with an incidence of roughly 1 in 20,000 live births, its clinical features and the distinct

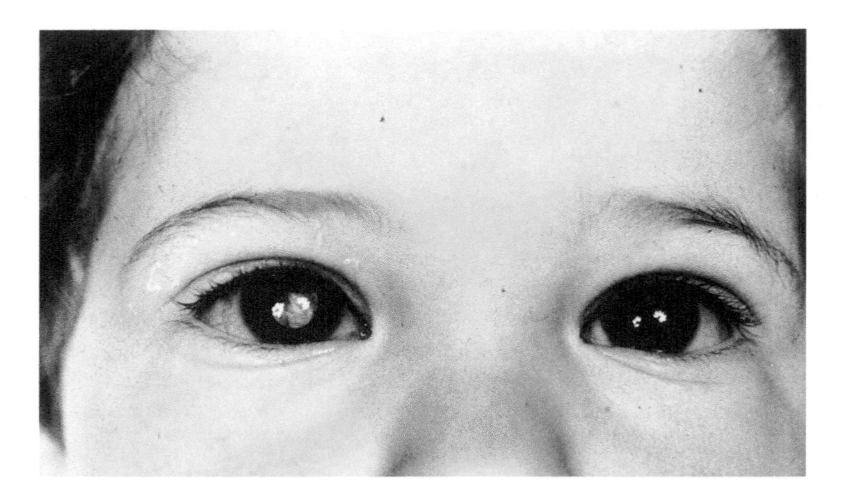

Fig. 3.2 Retinoblastoma. A pediatric malignancy of the retina, retinoblastoma occurs in hereditary and sporadic forms. Shown is a unilateral tumor in the patient's right eye. Image from the National Cancer Institute

characteristics of sporadic and heritable tumors have provided a model for understanding how tumor suppressor genes work.

Retinoblastoma occurs during infancy and early childhood, and accounts for 11 % of all cancers that occur in the first year of life. Ninety percent of patients have no family history of the disease.

The cells of the retina are nearly fully differentiated at birth and have a limited capacity for further proliferation. The early differentiation of the blast cells of the retina provides, in effect, a temporal window of cancer susceptibility. Somatic mutations that occur within this proliferative window can potentially contribute to the subsequent growth of tumors.

Retinoblastoma has distinctive clinical features that allow it to be diagnosed with a high degree of accuracy. These cancers occur in two distinct patterns. Examination of epidemiological data by Alfred Knudson in the early 1970s revealed that retinoblastomas that occur in individuals with a family history of the disease frequently affect both eyes and exhibit multifocal tumors in a single eye. However, the more common presentation, which accounts for about two thirds of all cases, is a tumor that is unifocal and restricted to one eye. While there is considerable overlap in the age at diagnosis, the bilateral form of the disease is, on average, diagnosed at 1 year of age. The unilateral cases peak at about 2 years. Rare cases have been reported in older children and even in young adults.

Building upon these data, Knudson formulated what would come to be known as the two-hit hypothesis (Fig. 3.3). Knudson deduced that two genetic alterations, or 'hits', are necessary for retinoblastoma development. In individuals with the bilateral form of the disease, the first hit is always in the germline and thus present in every cell. The second hit required for the disease in these predisposed individuals

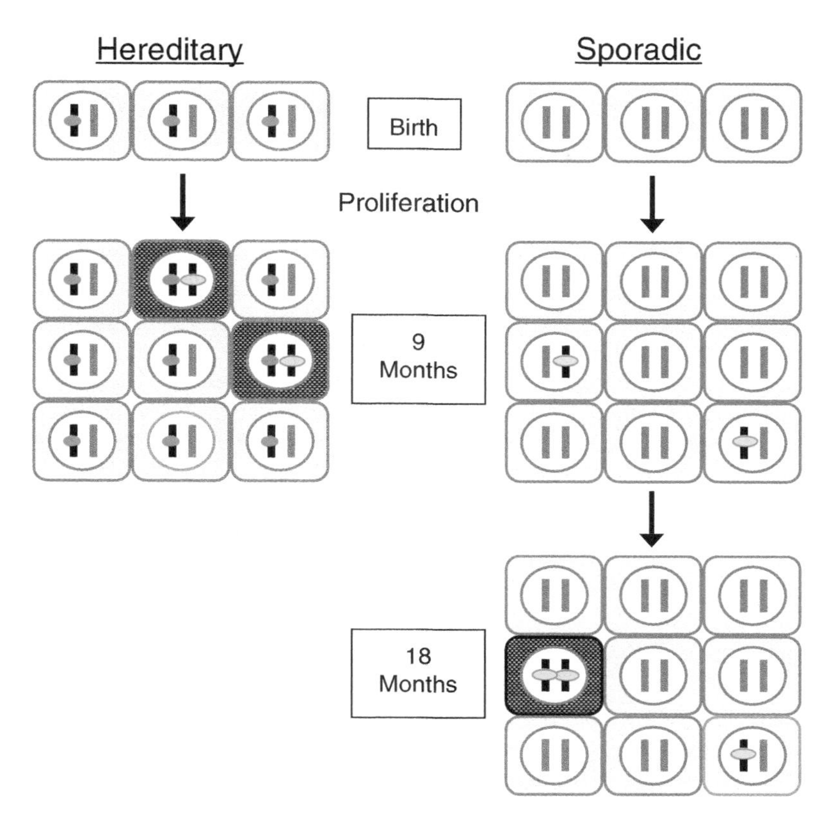

Fig. 3.3 The 'two-hit' hypothesis. At birth, individuals predisposed to retinoblastoma harbor a mutant allele (shown in *red*) in every cell, including the blast cells of the retina. These cells continue to proliferate during the first 9 months of life. During this time, somatic mutations at the retinoblastoma locus (shown in *yellow*) occur at a low frequency. In individuals predisposed to retinoblastoma, the somatic inactivation of a single allele is sufficient to provide the second hit required for tumor formation. Multiple tumor precursor cells (shown as *dark cells*) are thus generated. These develop into bilateral and multifocal tumors. In contrast, non-carriers require two independent somatic hits for tumor development. Because of the requirement for two sequential somatic hits, sporadic retinoblastomas are usually diagnosed at a somewhat older age than heritable retinoblastomas caused by germline mutations

is a somatic mutation in a single precursor cell, which then expands into a tumor. In unilateral cases of retinoblastoma, both of the required hits were acquired via somatic mutations in a single precursor cell. Notably, most bilateral cases of retinoblastoma occur in the absence of a family history of the disease, suggesting the *de novo* appearance of new germline mutations.

The Knudson model explains why bilateral and multifocal tumors occur only in the heritable form of the disease. The rate limiting event is the somatic mutation, which occurs at random and at a very low frequency during the limited temporal window of susceptibility. Individuals predisposed to retinoblastoma, whether from an inherited allele or a new germline mutation, already harbor the first mutational hit in every cell. Each proliferative cell in the retina is thus a potential precursor to a tumor. The onset of disease requires only one rate-limiting step. In cases arising from somatically acquired mutations, two rare events must have occurred within a single cell within a brief window of time. Such cases are always unilateral because of the improbability that more than one precursor cell will independently acquire two hits.

The formulation of the two-hit hypothesis by Knudson was contemporary with the somatic cell genetic studies undertaken by Harris. These two very disparate lines of inquiry converged on a common principle: recessive genetic determinants play a significant role in cancer. While these studies laid the framework for understanding the roles of tumor suppressor genes, the actual loci that possessed these properties remained to be identified. Only upon the actual cloning and characterization of prototypical tumor suppressor genes, did the extent of their involvement in cancer become apparent.

Chromosomal Localization of the Retinoblastoma Gene

Based on epidemiology alone, the two hits required for retinoblastoma could have been accounted for by mutations in two separate genes, perhaps two oncogenes that were sequentially activated. However, the experiments by Harris had shed light on a completely novel and uncharacterized type of cancer gene that was recessive in nature. Knudson suggested that both hits could occur in the two alleles of a single locus, and thereby cause the total inactivation of a recessive cancer gene. Knudson's hypothesis was supported and extended with the cloning and identification of the retinoblastoma susceptibility gene, *RB1*.

The genetic basis of retinoblastoma was inferred from its distribution among sporadic and familial cases. However, the identity of the actual gene or genes that might be the target of Knudson's hits was completely unknown. The progressive mapping and ultimately the identification of the retinoblastoma gene was a landmark discovery that not only revealed the molecular basis of retinoblastoma susceptibility, but also shaped a general and central principle of cancer genetics.

Retinoblastoma tumor cells had no known biochemical or signaling defect. There was therefore no basis to suspect that the causative gene might encode any particular enzyme or regulatory protein. Ultimately, the retinoblastoma gene was not identified by virtue of its function, but rather on the basis of its location.

The first clue as to the location of the retinoblastoma locus arose from cytogenetic studies in the late 1970s. Improvements in chromosome banding techniques facilitated the detailed analysis of karyotypes from normal and tumor-derived cells. Microscopically visible deletions within one copy of chromosome 13 were observed in the normal blood cells of a small proportion of individuals with the inherited form of the disease. A cytogenetic aberration that is found in the normal cells of an individual is known as a *constitutional* alteration.

While the extent of the constitutional deletion varied among retinoblastoma-prone individuals, one particular chromosomal band on the short arm of chromosome 13, designated 13q14, was consistently missing. Somatic deletions involving band 13q14 were also found in about 25 % of retinoblastoma tumor samples from patients with the non-heritable form of the disease. In these cases, examination of blood cells from the same patient revealed two normal homologs of chromosome 13, indicating that the 13q14 deletions found in the tumors were somatic mutations that occurred during tumor development. Thus, a defined chromosomal deletion within the body of a chromosome, known as an *interstitial* deletion, appeared to be associated with at least some cases of both heritable and non-heritable retinoblastoma.

The pattern of these interstitial deletions in normal and cancer cells was consistent with the 2-hit model proposed by Knudson. The constitutional deletion found in patients with heritable retinoblastoma was present in all cells and consistent with a first hit in the germline. The deletions present in the cancer cells obtained from the unilateral, sporadic cases were clearly somatic hits that had occurred during tumorigenesis, though it was not yet clear that they had initiated the process.

The recurrent nature of the 13q14 interstitial deletion suggested that a gene within the 13q14 band might be the target of the two hits required for retinoblastoma development. However, in the majority of retinoblastoma cases, no obvious karyotypic abnormalities were observed. It remained a possibility that a smaller deletion, undetectable by cytogenetic approaches, might constitute a genetically equivalent hit in these cases. Deletions that can be appreciated by microscopy are large, typically extending over regions that can span hundreds of kilobases. No abnormalities in this size range could be observed in the majority of retinoblastoma patients. Additional evidence was required to establish that the retinoblastoma susceptibility locus was located within the cytogenetically-defined 13q14 region.

The mapping of the retinoblastoma susceptibility gene to the 13q14 region was confirmed by a meticulous process known as *linkage analysis*, whereby a previously mapped gene is used as a physical point of reference. The *ESD* gene, which encodes an enzyme known as esterase D, had recently been localized to the 13q14 band by William Benedict and his colleagues. While the biochemical function of esterase D was irrelevant to the pathogenesis of retinoblastoma, *ESD* could be used as a genetic marker to assess smaller 13q14 deletions in individuals that did not exhibit gross karyotypic abnormalities.

Esterase D exists in two distinct forms that are encoded by two common *ESD* alleles. The two forms of esterase D protein could be resolved by protein electophoresis, and thus heterozygous individuals could be identified. Heterozygosity at the *ESD* locus allowed the tracking of each allele through the pedigrees of families with inherited retinoblastoma. Benedict and his coworkers determined that, within a disease-prone family, children that inherited one allele of *ESD* invariably developed retinoblastoma while children that inherited the other *ESD* allele remained disease-free (Fig. 3.4). In genetic terms, the *ESD* alleles co-segregated with the retinoblastoma susceptibility trait. These studies revealed that *ESD* and the as-yet undiscovered retinoblastoma gene were tightly linked and therefore in close physical proximity to one another.

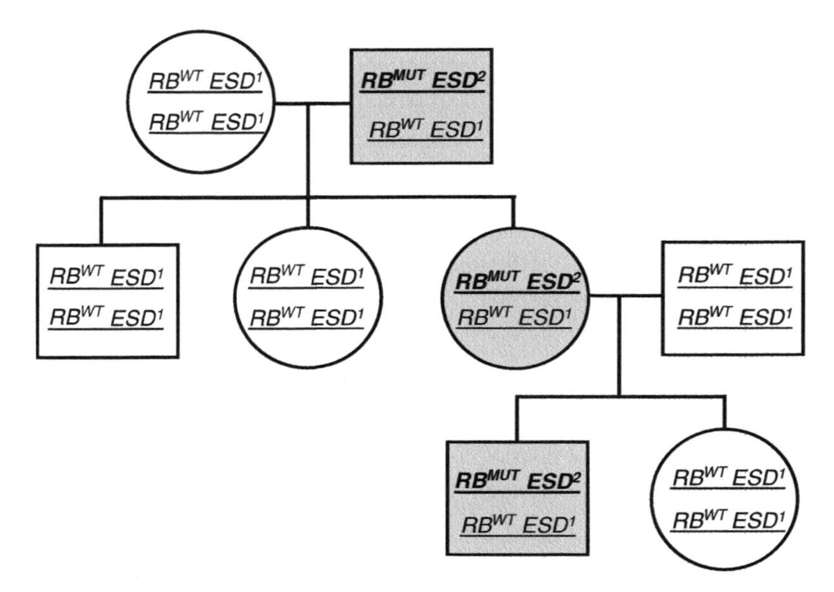

Fig. 3.4 Linkage between the retinoblastoma disease locus and *ESD*. Distinct alleles of the *ESD* gene (denoted ESD^1 and ESD^2), encode proteins that can be resolved by protein electrophoresis. Evaluation of *ESD*-encoded proteins thus provides an assessment of *ESD* allelotype. In retinoblastoma kindreds, allelic variants of *ESD*, when present in the heterozygous state, invariably co-segregate with disease. In the pedigree shown, *circles* represent females, *squares* represent males. *Shaded circles* and *squares* represent individuals affected by retinoblastoma

The Mapping and Cloning of the Retinoblastoma Gene

The linkage between the retinoblastoma susceptibility locus and *ESD* provided a means of exploring the nature of the hits that involved a putative retinoblastoma gene in the 13q14 region. Cases were identified in which normal cells of a retinoblastoma patient were heterozygous for *ESD*. Heterozygosity of the nearby *ESD* locus did not affect retinoblastoma predisposition *per se*, but rather created a situation in which the two chromosomal loci could be distinguished. Heterozygosity was thus informative; no additional information could be extracted from homozygous cases wherein the *ESD* alleles were indistinguishable.

In several informative, heterozygous cases, both *ESD* alleles were present in normal blood cells, while only one of the two *ESD* genes was present in the cells of the tumor (Fig. 3.5). The tumor cells thus exhibited a *loss of heterozygosity* – a state that is often used in the abbreviated form LOH – in the region adjacent to the susceptibility locus. LOH was also detected in inherited cases of retinoblastoma. In these cases, the allele of *ESD* retained in the tumor cells was invariably the one that

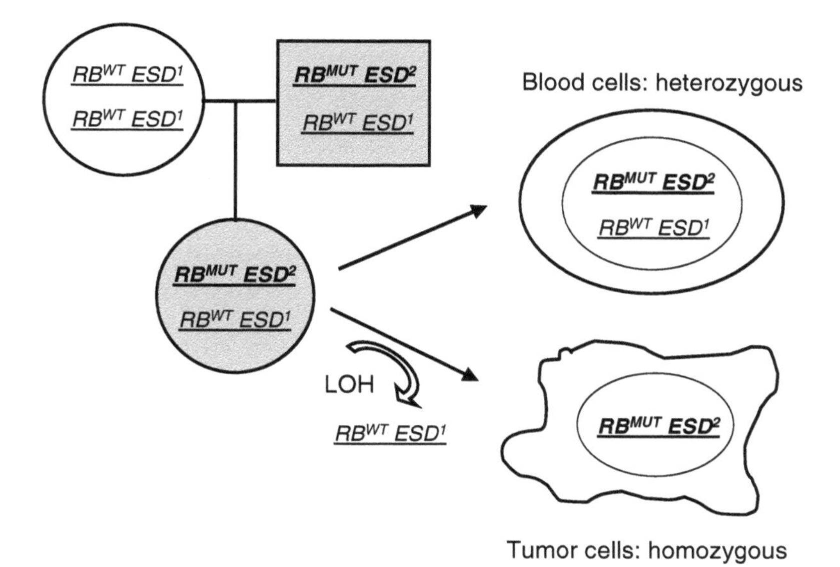

Fig. 3.5 Loss of heterozygosity in the region of the retinoblastoma disease locus. The mutation that causes heritable retinoblastoma (RB^{MUT}) is present in the germline of an affected individual. In this example, RB^{MUT} co-segregates with a distinguishable *ESD* allele, ESD^2. During tumor development, the single normal allele and the ESD^1 allele to which it is linked are invariably lost. Only ESD^2 is detectable in tumor cells. In contrast, both alleles are retained in normal blood cells

was inherited from the affected parent. The reduction of the *ESD* locus to homozygosity was an important piece of evidence that a somatic mutation resulting in a loss of genetic material had functionally inactivated the single normal copy of the putative retinoblastoma gene in susceptible individuals. Thus, the link between the retinoblastoma locus and *ESD* provided an indirect means of assessing genetic losses in that region. While the broad 13q14 region was lost in only a small fraction of retinoblastoma patients, the LOH at *ESD* suggested that smaller, submicroscopic deletions could account for the loss of a neighboring gene in many additional patients.

The precise location and the identity of the actual retinoblastoma gene remained to be determined. The fact that a tumor suppressor locus was strongly linked to a polymorphic gene that encodes readily distinguishable proteins was highly fortuitous. In most cases, tumor suppressor loci cannot be evaluated for losses by examining expressed proteins. A more versatile mapping strategy was to link unknown genes with known DNA polymorphisms using available methods for DNA analysis.

One type of polymorphism that could be detected with the information and technology available during the 1980s was the *restriction fragment length polymorphism*, or RFLP. Restriction enzymes are enzymes that cut DNA at sites that have defined and highly specific recognition sequences. Some DNA sequence polymorphisms result in changes in the pattern at which these recognition sequences occur in a chromosomal region. Differences between homologous chromosomal loci could therefore be detected by examining the lengths of the polymorphic restriction fragments produced by the digestion of genomic DNA. Specific fragments could be visualized by the technique of Southern blotting, in which a defined, locus-specific probe is hybridized to a restriction fragments that are fractionated by length.

In 1983, RFLP analysis performed by Webster Cavenee, Ray White and their colleagues confirmed and more exactly defined the linkage between *ESD* and the putative retinoblastoma gene. They were able to track specific heterozygous restriction fragments from affected parents to affected children, and were able to detect LOH in tumor cells. With the use of additional probes, Thaddeus Dryja and his coworkers were able to detect relatively small regions within the 13q14 region that were homozygously deleted in retinoblastoma tumor cells. Thus, two significant milestones had been simultaneously attained. First, the direct relationship between genetic loss and retinoblastoma cancer development was firmly established. Second, the location of the putative retinoblastoma locus had been narrowed down to a relatively short region on chromosome 13. The technique of using a series of adjacent probes to systematically examine loss patterns along lengthy regions was a powerful technique that became known as '*walking the chromosome*'.

The retinoblastoma gene, *RB1*, was identified in late 1986 and early 1987 by three independent groups. In collaboration with Robert Weinberg and his laboratory, the Dryja group cloned the retinoblastoma gene by hybridizing cloned genomic DNAs from within the known region of loss with fractionated RNA transcripts from normal retinal cells and retinoblastoma cells. A 4.7 kilobase RNA transcript was identified that was present only in normal cells and not in tumor cells. The laboratory of Wen-Hwa Lee and that of Yuen-Kai Fung and William Benedict also cloned the *RB1* gene using the same general strategy. The approach of using localized markers to identify physically-linked disease genes came to be known as *positional cloning*.

The cloning and characterization of *RB1*facilitated detailed mutational analysis in large tumor panels. *RB1* consists of 27 exons that span a genomic region that is approximately 178 kb in length. Subsequent mutational studies detected frequent deletions that eliminate all or part of the coding region. Other types of mutations that result in *RB1* inactivation occur at lower frequencies.

Functional analysis of *RB1* has revealed a central role for its encoded protein in the regulation of the cell cycle. Homozygous inactivation of *RB1* results in a cell that is completely deficient in the expression of Rb protein, with a corresponding lack of cell cycle regulation. This loss of regulation is apparently sufficient to initiate tumor growth in the immature cells of the retina. The role of *RB1* in the regulation of the cell cycle will be described in detail in Chap. 6.

Tumor Suppressor Gene Inactivation: The Second 'Hit' and Loss of Heterozygosity

One of the key observations that guided the discovery of the *RB1* gene and confirmed its recessive nature was LOH, the reduction to homozygosity in tumor cells of a locus that is heterozygous in normal tissues. LOH is the second 'hit' predicted by Knudson, and represents the loss of the remaining wild type allele of a recessive tumor suppressor gene. With more refined methods, LOH at subsequently discovered tumor suppressor loci could be more rapidly assessed by the examination of known single nucleotide polymorphisms (SNPs), which represent plentiful and easily detectable genetic markers (see Chap. 1).

During the process of tumorigenesis, LOH can occur by several mechanisms (Fig. 3.6):

Loss of a Whole Chromosome Chromosome nondisjunction during mitosis can cause an imbalance in chromosomal segregation, resulting in a chromosome loss in one daughter cell. Nondisjunction is sometimes followed by reduplication of the

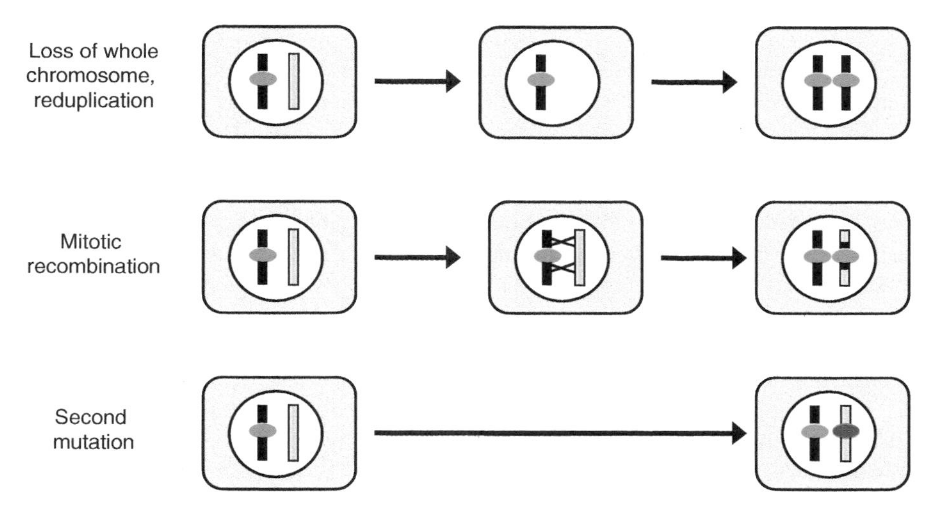

Fig. 3.6 Mechanisms of Loss of Heterozygosity (LOH). A cell contains two homologous chromosomes, one of which is shown in this illustration to contain a genetic alteration (*red*). Loss of the remaining allele, measured as LOH of linked markers, can occur by several mechanisms: (1) complete loss of the "wild type" chromosome, followed by reduplication of the "mutant" chromosome, will result in LOH across the entire chromosome (*top*); (2) Recombination during mitosis results in the replacement of wild type sequence with a region containing the mutation on the homologous chromosome-, resulting in regional LOH (*middle*); (3) A second mutation (*blue*), such as a deletion, can spontaneously arise in the second allele, resulting in a very localized region of LOH confined to the region encompassing the second mutation. In the case of a point mutation, there will be no detectable LOH at other markers (*bottom*)

remaining unpaired chromosome. In these cases, the overall number of alleles is preserved. Following chromosome loss, heterozygosity of all genes and markers on a chromosome is also lost, regardless of whether reduplication takes place.

Mitotic Recombination The pairing of homologous chromosomes during mitosis results in crossing over and physical exchange of genetic material. Recombination of this type occurs most frequently during meiosis, but also occurs at a lower rate during mitosis. The transfer of a region of DNA from one paired chromosome to another by homologous recombination is known as *gene conversion*. LOH resulting from gene conversion is restricted to a portion of a chromosome.

Localized Mutations The remaining wild type allele of a tumor suppressor gene can be lost by a second mutation that does not involve a large chromosomal region, but is rather more local in nature. In retinoblastomas, for example, deletions have frequently been found to inactivate both *RB1* alleles. In such cases, the first and second 'hits' occur via the same mechanism but independently of one another, resulting in a homozygous deletion that disrupts both *RB1* alleles. Other types of mutations can also confer the second 'hit' predicted by the Knudson hypothesis, without necessarily causing LOH.

These processes occur at a higher rate in many tumor cells than they do in normal cells. Correspondingly, the rate of tumor suppressor gene loss is frequently higher in early stage cancers than in their pre-cancerous precursors. The inherent genetic instability of cancer cells and the contribution of instability to LOH will be described in Chap. 4.

Two mechanisms of LOH – chromosome loss and mitotic recombination – involve very large regions of the chromosome. In such cases, detection of LOH was a very low resolution method of tumor suppressor gene mapping. More localized mutations were usually needed to finally pinpoint a region that contained a putative tumor suppressor locus. In the case of *RB1*, it was the analysis of homozygous deletions that provided this crucial information.

In summary, the inactivation of a tumor suppressor gene occurs in two distinct steps that correspond to Knudson's two 'hits'. The first step is the mutational inactivation of one allele. An individual can acquire an inactivated tumor suppressor allele by somatic mutation. Alternatively, an individual can inherit a predisposition to cancer by inheriting a mutated allele via the germline, thereby bypassing a rate-limiting step. This inactivated allele does not, in most cases, directly confer any cellular phenotype, but merely heightens the risk that the gene will subsequently become biallelically inactivated. While the first step varies in heritable and non-heritable, sporadic cancers, the second step to total gene inactivation is always the same: the somatic loss of the remaining normal allele.

Recessive Genes, Dominant Traits

The cloning of the retinoblastoma gene was a landmark in cancer genetics. The incremental localization of *RB1* by virtue of its linkage to known genetic markers provided a highly successful paradigm for tumor suppressor gene discovery. In more recent years, the sequencing of the human genome and the identification of many defined polymorphisms have greatly streamlined the search for tumor suppressors. As a result, the laborious methods that were used to clone the first tumor suppressor genes have become obsolete. Nonetheless, the principles forged by these early efforts have largely informed our current understanding of how tumor suppressor genes contribute to tumorigenesis and cancer susceptibility.

The identification of *RB1* was a considerably more complex, laborious, time consuming and costly process than the isolation of the first oncogenes had been less than a decade earlier, despite dramatic improvements in molecular technology. This is because tumor suppressor genes were inherently more difficult to identify. Tumor suppressor genes are recessive while oncogenes are dominant. It is simpler to assess the one-step gain of a dominant gene than the two-step loss of a recessive gene. A dominant gene such as an oncogene can in many cases recapitulate its cancer phenotype upon experimental introduction into normal cells. In contrast, the cancer-related effects of a mutated tumor suppressor gene are masked by the presence of a normal allele. Recessive phenotypes can be clearly attributed to a given gene only upon the experimental inactivation of all normal alleles.

The relationship between cancer susceptibility as an organismal trait and the cellular phenotypes of tumor suppressor genes can be confusing. Individuals are strongly predisposed to retinoblastoma if they inherit a single defective *RB1* allele. Cancer predisposition is the trait caused by the germline mutation, and because it is caused by the inheritance of a single allele located on an autosome it is by definition an *autosomal dominant* trait. However, at the cellular level tumor suppressor genes behave in a recessive fashion. The cellular phenotypes of a mutated tumor suppressor allele are only manifest when the remaining normal (wild type, non-mutated) allele is lost. In a strictly numerical sense, these second hits are rare. However there are many cellular targets in which they can occur. In the infant retina, for example, there are more than 10^6 cells, many of which proliferate during the window of susceptibility. Even a rare genetic event is likely to occur in a sufficiently large population of cells. Importantly, tumor suppressor traits such as retinoblastoma are highly penetrant. Thus, even rare events occurring in only a few proliferating cells can give rise to multiple tumors.

APC Inactivation in Inherited and Sporadic Colorectal Cancers

Colorectal cancer occurs in both heritable and sporadic forms (see Chap. 1). As in the case of retinoblastoma, the heritable forms of colorectal cancer are caused by germline tumor suppressor gene mutations. Sporadic tumors arise as a result of either germline mutations that arise *de novo*, in the absence of a family history of disease, or two somatically required mutations in the same gene. In colorectal cancer, a gene that plays a role analogous to that of *RB1* is *adenomatous polyposis coli*, now designated *APC*.

APC is a tumor suppressor gene that is critically involved in the development of colorectal cancers. Like *RB1*, *APC* was cloned by virtue of its chromosomal location. The identification of the *APC* locus arose from intensive studies of familial adenomatous polyposis (FAP), a heritable form of colorectal cancer in which predisposed individuals develop a large number of polyps and cancers. Upon cytogenetic analysis of normal blood cells, one FAP patient was identified that had an interstitial deletion within the long arm of chromosome 5. This chromosome had been inherited from an affected parent. As was the case with retinoblastoma, the finding of a constitutional chromosomal deletion in a susceptible individual provided the first clue as to the location of the gene that was the primary cause of the disease.

A second, independent line of evidence implicating the 5q region in colorectal tumorigenesis arose from the study of LOH in sporadic colorectal cancers. These studies showed that chromosome 5 losses occurred frequently in sporadic tumors. Importantly, LOH on chromosome 5 was found in both small adenomas and in large carcinomas, suggesting that inactivation of a tumor suppressor gene on chromosome 5 was an early event, and thus possibly required for tumor initiation.

A total of four genes were mapped to the common region of loss at chromosome band 5q21–22 by the laboratories of Ray White, Yusuke Nakamura and Bert Vogelstein. Each of these genes was interrogated by DNA sequence analysis. One gene within the defined region, *APC*, was found to be mutated in sporadic tumors and in the germline of FAP patients. In tumor samples from sporadic and inherited cases alike, LOH had resulted in the complete loss of wild type *APC* alleles.

The cloning of the *APC* gene and the characterization of *APC* mutations in inherited and sporadic colorectal cancers reinforced and extended many of the basic principles of tumor suppressor genes originally established by the cloning of *RB1*. The fact that colorectal cancer is much more common than retinoblastoma and occurs in more diverse forms revealed several important facets of tumor suppressor gene mutations.

The *APC* mutations that are present in the germline of FAP kindreds and those that occur somatically in sporadic cases are similar in type. Single nucleotide substitutions within the open reading frame cause nonsense codons and splice site mutations, while small insertions or deletions lead to frameshifts. In contrast to the mutations that inactivate *RB1* in retinoblastoma, which are most commonly deletions, the mutations that inactivate *APC* result in the truncation of the expressed APC protein.

The clinical features of FAP vary among affected families, depending upon the specific *APC* mutant in the germline (Fig. 3.7). Truncating mutations that occur between codons 463 and 1387 cause retinal lesions called congenital hypertrophy of the retinal pigment epithelium (CHRPE). In contrast, truncating mutations between codons 1403 and 1578 are associated with desmoid tumors and mandibular osteomas, a condition known as Gardner's syndrome – but do not cause CHRPE. Other *APC* mutants are associated with increased or decreased numbers of tumors. While a variety of germline *APC* cause colorectal tumors, these different alleles are clearly not equivalent. FAP thus illuminates the general principle that the genotype/phenotype relationship involving a tumor suppressor gene and a cancer can be highly specific. Even patients that carry identical *APC* mutations can have differing disease manifestations. For example, while one individual with a mutation near codon 1500 may develop the extra-colonic tumors associated with Gardner's syndrome, another individual with the same mutation may not. Other genetic differences, not directly involving the *APC* locus, are likely to play a role in the types of cancer that ultimately arise in predisposed individuals. Genetic factors that affect the diseases caused by known tumor suppressor mutations are referred to as *modifiers*.

Colorectal polyps are common in the general population. About one half of all individuals will develop an adenomatous polyp, a precursor lesion to an invasive cancer, by the age of 70. Interestingly, as many as 25 % of individuals with multiple polyps carry variant *APC* alleles in their germline, that are present in only 12 % of normal controls. These allelic variants are not truncated *APC* alleles, but contain

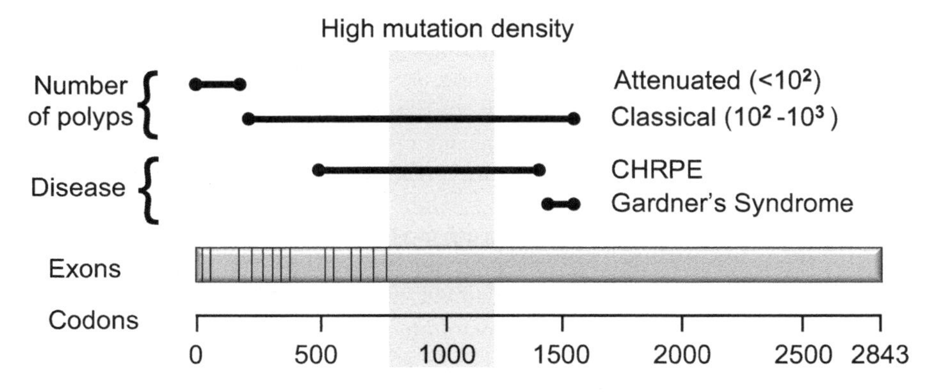

Fig. 3.7 Inherited mutations of the *APC* gene. In many cases, specific *APC* mutations can be correlated with distinct phenotypes and disease subtypes. The *APC* gene is composed of 15 exons that in total contain a 8538 bp open reading frame that normally encodes a protein of 2843 amino acids. The last exon is unusually large. Approximately two-thirds of all *APC* mutations found are clustered in the 5′ region of exon 15. An attenuated form of FAP is associated with mutations within the first 157 codons, whereas more typical pronounced levels of polyposis are associated with mutations occurring between codons 169 and 1600. Mutations within distinct domains cause CHIRPE and Gardner's syndrome

single nucleotide substitutions that may cause subtle variations in APC protein function. It thus appears possible that some relatively common variants of *APC* carry an increased risk of polyps and cancer. The contributions of common alleles to this common type of tumor remain to be firmly established.

While the majority of cancer-associated *APC* mutations give rise to truncated and highly dysfunctional proteins, other rare mutations appear to affect cancer predisposition in more subtle ways. These types of mutations do not appear to account for a large proportion of colorectal cancers, but they nonetheless illustrate the remarkable and varied ways that heritable tumor suppressor gene mutations alter the overall cancer risk.

Mutations Causing Altered Gene Expression An FAP kindred was identified in which no obvious mutation could be detected within the *APC* open reading frame. However, detailed analysis of one affected individual revealed markedly reduced expression of one *APC* allele. Presumably, an unidentified mutation in a regulatory region outside the open reading frame had altered the expression of *APC*. As is typically the case with FAP, LOH involving the *APC* locus was detected in the majority of the tumors removed from this patient. In every lesion, the *APC* allele lost was the wild type allele that was expressed at normal levels. Linkage of a low-expressing *APC* allele with polyp formation thus suggests that even partial loss of function of this gene is sufficient to confer cancer predisposition.

'Pre-mutations' in APC Distinct germline *APC* mutations cause less penetrant predispositions to colorectal cancer that are distinct from FAP, a highly penetrant syndrome. An *APC* allele that contains a missense mutation in codon 1307 – changing the encoded amino acid from an isoleucine (I) to a lysine (K) – is found at a relatively high frequency among individuals of Ashkenazi Jewish ancestry. This allele, designated I1307K, is present in approximately 6 % of individuals in this ethnic group, but is rare in the general population. Among the Ashkenazim, the I1307K allele is overrepresented in patients with colorectal cancer and in individuals with a family history of colorectal cancer. Molecular epidemiology shows that the I1307K allele is associated with a twofold increased risk of developing cancer. The I1307K allele predisposes carriers to cancer by a unique mechanism. Sequence analysis of the codon 1307 region in tumors occurring in I1307K carriers revealed a high frequency of somatically-acquired truncating mutations. These somatic changes were restricted to the I1307K allele; the normal APC allele was not mutated in the tumors analyzed. The surprising conclusion drawn from these studies is that the 1307 germline variant is a genomic sequence that is uniquely prone to somatic mutations. The 1307 mutation has been accordingly referred to as a pre-mutation, which alone does not alter the encoded protein in a functionally significant way, but instead raises the probability of a subsequent mutation.

Germline Mutations in MUTYH A rare, genetically distinct form of familial colorectal polyposis is caused by recessive mutations in the gene *MUTYH*, which encodes an enzyme involved in DNA damage repair. The polyps caused by loss of MUTYH activity occur later in life and are less numerous than those caused by *APC* heterozygosity. The overall risk of cancer is therefore lower than for the classic type of FAP caused by truncating mutations in *APC*.

TP53 Inactivation: A Frequent Event in Tumorigenesis

While *APC* is a very frequent target of mutation during the early development of colorectal cancer, it was not the first tumor suppressor gene discovered to be involved in colorectal tumorigenesis. That distinction belongs to *TP53*, the mutant forms of which are highly prevalent cancer genes found about one half of all colorectal cancers and in a large proportion of many other human malignancies. *TP53* mutations are associated with almost every type of human cancer.

Unlike *RB1* and *APC*, *TP53* was cloned only after the discovery and characterization of its encoded protein. The p53 protein was independently discovered by David Lane and Arnold Levine, and their colleagues, in 1979. Both groups detected a 53 kDa protein that was physically associated with an oncogenic, DNA tumor virus-encoded protein called large T antigen. Because the identity and function of this cellular protein were completely unknown, the protein was named for its molecular weight. Specific antibodies raised against p53 were used to screen gene expression libraries, resulting in the isolation of cDNAs derived from *TP53* transcripts. A *TP53* cDNA was then used to isolate a genomic DNA fragment that mapped to the short arm of chromosome 17.

Several attributes of this new gene suggested that it might play an important role in cancer cells. The most compelling finding was that p53 protein levels were elevated, sometimes to a great extent, in a wide range of cultured cancer cells and tumors. Furthermore, the experimental overexpression of p53 protein in primary cells contributed to changes in their growth and enhanced their ability to form tumors in mice, an attribute known as *tumorgenicity*.

At the early stages of *TP53* gene characterization, the oncogene hypothesis was well established while evidence favoring a major role for tumor suppressor genes was still very limited. The overexpression of p53 protein in cancer cells immediately suggested a gain-of-function, consistent with a role for *TP53* as a proto-oncogene. The detection of p53 in virus-infected cells was reminiscent of the earlier isolation of the first oncogenes. However, inconsistencies arose in these early studies, leading to their reevaluation. It became apparent that *TP53*-derived cDNA clones isolated by different laboratories had slightly different sequences. Further analysis of more primary samples revealed that the gene sequences thought to be wild type (non-mutated) were actually tumor-associated mutants. These mutated alleles had been inadvertently isolated because *TP53* mutations are very prevalent in human cancer, a fact that was not yet known at the time.

The confusion over the role of *TP53* was resolved with the discovery that the gene mapped to a common region of allelic loss in colorectal cancers, located at 17p13. In a colorectal tumor that had undergone LOH at this region, the remaining *TP53* allele contained a missense mutation. This single nucleotide substitution was not present in the normal tissue of the same patient and was therefore the result of a somatic mutation. These findings, by Bert Vogelstein and colleagues, perfectly conformed to Knudson's hypothesis and thus provided conclusive evidence that *TP53* was in fact a tumor suppressor gene.

Subsequent analysis of large numbers of tumors has revealed that mutational loss of *TP53* function is a very frequent event in many human cancers (Fig. 3.8). Inactivated *TP53* is a cause of some of the most common and lethal types of cancer.

In contrast to *RB1*, which tends to be inactivated by large deletions, *TP53* is typically inactivated by subtle alterations to the DNA sequence (Fig. 3.9). A smaller proportion of mutations inactivate *TP53* by truncating the open reading frame, either by a nonsense point mutation or by a small insertion or deletion that causes a

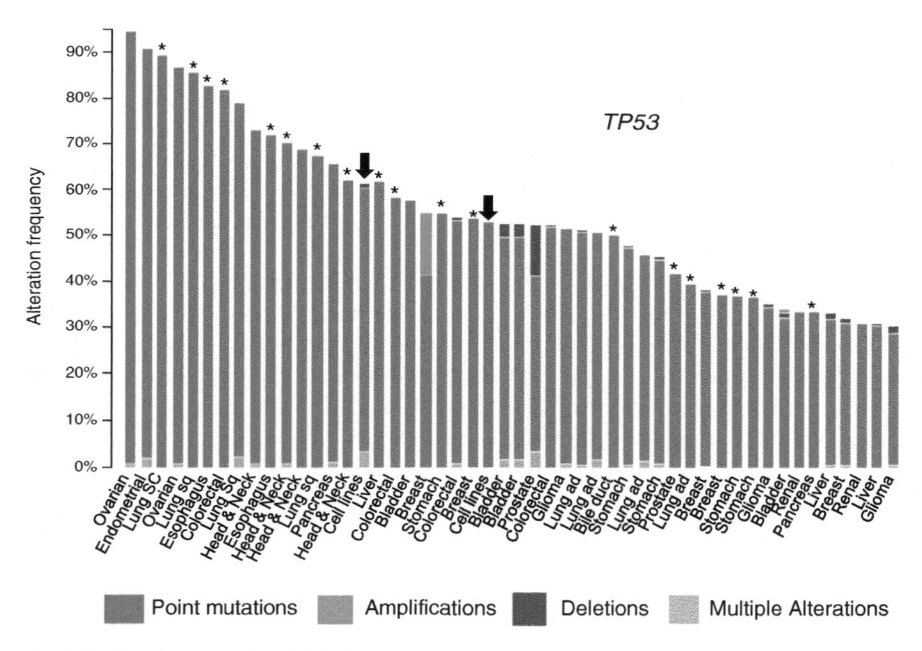

Fig. 3.8 A meta-analysis of *TP53* across tumor types reveals a high frequency of loss-of-function point mutations. *TP53* was first definitively established as a tumor suppressor because it is functionally inactivated during colorectal tumorigenesis. Subsequent analyses have shown that *TP53* is mutationally inactivated at high frequency in many types of human cancer, including most of those that occur at a high incidence. Nearly all of these mutations are single nucleotide substitutions; deletions are observed at low frequencies in several tumor types. *, denotes a study in which amplifications were not assessed. ↓, denotes a study of cell line collections that were derived from various tumor types. The results shown here are based upon data generated by the TCGA Research Network: http://cancergenome.nih.gov/

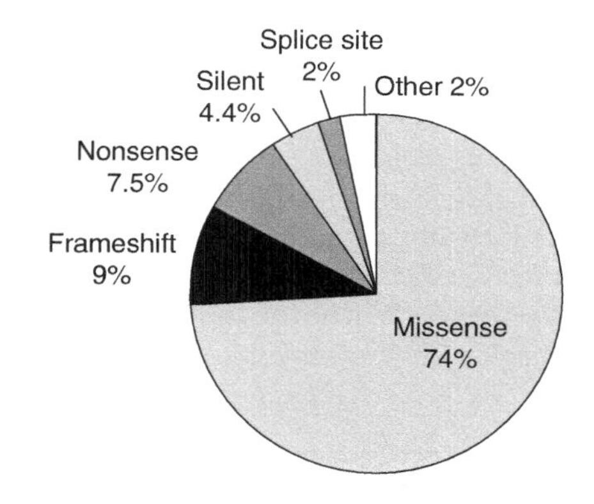

Fig. 3.9 Spectrum of somatic *TP53* mutations. The majority of *TP53* mutations detected in tumors are single nucleotide substitutions that result in missense codons

frameshift. In some cancer types, specific mutations in *TP53* are associated with environmental mutagens (see Chap. 1). Ultraviolet radiation, food-borne toxins, and cigarette smoke have all been found to leave highly characteristic molecular signatures in *TP53*.

Mutations in *TP53* do not occur with equal frequency throughout the coding sequences, but rather typically occur in a central region that interferes with the primary function of the encoded protein. The *TP53* gene encodes a 393 amino acid protein. About 20 % of all somatic mutations alter one of three codons, 175, 248 and 273, which are thus mutational hotspots. As will be described in detail in Chap. 6, *TP53* is a trans-regulatory element that encodes p53, a transcription factor that binds to specific sites within the promoters of growth inhibitory genes. The majority of *TP53*-inactivating mutations occur in exons that encode a large, centrally located, DNA binding domain that spans codons 100–300. Mutant p53 proteins fail to specifically bind DNA and thus lose their ability to transactivate transcription.

Functional Inactivation of p53: Tumor Suppressor Genes and Oncogenes Interact

In a significant number of cancers, *TP53* is not inactivated by mutation, but is instead functionally repressed by the activation of an antagonistic oncogene. This form of inhibition occurs at the posttranslational level and is mediated by protein-protein interactions. There are two highly illustrative oncoproteins that inhibit p53 and contribute to tumorigenesis:

MDM2 In normal cells, the level of p53 protein is highly regulated. A central mechanism of regulation involves the physical interaction of p53 with a protein encoded by *MDM2*. *MDM2* is a proto-oncogene that was originally found in double minutes in tumorigenic mouse cells (see Chap. 2). The human homolog (previously referred to as *HDM2*) is an enzyme that covalently modifies proteins by the addition of a peptide moiety called ubiquitin. The ubiquitination of proteins by ubiquitin ligases like MDM2 can target those proteins for degradation by the proteasome. The interaction of p53 with MDM2 leads to continuous p53 degradation, keeping p53 protein levels within a narrow range of intracellular concentration. In several types of cancers, principally soft-tissue sarcomas and gliomas, the *MDM2* gene is amplified, leading to increased expression of MDM2 protein and decreased expression of p53. The increased levels of MDM2 are therefore oncogenic. MDM2 amplification thus causes functional, rather than a mutational, loss of p53. *MDM2* is amplified in roughly 25 % of sarcomas and in 10–15 % of brain tumors known as gliomas. The *MDM2* locus is often amplified 50-fold or greater in these cancers.

More subtle alterations in *MDM2* can also affect p53 function. A common allele of *MDM2* contains a single nucleotide polymorphism (SNP) that affects gene expression. A T → G change found at the 309th nucleotide of the first intron, within the gene promoter region, increases the binding of a transcriptional activator and results in higher levels of *MDM2*-encoded RNA and protein. As in the case of *MDM2* amplification, the increased level of Mdm2 causes a corresponding attenuation of p53 function. Known as the SNP309 allele, this *MDM2* variant is very common; approximately 40 % of individuals in the general population are heterozygous and 12 % are homozygous for SNP309. Studies of patients with sporadic soft tissue sarcomas revealed that SNP309 is found at a higher frequency in younger patients, and that homozygosity of SNP309 was associated with a significantly earlier onset of disease. These findings suggest that attenuation of p53 function can accelerate tumor formation. SNP309 has been associated with increased incidence of cancer, including breast cancer, melanoma, and non-small cell lung cancer.

Human Papillomavirus Oncoprotein E6 (HPV E6) A second oncogene that affects p53 is not a cellular gene, but a viral gene that is introduced upon infection by the human papillomaviruses (HPV). While the vast majority of cancers arise solely as a result of germline and/or somatically-acquired mutations, an important exception is cancer that arises in HPV-infected tissues, including the uterine cervix and the epithelia of the head and neck. In such cancers, p53 is functionally inactivated by the inhibitory binding of an HPV-encoded protein known as E6. The role of HPV and the E6 protein in tumorigenesis will be described in Chap. 6.

Mutant *TP53* in the Germline: Li-Fraumeni Syndrome

Like *RB1* and *APC*, *TP53* mutations are involved in both sporadic and inherited cancers. *TP53* mutant alleles are the cause of a heritable susceptibility to cancer known as Li-Fraumeni syndrome (LFS). LFS is an autosomal dominant disorder characterized by the early onset of bone or soft tissue sarcomas, and by a significantly increased risk of several other cancers, including breast cancer.

LFS was first recognized as a clinical entity by Frederick Li and Joseph Fraumeni, in 1969. Five kindreds were identified in which childhood sarcomas affected siblings or cousins. Soon after the initial report by Li and Fraumeni, Lynch and colleagues similarly described pedigrees with unusual clusters of diverse cancers, including sarcomas, breast, lung, laryngeal and brain cancers, and leukemias.

Cancer predisposition syndromes that involve diverse types of cancer can be difficult to classify. Such was the case with LFS, which for a time was known by varying terminology. The precise clinical criteria for LFS took years to firmly establish largely because of inherent biases in the ways that clinical syndromes come to the attention of epidemiologists. Known as *ascertainment bias*, factors that complicate the classification of cancer syndromes include the preferential attention paid to kindreds that are most dramatically affected, the clustering of common cancers in families purely by chance, and uncertainty regarding the prevalence of the syndrome and the penetrance of the underlying genetic defect. In the case of LFS, these factors were eventually mitigated by the establishment of rigorously defined diagnostic criteria and, ultimately, by the identification of the inherited cancer genes.

As was observed in the heritable form of retinoblastoma, many patients with LFS were found to develop multiple primary tumors. Additionally, cancer was often found to strike at several times throughout life in many LFS patients, in many cases years apart. The later-onset cancers were often causally related to previous rounds of DNA-damaging cancer therapy. While the epidemiological data were strongly suggestive of a heritable predisposition to cancer, the molecular basis of this predisposition was unknown.

The discovery of *TP53* mutations in many different types of cancer, including those that commonly affect LFS patients, prompted the examination of the *TP53* alleles in LFS kindreds. Mutations in *TP53*, primarily single nucleotide substitutions, were found in the germline of all of the affected individuals from the initial five kindreds tested. Analysis of tumors from these patients confirmed that the normal allele had been lost during the process of tumorigenesis; tumors were homozygous for the mutant *TP53* allele. Not all individuals that carried the mutant *TP53* allele had been affected by cancer at the time that they were tested. But these individuals were clearly at high risk for developing cancer in the future. The identification of *TP53* mutations as the genetic defect that underlies LFS was a watershed development: for the first time, cancer predisposition could be predicted by genotype analysis.

Study of many LFS kindreds has revealed that the spectrum of *TP53* mutations found in this cancer predisposition syndrome is similar to that found in sporadic cancers; about three quarters are missense mutations (Fig. 3.10). Similarly, the germline *TP53* mutations associated with LFS typically affect the central, DNA binding domain of the encoded protein. There is considerable overlap: codons 248 and 273 are most commonly mutated in both sporadic cancers and in LFS. However some of the codons mutated in LFS, such as codon 337 which is mutated in about 10 % of disease kindreds, are rarely mutated in sporadic cancers.

The patterns of cancer in that occur in LFS patients are partially dependent on the precise *TP53* mutation present in the germline. Mutations within the exons that encode the DNA binding domain of p53 are associated with a higher prevalence of brain tumors and an earlier onset of breast cancers, whereas the less common

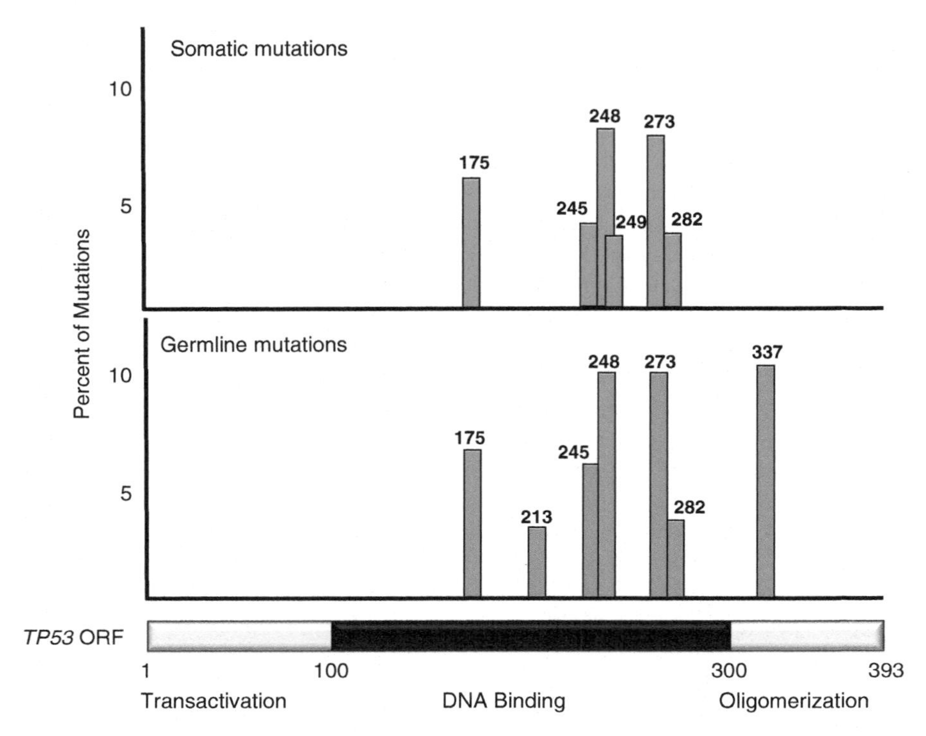

Fig. 3.10 Somatic and inherited mutations of *TP53*. The distribution of *TP53* mutations in Li-Fraumeni syndrome kindreds and in sporadic tumors is similar. Most mutations affect the central coding region that encodes a sequence-specific binding domain critical for protein function. A highly acidic domain that interacts with other transcription factors, located at the n-terminus, is rarely targeted by mutation. A c-terminal domain is important for the organization of p53 molecules into active, oligomeric complexes. A relatively common germline mutation in this coding region is rarely found in sporadic tumors. Note that only the most common mutations (>3 %) are shown. More rare mutations are generally clustered in the DNA binding domain

mutations outside the DNA binding domain are associated with a higher incidence of adrenal cancers.

Breast cancer eventually occurs in over a quarter of LFS patients (Fig. 3.11), whereas about 40 % of sporadic breast cancers have mutations in *TP53* (Fig. 3.8). The majority of these mutations were somatically acquired. *TP53* is mutated in more than 60 % of all colorectal cancers. However, this type of tumor does not occur at greatly elevated levels in LFS families. The initiating event of the colorectal cancers that do occur in LFS cases is loss of *APC* function, just as in the general population.

Mutations in*TP53* have not been found in all families that fit the clinical criteria for LFS. This lack of complete concordance between the *TP53* mutant genotype has several contributing factors:

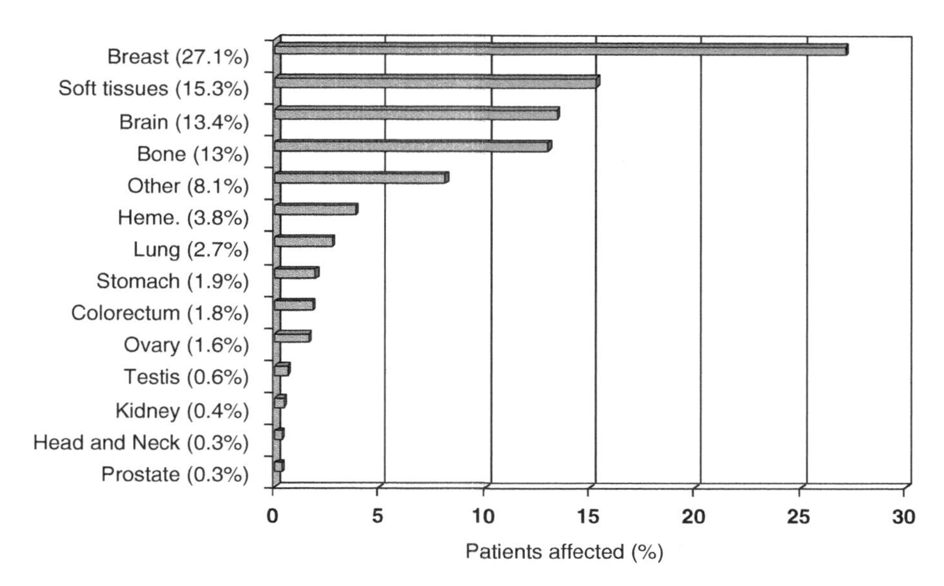

Fig. 3.11 Tumors associated with germline *TP53* mutations. Individuals with Li Fraumeni syndrome are predisposed to diverse cancers

False Negatives The techniques of analyzing patient-derived DNA samples have been in a state of constant development and refinement. The lack of sensitivity and the exclusion of large regions of genomic DNA in earlier DNA sequencing efforts contributed to an underestimation of germline *TP53* mutations in LFS kindreds. Many *TP53* mutations were simply missed.

Phenotypic Variability The aforementioned ascertainment bias complicates patient categorization, and has led to errors in identifying true LFS families. In recent years, the establishment of rigorous diagnostic criteria has minimized this problem. Careful diagnosis has resulted in the identification of a separate group of families in which the classic phenotype of LFS is incompletely expressed. This group has accordingly been termed Li-Fraumeni-like syndrome (LFLS). *TP53* mutations have been found in some of these kindreds as well, suggesting that the penetrance of *TP53* mutations can vary in different genetic backgrounds.

Other Mutations p53, like all cancer gene products, functions as part of a multi-protein signaling pathway (see Chap. 6). Mutations in other genes that contribute to the p53 pathway could theoretically phenocopy some of the effects of *TP53* mutation. Several genes have been proposed as putative tumor suppressor genes that might account for some LFS kindreds, but the mutational data has not been conclusive.

The variability of LFS, even in rigorously defined cases with validated *TP53* mutations, suggests that there are other genetic factors, known as modifiers, which can affect the *TP53* mutation-carrier phenotype. One modifier of *TP53* is the common SNP309 allele of *MDM2*. SNP309 occurs in LFS kindreds at a frequency that is similar to that in the general population. But LFS patients that also carry the SNP309 allele develop cancers at a significantly earlier age than FLS patients without SNP309. As described above, SNP309 increases the Mdm2 level and thereby reduces the level of p53.

Gains-of-Function Caused by Cancer-Associated Mutations in *TP53*

Among the many genes that are transcriptionally transactivated by p53 are several that function in the regulation of oxidative metabolism by the mitochondrion. Paul Hwang and colleagues have demonstrated that p53 directly induces the expression of a gene called *SCO2*. *SCO2* encodes a protein that assembles the cytochrome C oxidase, an enzyme complex that pumps protons across the inner mitochondrial membrane. The loss of SCO2 expression that occurs as a result of *TP53* inactivation has been shown to cause reduced levels of oxidative respiration. A constitutive increase in glycolysis is a common feature of many tumors known as the Warburg effect (see Chap. 1).

Unexpectedly, Hwang and colleagues found that many LFS-associated p53 proteins cause the *increased* expression of SCO2 and a corresponding increase in oxidative metabolism. This surprising gain-of-function apparently has metabolic consequences for LFS-affected individuals that harbor certain germline *TP53* mutations. Such individuals exhibit a measurably increased capacity for oxidative phosphorylation by their mitochondria, and improved recovery of metabolite levels in skeletal muscles after exercise. Other gain-of-function phenotypes have similarly been attributed to *TP53* mutant proteins.

Tumor suppressor genes are defined by the loss-of-function mutations that are found in cancers. Indeed, the loss-of-function is the *sine qua non* of a tumor suppressor locus, and this concept provides an explanation for the patterns of mutation and LOH that are recurrently found in cancers. However, studies of p53 suggest that in some cases, the losses-of-function inherent to some of the most frequently observed mutants can be accompanied by phenotypic gains-of-function. It is possible that the tandem loss- and gain-of-function phenotypes associated with some *TP53* mutant alleles might provide additional selective pressure for these mutations, and therefore be a reason they are found in so many cancers.

While somatic mutations that affect *TP53* are very common in cancers, the frequency of germline *TP53* mutant alleles within the human population is very low. LFS is accordingly rare. Overall, *TP53* mutations arise somatically, in tumors, much more often than they appear in the germline. Nonetheless, LFS serves to illustrate a central principle of cancer genetics. In familial retinoblastoma, FAP and LFS, inheritance of a mutated tumor suppressor gene is followed by loss of the single wild type allele in the cells of the developing tumor. Thus, the pattern of inactivating mutations in sporadic and inherited cancers conforms to the predictions of Knudson's hypothesis.

One interesting question that emerges from studies of LFS families: why have *TP53* mutations persisted in the human germline? *De novo* mutations that occur during embryogenesis may explain as many as 20 % of heritable cases, but it appears that the majority of germline mutations in *TP53* have been passed down through many generations. For any detrimental phenotype that affects individuals of child-bearing age, there is a question of why the frequency of that gene does not approach the low rate of *de novo* mutation.

An increase in oxidative respiration is a distinct bioenergetic advantage in some environments. It is unclear whether this metabolic phenotype caused by germline mutations in *TP53,* or other phenotypic gains-of-function, substantially counteracts the negative selective pressure caused by the increase in cancer incidence. Nonetheless, these studies of p53, metabolism and other gain-of-function phenotypes underscore the emerging view that p53, and perhaps other cancer genes, have roles in the human body that transcend tumor suppression.

Cancer Predisposition: Allelic Penetrance, Relative Risk and the Odds Ratio

That tumor suppressor genes are mutated in sporadic cancers and are also inherited in the germline of cancer-prone families is incontrovertible evidence of their central importance in tumorigenesis. Numerous well-defined cancer syndromes are understood at the genetic level (Table 3.1). Collectively, these syndromes account for about 5 % of all human cancers. Understanding the genetic basis of a cancer syndrome allows carriers to be firmly identified. Cancer syndromes also illuminate the etiology of the more common sporadic forms of the disease. With a few exceptions, the sporadic cancers in which a somatic mutated gene is predominantly found mirror those that are characteristic of the heritable syndrome associated with that gene. The relationship between heritable and sporadic forms of cancer thus provides important clues into the molecular pathogenesis.

Genetically-defined cancer syndromes illustrate how the risk of cancer is inherited via the germline. A germline cancer gene allows cancer cell precursors to bypass a step on the genetic path to tumor formation. For rate-limiting steps regulated by critical genes, the extent of cancer predisposition can be striking. Inheritance of an inactivated allele of *APC* confers a very high probability that, without prophylactic therapy, a carrier will develop malignant colorectal cancer at a young age. Germline alleles of other tumor suppressor genes confer lesser risks.

Table 3.1 Tumor suppressor gene mutations in heritable cancer syndromes and in sporadic, non-heritable cancers

Gene	Cancer syndrome	Penetrance[a]	Inherited cancers	Sporadic, non-heritable cancers
RB1	Familial retinoblastoma	**>95 %**	**Retinoblastoma**,	Retinoblastoma
			Osteosarcoma,	Endometrial Ca,
			Neuroblastoma	Bladder Ca,
			Melanoma	Osteosarcoma,
				Lung Ca
APC	Familial adenomatous polyposis	**Up to 90 % (lower for attenuated FAP)**	**Colorectal Ca**,	Colorectal Ca
			Osteosarcoma,	Gastric Ca.,
	Gardner's syndrome		Sm Intestine Ca,	Sm. Intestine Ca,
			Gastric Ca	Adrenal gland Ca,
				Pancreatic Ca
TP53	Li-Fraumeni syndrome	**90 % females; ~75 % males**	**Breast Ca**,	Ovarian Ca,
			Sarcoma,	Colorectal Ca,
			Brain tumors,	Esophageal Ca,
			Others	Head and Neck Ca,
				Pancreatic Ca,
				Lung Ca,
				Skin Ca,
				Breast Ca,
				Endometrial Ca,
				Lymphoma
				Others
BRCA1	Familial breast and ovarian Ca	**55–65 % breast, ~40 % ovarian**	**Breast Ca**,	Ovarian Ca,
			Ovarian Ca	

BRCA2, PALB2	Familial breast Ca	**~45 % breast, <20 % ovarian**	**Breast Ca, (inc. males)**	Melanoma,
			Ovarian Ca,	Ovarian Ca
			Pancreatic Ca	
			Prostate Ca	
CDKN2A, CDK4	Familial Multiple Mole and Melanoma (FAMMM)	**~100 % develop moles, ~70 % develop melanoma, <20 % develop pancreas ca**	**Melanoma**	Malignant nerve sheath tumors,
			Pancreatic Ca,	Brain Ca,
			Brain Ca	Melanoma,
				Pancreatic Ca,
				Esophageal Ca,
				Lung Ca,
				Head and Neck Ca,
				Bladder Ca
PTEN	Cowden syndrome	**6 % (melanoma) – 85 % (breast)**	**Breast Ca,**	Endometrial Ca,
	Bannayan-Riley-Ruvalcaba syndrome		**Thyroid Ca,**	Brain Ca,
			Endometrial Ca	Prostate Ca,
			Colorectal Ca	Stomach Ca,
			Renal Ca	Lung Ca.
			Melanoma	
SMAD4, BMPR1A	Juvenile Polyposis syndrome	**100 % develop polyps, <20 % develop cancer**	**Colorectal Ca,**	Bile duct Ca
			Gastric Ca,	Pancreatic Ca
			Sm intestinal Ca	Colorectal Ca
NF1	Neurofibromatosis Type 1	**>95 % develop benign lesions, ~5 % develop cancer**	**Brain Ca,**	Malingnant nerve sheath tumors, Brain tumors
			Neural tumors	

(continued)

Table 3.1 (continued)

Gene	Cancer syndrome	Penetrance[a]	Inherited cancers	Sporadic, non-heritable cancers
NF2	Neurofibromatosis Type 2	**>95 %**	**Neural tumors**	Rare.
PTCH1	Basal cell Nevus syndrome	**90 % develop basal cell carcinomas**	**Basal cell carcinoma of the skin,**	Basal cell carcinoma of the skin,
			Medulloblastoma	Malignant nerve sheath tumors,
			Rhabdomyosarcoma	Medulloblastoma
VHL	von Hippel-Lindau syndrome	**>90 %**	**Retinal Angioma,**	Renal Ca,
			Renal Ca, Hemangioblastoma	Hemangioblastoma
MEN1	Multiple Endocrine Neoplasia	**>90 %**	**Parathyroid tumors,**	Breast Ca
			Pancreatic islet cell tumors, Neuroendocrine tumors, Pituitary tumors	
MSH2, MLH1, MSH6, PMS1, PMS2	Hereditary nonpolyposis colorectal cancer, Turcot syndrome	**~60 % males, 50 % females**	**Colorectal Ca,**	Colorectal Ca
			Endometrial Ca,	Gastric Ca
			Ovarian Ca	Endometrial Ca
			Small Int. Ca	Bladder Ca
			Bladder Ca	
			Brain Ca	
			Biliary Tract Ca	

The predominant forms of inherited cancers are indicated in bold type
[a]Lifetime absolute risk for developing the predominant form of cancer

The consequence of inheriting or acquiring *de novo* a germline tumor gene mutation can be quantified in several ways. These figures are related to one another, but dependent on distinct variables:

Penetrance and Attributable Risk The penetrance of a mutant tumor suppressor gene and the absolute risk of cancer conferred by that mutation are one and the same. For example, inheritance of a hypothetical gene that has a penetrance of 50 % imparts an absolute risk that is also 50 %. One half of the carriers of that allele will develop cancer. In cases of incomplete penetrance, additional genetic and environmental factors, which can be difficult to quantify, will play an important role in determining if a given individual will eventually develop disease. When penetrance is near-complete, as is the case with familial retinoblastoma, other germline genes and somatically acquired mutations are less relevant to the absolute risk. In cases of incomplete penetrance and common cancers, a proportion of cancers in carriers will not necessarily be directly caused by the mutant allele, as some cancers would have been expected even in the absence of the gene. Thus, the penetrance of a given allele is not the same as the attributable risk, the calculation of which requires a consideration of the cancers that occur in non-carriers. Distinct germline mutations in the same tumor suppressor gene can be differentially penetrant, as is the case with the *APC* alleles that cause colorectal cancer, and the breast cancer susceptibility genes described below.

Relative Risk All human beings are at risk of cancer. In kindreds with germline tumor suppressor gene mutations, that risk is elevated. For a predisposing mutation, the relative risk (also known as the risk ratio) represents the probability of cancer in individuals harboring a specific germline cancer-associated mutation divided by the probability of cancer occurring in the general population.

Genotype	Cancer	No cancer
Mutation	a	b
No mutation	c	d

$$\text{Relative risk} = \frac{\text{Probability of cancer in carriers}}{\text{Probability of cancer in the general population}}$$

Therefore,

$$\text{Relative risk} = \frac{a/(a+b)}{c/(c+d)}$$

Odds Ratio Another comparison of risk between two genetic cohorts is the odds ratio. For a germline mutation associated with cancer, the odds ratio quantifies how strongly that allele leads to the outcome of cancer, as compared to the odds of cancer in individuals who do not harbor that mutant allele.

$$\text{Odds ratio} = \frac{\text{Odds that an individual with a mutation will develop cancer}}{\text{Odds that an individual without the mutation will develop cancer}}$$

Therefore,

$$\text{Odds ratio} = \frac{a/b}{c/d} = \frac{ad}{bc}$$

When applied to studies in which the specific type of cancer is rare and the allele has low penetrance, (ie, a<b), the odds ratio will be roughly equal to the relative risk.

A relative risk of 1 implies that the carriers of a given allele have no increased risk over the general population. As an example, consider a hypothetical cancer-causing allele that has a penetrance of 10 %. The absolute risk of cancer in these individuals is also 10 %. If the incidence of the same cancer in the general population is 1 in 1000, or 0.1 %, the relative risk is 0.10/0.001 = 100. Carriers of that allele therefore have a 100-fold increased risk of developing cancer compared to general population. The odds ratio in this scenario would be (10/90)/(0.1/99) = 0.11/0.01 = 110, which is similar to the relative risk. However, for a fairly common disease such as breast cancer the relative risks and odds ratios diverge. The lifetime risk of breast cancer among women in the US is about 12 %. The germline genes associated with heritable breast cancer are about 50 % penetrant, and therefore the relative risk and odds ratio for carriers are 4.2 and 7.1, respectively. In general, the relative risk yields a more intuitive result than an odds ratio. However, the odds ratio can more readily be determined from the data obtained from a case-control study that measure cancers as an endpoint.

Aside from the well-described cancer syndromes listed in Table 3.1 and described in this chapter, there are many familial clusters of cancer that are less well understood. While highly penetrant genes that cause readily discernable forms of hereditary cancer are most straightforward to classify, tumor suppressor genes with incomplete penetrance that contribute to common forms of cancer can be much more difficult to detect.

Breast Cancer Susceptibility: *BRCA1* and *BRCA2*

Breast cancer is among the most common malignancies. As in most cancers, most cases are sporadic and result from somatically acquired mutations. However, epidemiologic evidence has long supported a heritable component for a small proportion of breast tumors (approximately 5–10 %). The identification of *RB1* and *APC* created a paradigm for relating both sporadic and heritable forms of a cancer to a single tumor suppressor gene. It was anticipated that analysis of the small fraction of inherited breast cancers might be similarly informative.

For the discovery of germline susceptibility genes, breast cancer poses a major challenge. Unlike colorectal cancers and retinoblastoma, the clinical presentation of inherited and sporadic breast cancers is largely the same. Heritable breast cancers sometimes present as bilateral tumors, and the onset of disease often occurs prior to menopause, but these features are not universal. Because breast cancer occurs so frequently in the general population, it can be difficult to identify kindreds that unambiguously carry a predisposition. While a familial cluster of retinoblastoma is a reliable indicator of inherited susceptibility, multiple cases of breast cancer can occur in a single family solely by chance. The clinical finding of a large number of polyps is highly suggestive of a predisposition to colorectal cancer, but there is no analogous pre-cancerous condition that might alert a physician to the presence of a germline gene for breast cancer. Further complicating genetic analysis, sporadic breast cancers can and do occur within kindreds that carry a predisposing mutation in the germline; such cancers will occur in carriers and non-carriers alike. Unraveling the genetic basis of breast cancer required an approach that combined careful epidemiology with molecular genetic analysis.

TP53 was the first breast cancer gene to be described. *TP53* mutations are present in a significant proportion – but not the majority – of sporadic breast cancers. Breast cancer is a primary phenotype of Li-Fraumeni syndrome, but because breast cancer is common and Li-Fraumeni syndrome is relatively rare, Li-Fraumeni cases do not account for a significant proportion of the total cases.

In pursuit of more common breast cancer genes, investigators sought chromosomal markers that were genetically linked to early onset cases within familial clusters. Focusing on a large group of families cumulatively composed of thousands of cases of early-onset breast cancer, Mary-Claire King and her coworkers established linkage with a region on the long arm of chromosome 17 in 1990. Three years later, Mark Skolnick and colleagues identified a gene in this region, termed *BRCA1*, which was mutationally truncated in the germline of several kindreds. *BRCA1* mutations were subsequently found in a major proportion of previously identified families with high incidence of inherited breast and ovarian cancers. By examining the families that did not carry mutant *BRCA1*, a large consortium of investigators found linkage to a second breast cancer susceptibility locus on chromosome 13. The *BRCA2* gene was cloned in 1995. In total, mutations in either *BRCA1* or *BRCA2* are thought to contribute to more than one half of inherited breast cancers.

The two breast cancer susceptibility genes are structurally unrelated. *BRCA1* is composed of 24 exons that encode a 1863 amino acid protein. Almost one-half of the germline mutations are single base substitutions that include missense, nonsense and splice site mutations. The remaining *BRCA1* mutations are predominantly small deletions and insertions. Truncation of the open reading frame is a common consequence of cancer-associated *BRCA1* mutations. Mutations have been detected throughout the *BRCA1* coding sequences. *BRCA2* is a 27-exon gene that encodes a 3418 amino acid protein. As is the case with *BRCA1*, the mutations in *BRCA2* are often truncating mutations caused by single base substitutions and small insertions and deletions. Among *BRCA2* mutations, those in the central region of the gene appear to confer a higher risk of ovarian cancer. This region has been termed the *ovarian cancer cluster region*.

Both *BRCA1* and *BRCA2* are dominant cancer genes with relatively high penetrance. The exact penetrance of *BRCA1* and *BRCA2* mutations, and therefore the additional risk of cancer conferred by such mutations, has been difficult to ascertain for several reasons. Different mutations appear to confer somewhat distinct risks. Another complicating factor is that the average age of incidence can vary significantly among families with the same mutation. The patterns of cancer can also vary. Some families have increased incidence of breast cancer only, while other families with the same mutation can present with breast and ovarian cancers. The reasons for this high degree of variability in risk are unknown, but may relate to both modifying genes and to components of lifestyle and environment. The approximate lifetime risks of breast and ovarian cancer associated with *BRCA1* and *BRCA2* mutations are shown in Table 3.2. Carriers of either *BRCA1* or *BRCA2* have a 4–5-fold higher risk for developing breast cancer during their lifetimes.

This relative risk may seem somewhat low for a gene with relatively high penetrance, but this is a direct result of the high lifetime risk of sporadic, non-heritable breast cancers in the general population. Indeed, the relative risk associated with *BRCA1* and *BRCA2* mutations increases markedly if an analysis is restricted to younger women. Like most cancers, the risk of breast cancer increases with age. In the general population, only 1 in 68 women will be diagnosed by the age of 40. Among individuals with germline mutations in *BRCA1* or *BRCA2*, the risk of a breast cancer by age 40 is 10–15 %. The relative risk in this young group of mutation carriers is therefore approximately 10.

Breast cancer in males is rare, but has a significant heritable component. Male carriers of *BRCA1* and, particularly, *BRCA2* mutations are at an increased risk of breast cancer and possibly prostate cancer. Overall, male breast cancers account for less than 1 % of cancers in men. However, the relative risk of male breast cancer by the age of 70 is approximately 40 in *BRCA2* mutation carriers. These cancers account for about 15 % of all male breast cancers. Among the males that develop breast cancer in the absence of a known BRCA gene mutation, about 30 % have

Table 3.2 Cumulative risks for developing cancer associated with *BRCA1* and *BRCA2* mutations at age 70. The penetrance of distinct *BRCA1* and *BRCA2* mutations has been found to be variable

		Mutant *BRCA1* carrier		Mutant *BRCA2* carrier	
Cancer	General population	Risk	Rel. risk[a]	Risk	Rel. risk[a]
Breast Ca	12 %	60 %	5	45 %	3.8
Ovarian Ca	1.8 %	40 %	22	15 %	8.3
Male breast Ca	0.1 %	1.2 %	12	6.8 %	42

Figures shown were compiled by the National Cancer Institute, and are approximate
[a]Defined as the fold-increase in the overall risk attributable to the mutated gene

male or female relatives with breast cancer, suggesting that there are additional genetic factors involved.

While *BRCA1* and *BRCA2* germline mutations are diverse in terms of their precise positions within the genes, several mutations have been found to be present in multiple families. These recurrent mutations are typically restricted to specific ethnic groups and reflect what is known in genetics as a *founder effect* – a recurring trait in a growing population that originates from a small group of common ancestors. Founder mutations in *BRCA1*and *BRCA2* have been found in geographically or culturally isolated Jewish, Icelandic and Polish populations. Three different founder mutations have been found in individuals of Ashkenazi Jewish ancestry, and are present in about 2 % of that population.

Mutations in *BRCA1* or in *BRCA2* are found in approximately 1 in 400 women in the general population, which implies that about 400,000 women in the US are carriers. The relatively low frequency of mutations in the general population and the clustering of founder mutations in defined ethnic groups has significant implications for the use of genetic screens to identify individuals at risk for cancer.

In general, there is an inverse correlation between the allele frequency of genetic variants that are statistically associated with cancer and their penetrance (Fig. 3.12). Common cancer-associated alleles, which are found at a high frequency in the general population, tend to have lower penetrance than more rare alleles, like the mutant forms of *BRCA1* and *BRCA2* that are associated with breast and ovarian cancers,

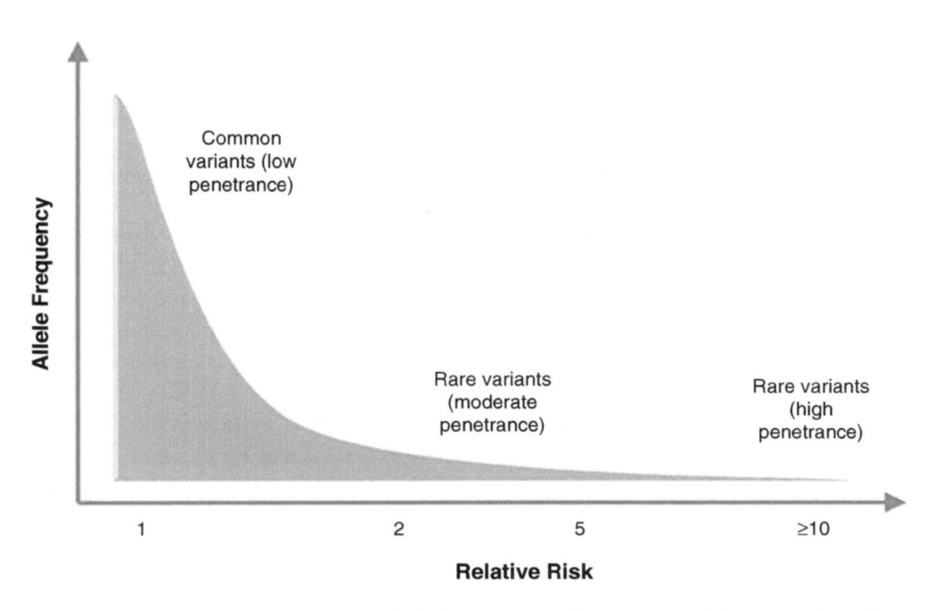

Fig. 3.12 The relationship between allele frequency and penetrance. Many genetic variants are statistically associated with an increased risk of cancer. However, alleles that occur frequently in the general population tend to have very low penetrance, and therefore confer a low or negligible relative risk. Figure from the National Cancer Institute

and the genes associated with heritable colorectal cancers. This relationship is intuitively apparent, as the majority of individuals in the population do not appear to inherit a strong predisposition to cancer.

BRCA1 and *BRCA2* are not widely mutated in sporadic breast cancers or other cancers. This finding came as a surprise and in some respects a disappointment. *RB1*, *APC* and *TP53* mutations are centrally involved in both heritable and sporadic forms of cancer, and it was widely assumed that solving the basis of familial breast cancer would similarly inform an understanding of the much more common sporadic cancers as well. This has not turned out to be the case. While the cloning of the *BRCA1* and *BRCA2* genes was a milestone in understanding and predicting cancer risk, the results of that successful effort have not been directly applicable to the pathogenesis of most breast tumors. Nonetheless, the functional analysis of *BRCA1* and *BRCA2* has provided useful insights into the biological basis of breast cancer, and has informed a unique mode of therapy for tumors that are BRCA1/2-deficient (see Chap. 8). The proteins encoded by *BRCA1* and *BRCA2* play central roles in the repair of damaged DNA, suggesting that their tumor suppressor function is based upon the suppression of spontaneous mutations. As epidemiological studies have pointed to strong links between breast cancer incidence and certain environmental mutagens, the involvement of *BRCA1* and *BRCA2* in hereditary forms of the disease suggest a compelling relationship between mutagenesis, DNA repair and breast tumorigenesis. The nature of DNA repair pathways and their role in breast cancer will be discussed in detail in Chap. 6.

Genetic Losses on Chromosome 9: *CDKN2A*

A frequent site of genetic loss in human cancers is the short arm of chromosome 9. Recurrent cytogenetic abnormalities affecting region 9p21 are found in numerous tumors, including melanomas, and brain and lung cancers. In 1994, a group led by Dennis Carson examined the patterns of loss of two known genes within this region that were variably deleted in cancer cell lines, and concluded that a tumor suppressor gene resided somewhere between them. Refined mapping and sequencing of candidate genes within this defined region eventually revealed a gene that was consistently deleted in sporadic cancers. An independent group, led by Mark Skolnick, isolated the same gene by mapping homozygous deletions in melanoma cell lines. In melanoma cell lines that had lost only a single allele, the remaining allele was frequently found to harbor a nonsense, missense or frameshift mutation. These pieces of evidence were a strong indication that a new tumor suppressor gene had been found.

The identified gene on 9p21 encoded a protein that was already known to play a central role in the regulation of cell growth. A year before the positional cloning of the 9p21 tumor suppressor locus, David Beach and his coworkers had discovered and characterized a 16 kDa protein, designated p16, that binds to cyclin-dependent kinase 4 (Cdk4), an enzyme that promotes the progression of the cell cycle (see

Chap. 6). The interaction between p16 and Cdk4 inhibits this pro-growth activity. Sequencing of the open reading frame of the 9p21 tumor suppressor gene revealed that p16 and the tumor suppressor gene-encoded protein were one and the same. The p16 proteins encoded by the tumor-associated mutant genes fail to inhibit Cdk4 and thus fail to block cell cycle progression. An important downstream substrate of Cdk4 is Rb, the product of the tumor suppressor gene, *RB1*, inactivated in retinoblastoma. The compelling functional link between p16 and Rb suggested that inactivation of their corresponding tumor suppressor genes might cause common cellular effects. The roles of p16 and Rb in the progression of the cell cycle will be described in detail in Chap. 6.

The tumor suppressor gene on 9p21 was designated *CDKN2A*, to reflect the role of the encoded protein as a specific inhibitor of Cdk4 and as a member of a family of genes that are cyclin-dependent kinase inhibitors. The protein encoded by *CDKN2A* is still referred to as p16.

CDKN2A is mutated in a wide range of tumors (Fig. 3.13). Melanomas are the form of cancer originally associated with *CDKN2A* loss. About 40 % of sporadic melanomas homozygously inactivate *CDKN2A*. Subsequent studies have revealed deletions involving *CDKN2A* in high proportions of peripheral nerve sheath tumors, brain tumors (predominately gliomas), and in cancers of the head and neck, lung, pancreas and bladder. *CDKN2A* inactivation occurs most often by genetic deletion, but significant proportions of missense, nonsense and insertion mutations also occur.

Exposure to UV is an important environmental risk factor for melanoma development. A significant number of the small mutations in *CDKN2A* are single base substitutions are of the C→T and CC→TT type, which are known UV signature mutations (see Chap. 1).

Approximately 10 % of all melanoma cases occur in individuals with a family history of the disease. Germline *CDKN2A* mutations account for about 20–40 % of these cases. Carriers of *CDKN2A* mutations typically develop benign pigmented moles, known as *nevi*, in the context of a syndrome known as Familial Multiple Mole and Melanoma, or FAMMM. Not all carriers will develop a malignant melanoma. Overall, carriers of germline *CDKN2A* mutations have an approximately 75-fold increased risk of developing melanoma, as compared to the general population (relative risk = 75). *CDKN2A* mutation carriers are also at a significantly higher risk of developing pancreatic cancer. An increased risk of pancreatic cancer is not apparent in melanoma-prone kindreds that do not have a mutation in *CDKN2A*. There are several distinct mutations that appear multiple times in ethnically-defined subpopulations, and are thus likely to represent founder mutations.

Within cancer prone kindreds, affected individuals are almost always heterozygous for germline mutant tumor suppressor genes. As we have repeatedly seen, the single wild type allele is lost during tumorigenesis, which upon molecular analysis is observed as LOH. Remarkably, two individuals with biallelically mutated *CDKN2A* alleles have been identified. These unusual individuals were homozygous for a known founder mutation in *CDKN2A* that was present in each of their parents. Every cell in the bodies of these two individuals had thus already sustained two

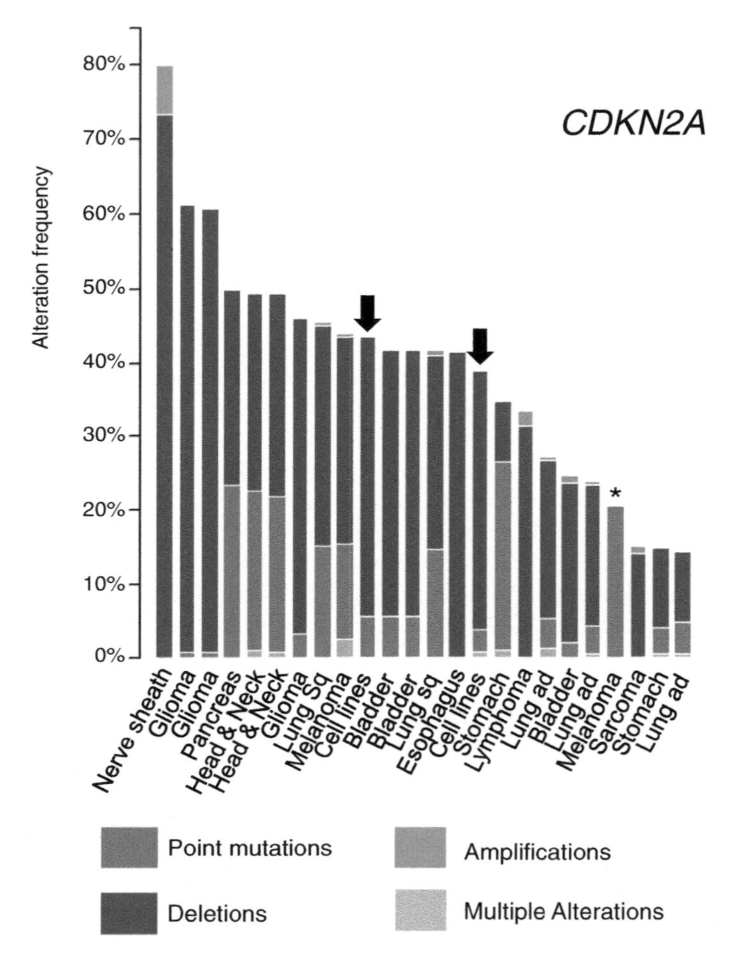

Fig. 3.13 A meta-analysis of *CDKN2A* across tumor types reveals a high frequency of deletions. *CDKN2A* was first identified as a tumor suppressor in melanomas. Subsequent analyses have shown that deletions involving *CDKN2A* occur at high frequency in many types of human cancer, including tumors involving the peripheral nerve sheath, brain, pancreas and epithelia of the head and neck. Inactivating point mutations are also observed at lower frequencies in several tumor types. The amplifications occasionally observed are probably incidental. *, denotes a study in which amplifications were not assessed. ↓, denotes a study of cell line collections that were derived from various tumor types. The results shown here are based upon data generated by the TCGA Research Network: http://cancergenome.nih.gov/

'hits' of *CDKN2A*. The homozygous patients were cancer-prone but otherwise healthy, indicating that expression of p16 protein is not essential for cellular viability or for normal development. One of these patients developed two primary melanomas by the age of 15, while the other was melanoma-free until she died at the age of 55 from an adenocarcinoma. The dramatically different onset of cancer in these two homozygous individuals clearly illustrates the variable phenotypes related to *CDKN2A* loss.

The typical penetrance of *CDKN2A* in well-defined melanoma-prone kindreds is about 70 %. As shown by the previous example, the same germline mutations can be variably penetrant in different individuals, depending on genetic modifiers and environmental exposures. Additionally, as was found to be the case with *BRCA1* and *BRCA2* in breast cancers, it has become apparent that some germline mutations of *CDKN2A* vary in their average penetrance.

Multiple primary tumors, in any cancer type, are a classic hallmark of an underlying predisposition. Melanomas, visible on the surface of the skin, can be diagnosed with relative ease compared with internal tumors, and patients with multiple tumors are readily apparent. It had long been noted that a subset of melanoma patients develop multiple lesions with no known family history of melanoma. These cases are sporadic, but the multifocal nature of their primary lesions suggested the germline presence of a low penetrance tumor suppressor gene mutation. Analysis of *CDK2NA* revealed a significant proportion of germline mutations in such patients, which were at first believed to have arisen *de novo*. However in several cases, analysis of other family members revealed the same mutations; closer investigation revealed evidence of previously obscure family history of the disease. Thus, the analysis of *CDKN2A* could be used to detect familial patterns of disease that were not previously apparent.

In summary, *CDKN2A* is a classical tumor suppressor gene, that is inactivated in many types of sporadic cancer, predominately via chromosomal deletion. Mutated *CDKN2A* alleles also arise *de novo* in the germline, and are then passed from one generation to another in nevus-prone and cancer-prone families.

Complexity at *CDKN2A*: Neighboring and Overlapping Genes

There are two idiosyncrasies that have complicated the analysis of the *CDKN2A* locus and its role in cancer. The first relates to its neighborhood on chromosome 9. The second is the highly unusual structure of the locus and the transcripts that are expressed from it. These features of *CDKN2A* illustrate some of the challenges that arose when examining chromosomal losses and mutations in at the 9p21 region in cancers.

The *CDKN2A* locus is located immediately adjacent to another gene, called *CDKN2B*, that encodes a distinct inhibitor of cyclin-dependent kinases. While the proximity of these two genes may seem to be a highly improbable coincidence, there are in fact numerous instances of physical linkage between genes with related primary structure and function. A well-known example is the cluster of major histocompatibility genes that encode cell surface molecules involved in immune recognition, on the short arm of chromosome 6. The evolutionary basis for this type of physical clustering of related genes remains incompletely understood, but is likely to involve past gene duplication events.

Allelic losses affecting the 9p21 region are commonly observed in many cancers. Kindreds have been identified that exhibit 9p21 loss, but the tumors from affected individuals retain wild type, non-mutated *CDKN2A*. One possibility is that a neighboring locus was the primary target of the first 'hit'. Is *CDKN2B* also a tumor suppressor gene? The indirect evidence is compelling. The *CDKN2B* locus expresses a 15 kDa protein that bears considerable similarity to p16. Both proteins function in cancer-related pathways that inhibit the progression of the cell cycle. Many of the larger genomic deletions that inactivate *CDKN2A* in malignant peripheral nerve sheath tumors, gliomas and bladder cancers also affect *CDKN2B*. In one large-scale analysis of sporadic cancers, many deletions were found to affect both genes, and several affected *CDKN2A* but left *CDKN2B* intact. Notably, there were no mutations that deleted *CDKN2B* and left *CDKN2A* intact. While inactivating point mutations were found in *CDKN2A*, none were detected in *CDKN2B*. Critically, no cancer-associated germline mutations solely involving *CDKN2B* have been reported. Lacking these types of direct evidence, it is difficult to definitively characterize *CDKN2B* as a tumor suppressor gene.

Another interesting and unique feature of the *CDKN2A* locus was reported in 1995, when several groups observed that two distinct transcripts are encoded by *CDKN2A* (Fig. 3.14). A previously unrecognized exon, designated exon 1β, was found upstream of the first coding exon that encodes p16, exon 1α. Exon 1β is spliced to the same downstream exons that encode p16, but defines an alternative reading frame. This second transcript encodes a 132 amino acid, 14 kDa protein designated p14ARF. Because they are encoded by two different reading frames, p16 and p14ARF are structurally unrelated. The expression of the transcripts that separately encode p16 and p14ARF is controlled by separate promoters.

Functional analysis of p14ARF has shown that it can play a role in the regulation of the cell cycle, in a manner that is mechanistically distinct from p16. The p14ARF protein can physically bind MDM2 protein and thereby indirectly increase the stability and abundance of the p53 tumor suppressor. Thus, p14ARF provides a functional link between two commonly mutated tumor suppressors, p16 and p53.

Does the mutational loss of p14ARF confer a distinct selective advantage during tumorigenesis? The overlapping nature of these two genes prompted a re-evaluation of the primary mutation data. Most of the point mutations and deletions that affected the p16-encoding exons also affected the expression of p14ARF. Exon 1β was found to be selectively deleted in several melanoma cell lines. These deletions left the p16 coding exons intact, suggesting that p14ARF might have been the primary target. This finding would be highly suggestive of a role for p14(ARF) in tumor suppression, but there was some debate as to whether deletions of 9p21 might spontaneously occur during cell culture, following tumor explantation. The exon 1β deletions observed could therefore represent an artifact. Interestingly, one study reported a small germline insertion in exon 1β that altered p14ARF, but did not affect p16 expression, in a patient with multiple primary melanomas. In contrast, both germline and somatic mutations of exon 1α, specific to the p16 coding region, have been observed in many cancer-prone individuals and tumors, respectively.

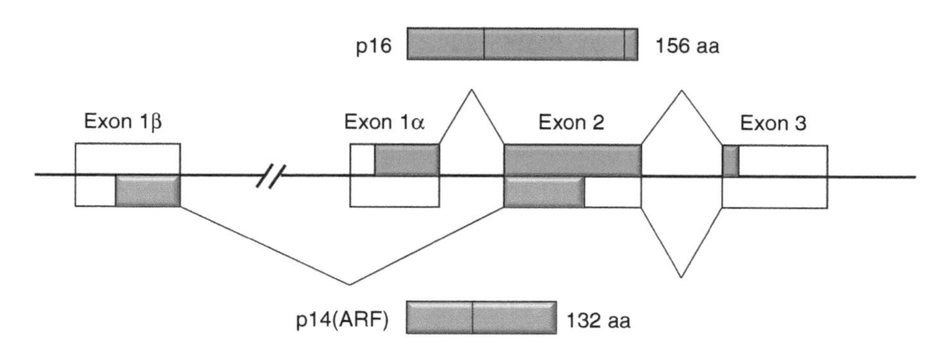

Fig. 3.14 One gene, two proteins. The *CDKN2A* locus encodes two distinct proteins, p16 and p14ARF. The two transcripts originate from two different first exons and use different reading frames within a common second exon. For these reasons, the two proteins encoded by the two respective transcripts do not share sequence homology

The complexity of the *CDKN2A* locus is striking: two unrelated proteins are expressed, via two distinct and independently regulated promoters, by two transcripts with an common exon that is translated in two different reading frames. From an evolutionary perspective, it is difficult to guess how such a locus might have arisen. The p16 protein is evolutionarily conserved, as are many cancer genes. The p14ARF open reading frame, in contrast, is not more highly conserved between mammals than arbitrary open reading frames, and thus there is little evidence for evolutionary selective pressure on p14ARF.

Genetic Losses on Chromosome 10: *PTEN*

The loss of tumor suppressor loci represents an important quantitative difference between cancer cells and their normal precursors. Linkage analysis can best identify these relatively small differences against a background of 'sameness'. For this reason, positional cloning approaches generally required a high frequency of mutation in a clearly defined type of cancer. Mutations in *APC*, *RB1* and *BRCA1* and *BRCA2* are highly specific to colorectal cancers, retinoblastomas and breast cancers, respectively. This tumor-specificity, combined with extensive epidemiological data and the identification of affected families, greatly facilitated their precise mapping and eventual sequence identification of the culprit mutations. Mutations in *TP53*, which was cloned via a more roundabout protein-based approach, are found in a more diverse spectrum of cancers. Paradoxically, more ubiquitous tumor suppressor gene mutations are more difficult to detect by positional approaches.

New techniques were devised to specifically isolate the DNA sequences that were lost in genetic deletions during tumorigenesis. The rationale for this new approach was that chromosomal regions that were recurrently lost in cancers were likely to contain tumor suppressor loci. Though this rationale was simple, the technology for comparing cancer cell genomes with their normal cell counterparts remained laborious. The haploid human genome is 3.4×10^9 bp in size; regions of loss can be large and diverse. In the early 1990s, methods of high throughput DNA sequencing and SNP analysis were at early stages of development.

An ingenious method to compare cancer and normal cell genomes was developed by Michael Wigler and his colleagues and published in 1993. Termed *representational difference analysis*, this subtractive method allowed the enrichment of lost sequences that were present in one genome but absent in another. In the first step of this complex method, representative regions of both genomes were amplified by PCR. The second step involved iterative cycles of DNA melting, annealing, amplification of rare, hybridized sequences and the degradation of common representations. The final product of this experimental method was a small set of short DNAs that were unique to one genomic DNA sample. The analysis of cancer genomes by this approach could amplify regions that were homozygously deleted in cancers. Employed in reverse, to assess genetic gains, representational difference analysis was successfully used to isolate small regions of herpesvirus DNA that are often integrated in the tumor cells of Kaposi's sarcoma, a cancer found in patients with AIDS.

In 1997, Ramon Parsons and his coworkers used a DNA probe derived by representation difference analysis to identify a specific region of loss on chromosome 10. The Parsons group found biallelic loss of their probe sequence in two different breast cancers. The same probe was used to isolate a genomic clone that spanned this homozygous deletion. Sequencing and mapping of the deleted region revealed a previously uncharacterized gene that encoded a 403 amino acid protein. Analysis of the protein sequence revealed several conserved motifs, including a protein tyrosine phosphatase domain and a region to a chicken cytoskeletal protein called tensin. Because of these homologies and the mapping of the gene to chromosome 10, the gene was designated *PTEN*. Independently a collaborative effort by the laboratory of Peter Steck and the company Myriad Genetics found that four brain tumor cell lines that had similarly deleted the same locus, which they designated *MMAC1* for *mutated in multiple advanced cancers*. In addition to homozygous deletions, the Steck/Myriad group also detected other mutations in prostate, kidney and breast cancers. Finally, a third group, Da-Ming Li and Hong Sun, used similarities shared by protein phosphatase genes, thought to have broad roles in cancer cells, to isolate a gene at 10q23 which they designated *TEP1*. *PTEN*, *MMAC1* and *TEP1* all refer to the same locus; the gene is now designated *PTEN*.

Losses of chromosome 10 sequences had previously been detected by cytogenetic analysis of several types of cancer, including brain, bladder and prostate cancer. LOH analysis was then used to map a common region of loss to chromosome band 10q23. These studies had been highly suggestive of a tumor suppressor gene within a relatively large region that contains many genes. The homozygous deletions located and mapped by the Parsons and Steck/Myriad groups confirmed this prediction. Additionally, it had been determined that the locus for Cowden disease, a rare autosomal dominant familial cancer syndrome, was located on chromosome 10. Cowden disease (also called Cowden syndrome) is typified by the presence of benign lesions, called *hamartomas*, that affect the skin, breast, thyroid, and the oral and intestinal epithelia. Breast and thyroid cancers are also components of Cowden disease. Prior to the cloning of *PTEN*, high resolution mapping by Charis Eng and her colleagues had demonstrated linkage to the 10q23 region.

The identity of the Cowden disease locus and *PTEN* was soon confirmed. Mutations of *PTEN* were found in over 80 % of the Cowden disease families. The mutations found in these families were missense and nonsense point mutations, insertions, deletions, and splice-site mutations, nearly one half of which affected the phosphatase domain at the N-terminus of the encoded protein. The mutated allele was often found to be retained after LOH in tumors, confirming the role of *PTEN* as a tumor suppressor in this syndrome.

Three rare, autosomal dominant diseases with clinical features that partially overlap those of Cowden disease are also caused by germline mutations in *PTEN*: Bannayan-Riley-Ruvalcaba syndrome, Proteus syndrome and Proteus-like syndrome. Collectively, these inherited cancer syndromes and Cowden disease are referred to as the PTEN Hamartoma Tumor Syndromes (PHTS). Affected individuals with Bannayan-Riley-Ruvalcaba syndrome develop the benign tumors associated with Cowden disease, but do not typically develop malignancies. Interestingly, one mutation found in a Bannayan-Riley-Ruvalcaba family was identical to a *PTEN* mutation previously found in a Cowden disease family. This suggests that variable penetrance of *PTEN* mutations can alternatively lead to two clinically distinct syndromes. It is possible that modifier loci might play a significant role in *PTEN* mutation-associated phenotypes.

Overall, about 80 % of individuals affected by Cowden disease harbor germline mutations in *PTEN*. The genetic basis for the remaining 20 % of cases is not yet known. It remains possible that additional mutations in *PTEN* exons or regulatory regions remain undetected or that additional loci play a significant etiologic role. The overall incidence of Cowden disease has been estimated to be 1 in 200,000, but the subtle manifestations of the disease and the variable penetrance of *PTEN* mutations suggest that this may be an underestimate.

PTEN is frequently mutated in diverse types of sporadic cancers. The two cancers that most commonly harbor mutated *PTEN* genes are glioblastomas, a type of brain cancer in which about 40 % of tumors are *PTEN*-mutant, and endometrial cancer, in which *PTEN* is mutated in over one half of the samples tested. While germline *PTEN* mutations predispose to breast, prostate and thyroid cancers, only a small percentage of sporadic forms of these cancers involve *PTEN* mutations. *PTEN* mutations have also been detected in smaller numbers of stomach and lung cancers and melanomas. In some cancer types, *PTEN* mutations are found in a greater proportion of larger, more malignant cancers, suggesting that *PTEN* loss can affect cellular phenotypes related to tissue invasion and motility.

Studies of prostate cancers have revealed that approximately one half exhibit LOH in the 10q23 region, while about 15 % have defined homozygous deletions at the *PTEN* locus. Similarly, breast cancers also have a high rate of LOH at 10q, while *PTEN* is actually found to be specifically mutated in only about 5 % of specimens analyzed. It thus appears to be fairly common that specific *PTEN* mutations are not found in tumors with LOH at 10q23. Why might this be the case? Similar to *RB1*, *PTEN* appears to be the frequent target of homozygous deletion. Historically, this type of mutation was difficult to ascertain by routine methods of genetic analysis. Point mutations are typically detected against a background of normal, wild type sequence. In contrast, the absence of signal that arises from attempts to amplify a deleted region can be difficult to quantify and verify. Thus, a lack of complete concordance between LOH and clear evidence of a first 'hit', as predicted by Knudson, was likely the result of technical difficulties inherent in the detection of unequivocal homozygous deletions.

The phosphatase activity of the PTEN protein plays a prominent role in the regulation of cell growth and cell death. Interestingly, the frequently mutated proto-oncogene *PIK3CA* also plays an antagonistic regulatory role in this enzymatic process. How *PTEN* and *PIK3CA* mutations affect the phenotype of the developing cancer cell will be discussed in Chap. 6.

SMAD4 and the Maintenance of Stromal Architecture

Polyps within the gastrointestinal tract occur frequently in the general population, and even in occur in younger individuals. The majority of these are sporadic lesions of no consequence that are sloughed into the lumen and excreted in the stool. In a small number of individuals, non-neoplastic, hamartomatous lesions known as *juvenile polyps* occur as part of a familial disorder known as Juvenile Polyposis Syndrome (JPS). The relationship between JPS-associated polyps and cancer illustrates the relationship between tissue architecture, development-associated genes and the risk of malignancy.

The polyps that occur in JPS patients are histologically distinct from the adenomas that are characteristic of FAP. Juvenile polyps are hamartomas, which are focal growths thought to result from faulty developmental processes. (The term 'juvenile' in this context refers to the histological appearance resembling immaturity, rather than the age of the patient population.) Hamartomas within the gastrointestinal tract are composed of a mixture of glandular and stromal elements. Though they resemble neoplasms, hamartomatous polyps grow at the same rate as the normal adjacent tissue and do not invade or otherwise alter the surrounding tissue structure. They therefore represent more of a structural defect, a malformation of the normal architecture of the mucosae, than a growth defect *per se*. Juvenile polyps are benign, but about 40 % of individuals with JPS will develop a malignancy. While the adenomas that occur in FAP patients are restricted to the colon and rectum, the hamartomas that occur in individuals affected with JPS occur throughout the upper and lower gastrointestinal tract.

Recognized as an autosomal dominant disorder in 1966, JPS is rare, with an incidence that has been estimated at 1 in 100,000. Though JPS appears to be genetically heterogeneous, linkage to markers on chromosome 18 has been found in approximately one half of known JPS kindreds. Within the interval of linkage on chromosome band 18q21 is a tumor suppressor gene cloned by Scott Kern and his coworkers in 1996.

Allelic loss involving the 18q21 region can be found in about 90 % of pancreatic adenocarcinomas. The Kern group mapped homozygous deletions within this region in a large panel of sporadic pancreatic tumors. These deletions were found to commonly include a locus that they designated *DPC4* (as it was the fourth gene that had been reported to be deleted in pancreatic carcinoma). Additional evidence for *DPC4* as a tumor suppressor gene was the finding of inactivating single base substitutions and a small deletion in pancreatic tumors that did not have homozygous deletions. *DPC4* was found to contain significant homology to the *Drosophila* gene Mothers against decapentaplegic (*MAD*) and the *C. elegans SMA* gene family, which are both involved in development. *DPC4* became known as SMA- and MAD-related gene 4, or *SMAD4*.

Germline mutations in *SMAD4* have been found in most of the JPS kindreds in which linkage to 18q markers had been established. Among sporadic cancers that occur in the general population, *SMAD4* is inactivated but point mutations or deletions in 15–30 % of pancreatic cancers, as well as in other cancers of the gastrointestinal system including bile duct cancers and colorectal cancers. *SMAD4* mutations are uncommon in tumors that occur outside the gastrointestinal tract.

SMAD4 and homologs of *SMAD4* in other species are important regulators of development and adult tissue homeostasis. Human *SMAD4* is a member of a *SMAD*-gene family that composes an intracellular communication network. The role of the *SMAD4* encoded protein in this network is to both receive signals communicated from the cell surface and transduce them to the cell nucleus, where gene expression is regulated. The SMAD signaling network is an important mechanism that allows cells to sense changes in their environment, such as those that naturally occur during development and normal growth of tissues, and to orchestrate a measured response to these changes. The role of *SMAD4*-dependent communication in the response of cells to their environment will be described in detail in Chap. 6.

Although hamartomas are benign lesions, the presence of large numbers of hamartomas is a significant risk factor for the development of carcinomas. In the preceding section, we have seen how germline mutations in *PTEN* cause the hamartomatous syndromes Cowden disease and Bannayan-Riley-Ruvalcaba syndrome and a corresponding increase in the risk of many types of cancer. Approximately one half of individuals with Cowden disease have gastrointestinal hamartomas. The extent of clinical overlap between Cowden disease and JPS is significant, and therefore the conclusive diagnosis of JPS largely depends on the exclusion of the other hamartoma syndromes. Correctly categorizing and diagnosing the patient with gastrointestinal hamartomas is challenging, but important. Individuals with Cowden disease must be monitored carefully for the development breast and thyroid cancers, while JPS does not carry these risks. Knowledge of the distinct genetic basis for both of these syndromes will be a useful tool for conclusive diagnosis and risk analysis.

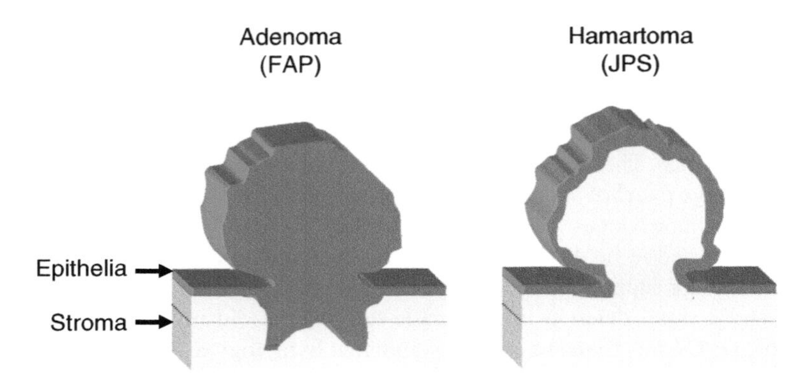

Fig. 3.15 Two types of colorectal polyp. In patients with FAP, germline mutations in *APC* lead to the development of hundreds of adenomas. Adenomatous polyps are composed primarily of epithelial cells (*red*). Mutant epithelial cells carry a significant risk of further clonal evolution, and eventual growth into a malignancy. The hamartomatous polyps characteristic of JPS are caused by germline mutations in *SMAD4*. In contrast to adenomas, hamartomas are composed primarily of stromal cells (*gray*). Stromal cells do not themselves evolve into cancers, but their proliferation alters the landscape of the colon epithelium. The resulting changes in the microenvironment provide selective pressure for the outgrowth of epithelial neoplasia

Can gastrointestinal hamartomas evolve into carcinomas? Histologic analyses of large numbers of sporadic and inherited juvenile polyps have revealed regions of adenomatous epithelium in a small proportion of these lesions. It therefore appears that each hamartoma associated with Cowden disease or JPS has the potential, albeit low, to progress to a carcinoma.

The adenomatous polyps associated with FAP are largely composed of epithelial cells. Analysis of these lesions has revealed clonal genetic defects that are associated with tumor progression (Chap. 1). In contrast with the adenomatous polyps of FAP, the hamartomas associated with JPS are composed largely of stromal cells (Fig. 3.15). Genetic losses have been detected in these stromal growths, suggesting that they are expanded clones. However, JPS does not predispose affected individuals to stromal cell cancer. The cancer associated with JPS is colorectal carcinoma, which, like all carcinomas, arises from epithelial tissue. The conclusion that can be drawn from these findings is that genetically-mediated changes in the stroma can create an environment that promotes the outgrowth of epithelial cell clones, a fraction of which progress to cancers.

The induction of tumors by the alteration of the stromal environment represents a distinct mechanism of tumorigenesis. Histological examination of hamartomas shows that epithelial cells become entrapped within abnormal stroma. These entrapped epithelial elements form dilated cysts and develop areas of local inflammation. As described in Chap. 1, inflammation creates a microenvironment in which the clonal growth of cancer cell precursors can be favored. Thus, early genetic changes that occur in stromal cells can promote tumorigenesis in neighboring epithelial cells.

Two Distinct Genes Cause Neurofibromatosis

Neurofibromatosis is a genetic disease that is characterized by numerous benign lesions. As in the case of juvenile polyps caused by inherited and *de novo* germline mutations of *SMAD4*, the mutations that cause neurofibromatosis lead to defects in tissue architecture and simultaneously cause a predisposition to cancer. The genetic alterations that cause neurofibromatosis are particularly devastating to affected individuals because the characteristic lesions are externally evident (Fig. 3.16).

The most common form of neurofibromatosis is Neurofibromatosis 1 (NF1), formerly known as peripheral neurofibromatosis or van Recklinghausen disease. Affected individuals exhibit varying numbers of pigmented lesions known as café-au-lait spots, freckling and hamartomas in the iris of the eye, called Lisch nodules. NF1 is strongly associated with cognitive dysfunction, including mental retardation and learning disabilities. Vision disorders, epilepsy, and scoliosis are also common symptoms. In addition to the diagnostic, disabling, features of the disease, patients affected by NF1 are prone to unusual malignancies in tissues that developmentally arise from the neural lineage. A small proportion of NF1 patients develop tumors in the fibrous sheath that envelops peripheral nerves (known as neurofibrosarcomas); such tumors are highly aggressive and metastatic. NF1 is also strongly associated with tumors in the optic nerve (optic gliomas) which rarely become symptomatic. Overall, patients affected by NF1 develop cancer at a higher rate than the general population.

The NF1 gene was cloned by the combined use of physical mapping and linkage analysis. A large-scale gene hunting effort used data derived from 142 families with

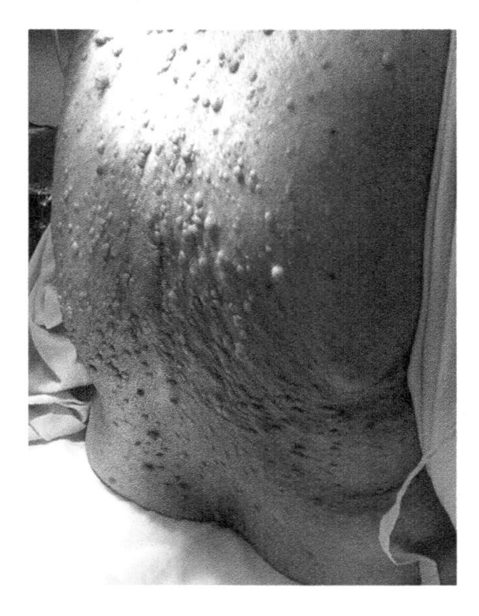

Fig. 3.16 Neurofibromatosis type 1. Severe disease is apparent on the back of an elderly woman. Café-au-lait macules and neurofibromas can be seen

over 700 affected individuals to localize the gene to17q11.2. Progress was accelerated by the analysis of two patients with balanced translocations involving defined breakpoints, which narrowed the search considerably. Candidate genes from the minimal region were evaluated by DNA sequencing. Ultimately, a large gene, spanning 300 kb and containing a 9 kb open reading frame was identified independently by groups led by Francis Collins and Ray White, and reported in 1990.

Germline alterations in the NF1 gene, designated *NF1,* include large deletions, small rearrangements and most frequently, point mutations. The latter type of mutation is distributed throughout the *NF1* coding region. *NF1* does not contain mutation hotspots. The protein encoded by *NF1*, called neurofibromin 1, bears significant homology to a family of signaling proteins that regulate cell size, shape and proliferation. The relationship of *NF1* to cell signaling pathways involved in cancer is described in Chap. 6.

Affecting 1 in 3500 in the US population, NF1 is one of the most common autosomal dominant disorders. A relatively large proportion of cases, approximately one half, arise from new germline mutations. This high rate of spontaneous mutation may be due in part to the large size of the *NF1* gene. Single mutated *NF1* alleles are dominant, and cause the clinical manifestations of NF1 with nearly complete penetrance. During the development of NF1-associated cancers, the remaining wild type tumor suppressor allele appears to be lost via LOH, as in other syndromes of cancer predisposition. In addition to its role in neurofibromatosis, the *NF1* gene has been found to be mutated in sporadic, non-heritable tumors including about 20 % of peripheral malignant nerve sheath tumors, and smaller proportions of gliomas, melanomas, ovarian cancers, and other more rare tumors that arise in cells of the neuroectodermal lineage.

A second, clinically-distinct form of neurofibromatosis is called NF2 or central neurofibromatosis. Affected individuals develop retinal hamartomas, but do not exhibit the other lesions associated with NF1. NF2 patients frequently develop bilateral tumors of the eighth cranial nerve, known as *vestibular schwannomas*, and other benign tumors that affect the central and peripheral nervous system. NF2 is considerably less common than NF1 and accounts for about one tenth of neurofibromatosis cases. Many NF2 cases occur in the absence of parental involvement. As is the case with *NF1*, *de novo* germline *NF2* mutations appear to account for up to one half of all cases.

The gene that causes NF2 was cloned independently in 1993 by groups led by James Gusella and Gilles Thomas. *NF2* mutations are found in the germline of NF2 patients and, rarely, in renal cancers, pancreatic adenocarcinomas and melanomas. *NF2*-associated schwannomas rarely develop into malignant lesions, but nonetheless cause significant morbidity and mortality. The overall rate of cancer is not significantly higher in NF2 patients than in the general population.

From Flies to Humans, Patched Proteins Regulate Developmental Morphogenesis

The development of a fertilized oocyte into a full term infant, replete with all of the spatially organized and highly specialized tissues that compose a functional human body, involves myriad interactions between embryonic cells as they proliferate and differentiate. Much of what we understand about the genetic basis of human embryonic development originated in seminal studies of the fruitfly, *Drosophila melanogaster*. This fundamental biological research has also illuminated the role of a tumor suppressor gene in heritable and sporadic cancers.

During the development of the fly, fertilized eggs gives rise to larvae with a segmented body plan characterized by the polarized distribution of tooth-like projections, known as denticles, that are organized along an anterior-posterior axis. In the late 1970s the developmental biologists Christiane Nusslein-Volhard and Eric Wieschaus isolated mutants in which proper body segmentation and patterning had been lost. These mutant larvae exhibited disorganized denticles and had a shortened anterior-posterior axis. The appearance of these larvae inspired the descriptive designation *hedgehog* for the underlying mutations.

Further investigation into the mechanisms of patterning during fly development revealed that the *hedgehog* gene encodes a secreted protein that facilitated intracellular communication. The hedgehog protein (hh) is distributed in an extracellular concentration gradient that establishes the anterior-posterior axis of the larval segments, and functions as a ligand that functionally binds a cell surface receptor encoded by the gene *patched* (*ptc*). The hh-ptc interaction triggers the downstream transcription of target genes that affect cell growth and developmental fates. These downstream activities are thus differentially controlled along the anterior-posterior axis by the graded distribution of hh ligand. Their identification of the genetic factors required for early embryonic patterning eventually lead Nusslein-Volhard and Wieschaus to shares in the 1995 Nobel Prize for Physiology or Medicine.

The hedgehog/patched signaling pathway was found by Matthew Scott and colleagues to be evolutionarily conserved in mammalian cells. The human genome encodes multiple hedgehog ligands and patched proteins, several of which appear to function in the respective roles of their orthologs in the fly. The discovery of hedgehog signaling in mammals helped delineate the developmental signaling pathways that are required for the proper development of many tissues and organs, a process known as *morphogenesis*. The most studied actors in human development are the hedgehog family member known as sonic hedgehog (SHH) and the patched protein encoded by *PTCH1*. Scott and a separate group lead by Phillip Beachy discovered that these genes, required for normal morphogenesis, can be postnatally reactivated in developing tumors.

Germline mutations in *PTCH1* cause basal cell nevus syndrome (BCNS), alternatively known as nevoid basal cell carcinoma syndrome or Gorlin syndrome. BCNS is a relatively rare, autosomal dominant condition that confers a predisposition for basal cell carcinoma, a very common non-melanoma skin cancer that rarely spreads beyond the skin. Affected individuals also develop cystic tumors within the mandible, and abnormalities of the cranium, ribs, vertebrae and facies are also common features. A greatly increased risk of pediatric brain tumors arising in the cerebellum (a tumor type known as a medulloblastoma) is the most life-threatening facet of the syndrome. Somatically-acquired mutations in *PTCH1* are found in sporadic basal cell carcinomas of the skin and sporadic medulloblastomas, and also in malignant peripheral nerve sheath tumors.

Most tumor suppressor genes were first discovered by positional approaches to identify the germline mutations that cause elevated cancer risk in cancer-prone kindreds (eg. *RB1*, *APC*, *BRCA1*, *BRCA2*). One prominent exception to this well-trodden path to discovery is *TP53*, which was first cloned after its encoded protein, p53, was observed to be overexpressed and associated with viral proteins. The discovery of *PTCH1* as a tumor suppressor also occurred by an indirect route. *PTCH1* only came to the attention to the cancer research community after it had been extensively studied in model organisms as a regulator of developmental morphogenesis.

von Hippel-Lindau Disease

von Hippel-lindau (VHL) disease is a cancer syndrome in which affected individuals develop multiple, bilateral kidney (renal) carcinomas and fluid-filled cysts at many different sites. Neoplastic growths made of newly formed blood vessels, known as hemangiomas, are also characteristic signs of the disease. Hemangiomas that form in the brain and spinal cord can cause headaches, gait disturbances and a loss of muscle coordination, dizziness and weakness. Hemangiomas in the eye can lead to loss of vision. This autosomal dominant disorder has an incidence estimated at 1 in 36,000 individuals.

About 10 % of VHL kindreds harbor constitutional chromosomal rearrangements at chromosome 3p25. The precise locus was delineated by three large, non-overlapping deletions. The *VHL* gene was cloned by a positional approach by a team led by W. Marston Linehan.

The cancers that develop in the kidneys of individuals with germline *VHL* mutations are of a histological subtype known as clear cell carcinomas. Sporadic clear cell renal carcinomas are similarly caused by somatic, non-heritable *VHL* mutations.

NOTCH1: Tumor Suppressor Gene or Oncogene?

The *NOTCH1* gene encodes an evolutionarily conserved[1] transmembrane receptor protein that regulates interactions between physically adjacent cells, and is involved in controlling cell fates during development. A role for *NOTCH1* in cancer was first

[1] Mutation of the orthologous gene in Drosophila causes a notched-wing phenotype.

proposed by Jeffrey Sklar and colleagues, who in 1991 observed the locus at the breakpoint of a translocation in T cell lymphoblastic leukemia. In subsequent years, sequence analysis of many diverse tumor types revealed *NOTCH1* mutations in a significant numbers of cancers. With over 600 mutations identified, *NOTCH1* appeared to be significantly involved in the process of tumorigenesis at many sites. But the nature of these mutations led to some confusion as to the primary role of *NOTCH1*.

Patterns of *NOTCH1* mutations differ significantly from one type of cancer to another. In lymphomas and leukemias, the mutations in *NOTCH1* are of the missense type, and are often recurrent. Such recurrent mutations, as well as the original translocation that linked NOTCH1 to a cancer, are highly suggestive of an oncogene (see Chap. 5). However, in solid tumors such as head and neck squamous cell cancer, the mutations in *NOTCH1* most often cause the functional inactivation of the encoded protein, and are generally not found to recurrently affect the same sites. These contrasting patterns initially led to some confusion as to whether *NOTCH1* was a proto-oncogene or a tumor suppressor gene.

The answer is that it is both. The patterns and quality of the mutations in *NOTCH1* suggest two distinct roles for this gene in different tissues. *NOTCH1* is a proto-oncogene in the cellular precursors of liquid tumors, activated by recurrent mutations during tumor evolution. However, this same gene functions to suppress neoplastic growth in the epithelia of the head and neck, and is accordingly functionally inactivated during tumorigenesis. A complete understanding of the role of *NOTCH1* in cancer would have been very difficult to achieve without the perspective gained by comparatively assessing the gene and its spectrum of mutations in many types of cancer. That a single gene can play such opposing cancer-associated roles in different tissues is highly unusual, but demonstrates the highly versatile functionality of developmental pathways in the diverse cellular lineages of the human body.

Multiple Endocrine Neoplasia Type 1

Multiple endocrine neoplasias are syndromes in which affected individuals are predisposed to benign and malignant tumors in various endocrine glands. There are two major forms with different genetic etiologies. Both are inherited as autosomal dominant traits. Multiple endocrine neoplasia type 1 (MEN1) is caused by the mutation of a tumor suppressor gene, *MEN1*. Multiple endocrine neoplasia type two (MEN2) is a more heterogeneous category of similar diseases; most cases can be attributed to germline mutations in the *RET* proto-oncogene (see Chap. 2).

MEN1, formerly known as Wermer syndrome, is most commonly characterized by tumors in the parathyroid glands and the anterior pituitary gland, islet cells of the pancreas, and carcinoid tumors in the gastrointestinal tract. The latter two types of tumors arise in tissues that are related developmentally to tissues of ectodermal origin. MEN1 is often associated with Zollinger-Ellison syndrome, a disorder causes by gastrin-secreting tumors of the pancreas and duodenum. Other, mostly benign, non-endocrine tumors are also found at elevated levels in affected individuals.

The *MEN1* gene was localized to chromosome 11 and positionally cloned in 1997 by Stephen Marx and colleagues. Sequence analysis revealed heterozygous inactivating mutations of *MEN1* in individuals with MEN1; the wild type copy of *MEN1* is subsequently lost via LOH during tumorigenesis. LOH of the *MEN1* locus at 11q13 is observed in sporadic endocrine tumors, But *MEN1* is mutated only rarely in non-heritable cancers, primarily in adrenal gland tumors.

The overall incidence of MEN1 is estimated to be approximately 1 in 30,000. Most multiple endocrine neoplasia cases occur in predisposed families, but about 10 % appear in the absence of a family history of endocrine tumors, and therefore probably result from *de novo* germline mutations.

Most Tumor Suppressor Genes Are Tissue-Specific

Tumor suppressor gene inactivation tends to be cancer-specific, particularly in the case of germline mutations. As we have seen, germline mutations in *APC* strongly predispose to pre-malignant lesions and carcinomas in the colorectal mucosa. FAP patients with mutant *APC* are not strongly predisposed to lung cancer or breast cancer, even though these malignancies similarly arise in epithelial cell populations. Loss of APC function obviously provides a unique selective advantage for cancer precursor cells in the colorectal mucosae, but does not appear to promote the clonal growth of precancerous lesions in other tissues. The basis of such tissue specificity is in most cases not apparent. But two factors to consider are the unique cellular architecture of colorectal crypts and the surrounding stroma, and the mechanism by which crypts are continually renewed. Presumably these distinctive characteristics of the renewable tissues of the large bowel somehow cause a reliance on APC protein activity for the maintenance of homoeostasis that is not as important in other epithelial tissues.

In some cases, the tissue compartment in which a given tumor suppressor gene is required to repress neoplastic growth can be precisely delineated. For example, tumors that arise as a result of the biallelic inactivation of *NF2* are largely confined to a single tissue and cell type: the nerve sheath that surrounds the eighth cranial nerve.

The relationship between tumor suppressor genes and specific tumors sometimes but not always extends to those genes that function in interconnected biological pathways. As will be described in detail in Chap. 6, the Rb and p16 proteins function in a common molecular pathway that regulates the progression of the cell cycle. This growth-inhibitory pathway can be disrupted by mutation of either *RB1* or *CDKN2A*. Despite this connecting molecular pathway, the types of tumors that occur in germline carriers of inactivating *RB1* and *CDKN2A* mutations are distinct and pathognomonic. Why does the same pathway tend to be disrupted by *CDKN2A* mutations in melanomas, but by *RB1* mutations in retinoblastomas? This interesting question remains difficult to answer. What is apparent is that these genetic alterations, although they affect a common pathway at different points, are not completely functionally equivalent. A deeper understanding of the molecular circuitry of the human cell will be needed to resolve these fundamental questions.

Another revealing facet of the various tissue-specific mechanisms of tumorigenesis arises from the comparison of tumor suppressor gene mutations in heritable and sporadic, non-heritable forms of cancer. Tumor suppressor genes that are mutated in familial cancer syndromes are sometimes – but not always – mutated in large proportions of sporadic cancers involving the same tissues (Table 3.1). For example, *APC* is mutated in nearly all FAP patients and also in sporadic colorectal cancers. In contrast, *TP53* is mutated in a large proportion of colorectal cancers, but the germline *TP53* mutations that cause Li-Fraumeni syndrome do not appear to strongly confer a predisposition to colorectal cancer. Conversely, germline *BRCA1* and *BRCA2* mutations account for the majority of heritable breast and ovarian cancers but these genes are mutated in only a minute proportion of sporadic breast and ovarian cancers that occur in the general population.

In some cases, somatic loss of a tumor suppressor gene contributes to sporadic tumors in one tissue, while germline mutations of the same gene confer a predisposition to tumors in a completely different spectrum of tissues. For example, germline mutations of *SMAD4* are found in some JPS kindreds, but *SMAD4* was cloned on the basis of its frequent loss in sporadic pancreatic cancers. Familial clusters of pancreatic cancer have not been found to involve *SMAD4*; some of these have instead been attributed to germline mutations in *BRCA2* or *CDKN2A*. One general conclusion that can be drawn from these disparate observations is that the same mutated gene may contribute to very different forms of cancer depending on whether the mutation was acquired somatically or via the germline.

The distinct effects of a germline versus a somatic mutation in a given tumor suppressor gene are probably related to stochastic factors as well as the cellular phenotypes that are required in different tissues for the distinct stages of tumor growth and maturation. *TP53* provides an interesting example of such stochastic and stage-specific effects. Germline mutations in *TP53* and LOH can apparently facilitate the earliest stages of tumor initiation in the breast, as breast cancer is a prominent feature of LFS. But LOH at *TP53* must either occur rarely or must be a relatively inefficient driver of neoplastic growth in the breast epithelia, as women affected by LFS harbor a mutant *TP53* allele in every cell, yet do not develop a multitude of breast tumors. In contrast, LOH at *APC* must strongly promote early-stage growth in the colorectal epithelia. FAP-affected individuals typically present with thousands of precancerous polyps. In more established colorectal tumors, somatic loss-of-function mutations in *TP53* occur at a relatively late stage of their evolution, just as tumor cells acquire the invasive properties that make them dangerous. Interestingly, *TP53* mutations are less prevalent among colorectal tumors that arise in the context of HNPCC, suggesting that these lesions acquire other alterations that lessen the selective pressure for inactivation of *TP53*. The differential requirements, and selective pressures, for other tumor suppressor gene mutations during the evolution of less common cancers are poorly understood.

Modeling Cancer Syndromes in Mice

Our understanding of tumor suppressor genes and their functions has been confirmed and expanded by studies of genetically-engineered mice. The effects of heritable cancer-associated mutations can be recapitulated in the mouse by the manipulation of the murine germline. In general, the experimental disruption of the murine orthologs of human tumor suppressor genes causes a significantly increased rate of cancers. Such studies provide an independent line of evidence that these mutations define *bone fide* tumor suppressors. They also provide valuable model systems that can be used for studying gene function and for the preclinical testing of new cancer therapies and preventive agents.

Genes can be selectively disrupted in mouse embryonic stem cells by a process known as *gene targeting*. Genetically modified stem cells are injected into mouse embryos. A small proportion of the resulting chimeric embryos will incorporate the modified stem cells into the germ cell lineage during subsequent development, thereby introducing the modified gene into the germline of the new strain. Animals with heterozygous disruptions are interbred to achieve homozygosity at the desired locus. A strain of mice with a heterozygous or homozygous loss of a gene (one copy altered, or both copies altered, respectively) by this gene targeting approach is informally known as a *knockout*.

Knockout mice are extremely powerful tools because they allow the effects of loss-of-function mutations to be directly assessed in a whole-animal model. In many cases, tumor suppressor gene knockouts result in dramatic phenotypes. Knockout mice that are homozygous for *Tp53*-mutant alleles (mouse gene symbols have only the first letter in upper case) develop tumors by the age of 9 months and typically succumb to cancer several months well before 1 year of age. Spontaneous cancers are rare in laboratory strains of mice that have wild type *Tp53* alleles, and these mice typically have a lifespan of about 2 years.

Heterozygous *Tp53*-knockout mice represent a model for the genetic and physiological study of Li-Fraumeni syndrome. These mice are prone to sarcomas and lymphomas. As expected they exhibit a longer latent period prior to cancer development and longer survival, compared to mice that harbor homozygous *Tp53* mutations. These mice also recapitulate the metabolic phenotypes that have been found in humans with the Li-Fraumeni trait, as described in Chap. 1. Only a small proportion of *Tp53*-heterozygous knockout mice develop carcinomas, the cancers that develop most frequently in Li Fraumeni syndrome patients. The spectrum of tumors that develop in *TP53*-mutant humans and orthologous mice thus overlaps significantly, but is not identical.

As in humans with FAP, heterozygous carriers of inactivating *Apc* mutations develop intestinal polyposis. These murine polyps exhibit LOH at the *Apc* locus, with retention of the mutant *Apc* allele. Many of these polyps become cancerous. Interestingly, the majority of polyps in *Apc* heterozygous knockout mice occur in the small intestine rather than the colon. This observation vividly demonstrates the important difference between knockout mice and the human patients they are designed to model, and underscores some of the limitations of such models.

Compound knockouts, in which two or more genes are simultaneously altered in a single strain of mice, can be particularly informative. Inactivation of one *Smad4* allele in mice does not lead to an increased rate of tumors. However, targeting of both *Smad4* and *Apc* leads to more rapid progression of tumorigenesis, and earlier lethality, than is observed upon *Apc* targeting alone. This finding complements human data suggesting that *Smad4* loss of function in stromal cells increases the rate at which epithelial cancers can arise.

In the study of *CDKN2A*, mouse models have provided answers but also framed additional questions. The design of the initial *Cdkn2a*-knockout mouse strain effectively eliminated the expression of both *Cdkn2a*-associated transcripts; these mice exhibited a cancer-prone phenotype. The discovery of the alternative p14ARF transcript in human cells led to subsequent attempts to specifically target the p14ARF mouse homolog, a transcript that encodes a somewhat larger protein known as p19ARF. It was found that knockouts that eliminated the expression of p16 but retained p19ARF expression were cancer-prone. Interestingly, the mouse knockout that eliminated p19ARF but retained p16 expression was similarly prone to cancer. The conclusion of these experiments is that, in mice, the genetic elements that encode both p16 and p19ARF are independently of critical importance in tumor suppression.

These results provide additional context in which to consider the data from humans. The region that uniquely encodes human p14ARF is not frequently mutated, if it is mutated at all, either in sporadic tumors or in the germlines of cancer-prone individuals. Nearly all of the validated mutations within *CDKN2A* that affect p14ARF also involve p16, suggesting that loss of p16 primarily provides the selective advantage for neoplastic growth. Notably, human p14ARF and murine p19ARF are only 50 % identical at the protein sequence level, but appear to be functionally similar. Based on the mouse data alone, one might conclude that p14ARF is a potent tumor suppressor, but the human data are more equivocal.

In cases where the data from human cancers and mouse models appear to support conflicting or divergent hypotheses, it is imperative to prioritize sources of information. From a biomedical standpoint, mouse models are important only because they provide insight into human cancer.

The results of these exemplary studies illustrate both the unparalleled strengths and limitations of mouse cancer models. Knockout mice have confirmed and extended the theory that inactivation of tumor suppressor genes are critical to tissue homeostasis and that their losses represent rate-limiting events during tumorigenesis. While mutated germline tumor suppressor genes clearly cause cancer in mice, the differences between human cancer syndromes and the phenotypes of knockout mice are in many cases significant. Perhaps these differences are not surprising at all, given the high degree of divergence between the two species. Cancers, particularly carcinomas, are strongly associated with human aging. Among many other differences, mice and humans have dramatically different lifespans. The relatively short life of the mouse may be too brief a period to allow the multi-step development of solid tumors, which in humans often grow and evolve for decades before their effects are clinically manifest. This limitation might also account for the relative paucity of carcinomas in *TP53* knockout mice, as other tumor types tend to develop more rapidly. More broadly, a short lifespan might explain why cancer is not observed at high rates in inbred strains of laboratory mice or in the feral mice found in the wild.

Some of the problems in comparatively evaluating cancer-relevant phenotypes that differ in mice and humans may be mitigated by examining other species. Indeed, complex cancer phenotypes have been rigorously investigated in diverse organisms, including zebrafish and rats. In general, non-human genetic models of cancer have contributed enormously to the progress of cancer research.

Genetic Variation and Germline Cancer Genes

The genetic mutations that cause cancer must be evaluated against a background of significant diversity. Distinguishing cancer genes from unrelated genetic variants can be a challenge. Unlike the inbred model organisms that have been widely used to study genes and cancer, humans are genetically diverse. The broad spectrum of phenotypic traits present within our species results from the genetic differences that, in part, define us as individuals. Our unique set of genes contributes much to who we are and what we look like, and in some cases affects our predisposition to diseases such as cancer.

By any measure, the human genome contains an enormous amount of information. The haploid maternal and paternal genomes within each diploid cell are composed of 3.4 billion base-paired nucleotides. As we have seen in the preceding chapters, germline alterations affecting a single base pair in a critical region of a gene involved with cell proliferation can confer a risk of cancer so high that eventual development of disease is essentially inevitable. Small genetic alterations in the human germline can have significant consequences.

At the DNA sequence level, each human is about 99.9 % identical to any other one. The genetic difference between any two unrelated individuals amounts to about 0.1 % of the genome, or from 3–12 million base pairs. Normal variations in the genome that are found in greater than 1 % of the population are known as *polymorphisms*. These can be in the form of single base variants, insertions, deletions, variations in repeat elements, and more complex structural rearrangements.

A common form of genetic variation between humans is the single nucleotide polymorphism, or SNP (pronounced "snip"). When the genomic DNA sequences of two individual, homologous chromosomes are compared, SNPs occur, on average, every 100–300 bp. More than 150 million SNPs have been identified in humans. The multitude of possible SNP combinations that can occur in a given individual accounts for a large proportion of human genetic variation.

No human carries a flawless set of genes. On average, each person carries 250–300 genetic mutations that would be predicted to alter the function of a protein-coding gene, and about 50–100 of these mutations are associated with a disease. However, we are protected by diploidy. With two copies of most genes in every somatic cell, defective genes are paired with a copy that functions normally and are therefore not phenotypically expressed.

Somatic mutations can readily be differentiated from SNPs by comparing cancer cells to normal cells from the same individual. In practice, this comparison can be facilitated by the microscopic dissection of biopsy samples that contain both cancer cells and the cells that make up the normal surrounding tissues, or by comparing a tumor sample with blood cells from the same patient, if the latter is available. Polymorphisms present in the germline will be found in every cell; somatic mutations will only be present in the cancer cells.

More problematic is the evaluation of genetic variants that are present in the germline of individuals with cancer. All variants originally arose by mutation of the genome, but of course not all mutations cause cancer. Most genetic variants are in fact unrelated to an individual's risk of developing cancer. Which variants contribute to disease and which are incidental to the cancer-prone phenotype? How can a cancer gene be distinguished from a benign variant? As described in previous sections, the isolation of genetic variants that cause increased cancer risk has been a difficult undertaking marked by remarkable triumphs.

There are several clues that might indicate that a given SNP or other variation measurably affects the risk of cancer. One important parameter is the *allele frequency*. It appears that inheritance of germline mutants accounts for a relatively modest proportion of all cancers. Most known cancer genes are acquired by somatic mutation rather than inheritance. These observations suggest that germline cancer genes should be relatively uncommon. Common SNPs probably do not impart large cancer risks. For example, if a SNP present in an individual from a cancer-prone family is also present in a large proportion of individuals that are not particularly predisposed to developing cancer, then that SNP is unlikely to define a penetrant cancer gene.

The pattern of inheritance within a family pedigree is a critical criterion for identifying a germline cancer gene. A germline cancer gene would be expected to *cosegregate* with cancer predisposition; the allele suspected to be a cancer gene should be present in family members who develop inherited cancers, and absent in those that do not.

The location of a variant sequence and the consequences of that variant on protein function are additional factors to consider. Mutations can occur anywhere in the genome. Many of these changes will have little obvious effect on gene function. In contrast, most known mutations that increase cancer risk have measurable effects on gene function or expression. Unlike the majority of mutations that occur in introns or intergenic regions of the genome, those that are known to contribute to cancer risk most often are located in or near exons and affect the structure and function of encoded proteins.

Much remains to be learned about how genetic variation contributes to cancer risk. Most of the heritable cancer genes described in this chapter are highly penetrant and therefore impart a significant predisposition to the development of cancer. Low penetrance cancer genes are inherently more difficult to identify and characterize. Mutant genes that may modify cancer risk in subtle ways are far more difficult to detect but may collectively cause a significant number of cancers if they occur at a sufficiently high frequency in the general population. Extensive statistical analysis of compiled genetic information will be required to fully understand the relationship of many sequence variants to cancer risk.

Tumor Suppressor Gene Inactivation During Colorectal Tumorigenesis

How does the mutational inactivation of tumor suppressor genes contribute to tumor development? The timing of common genetic losses during tumorigenesis provides considerable insight. The first and still most comprehensive genetic model for multistep tumorigenesis is based upon extensive data collected from colorectal cancers and their precursor lesions. In the colorectal mucosae, characteristic genetic alterations demarcate the stages of tumor growth.

Inactivation of *APC* is a very frequent event in both inherited and sporadic forms of colorectal cancer. *APC* mutants are accordingly prevalent in this type of cancer. Heritable germline mutants are highly penetrant. Even in the absence of other data, these observations strongly suggest that *APC* inactivation is a rate-limiting step in colorectal tumorigenesis. Further insight can be gained from examination of chromosomal lesions at different stages. Mutations of *APC* and losses of chromosome 5q, indicative of LOH at the *APC* locus, are found in the entire spectrum of colorectal neoplasia, from small adenomas to metastatic cancers. *APC* mutations are found in the majority of each of these lesions. As will be described in Chap. 6, the small proportion of colorectal tumors that have wild type *APC* often contain mutations in, *CTNNB1*, a gene that functions in cooperation with *APC*. Even the smallest and therefore earliest lesions analyzed, aberrant crypt foci, have been found to harbor *APC* mutations. The unifying model derived from these observations is that functional inactivation of *APC* triggers the first wave of clonal expansion of colorectal cancer precursors.

The pattern of *TP53* inactivation in colorectal cancers is different from that of *APC*, suggesting a distinct role for these two events. While *TP53* mutations and chromosomal losses involving the *TP53* locus on chromosome 17p are frequently, but not always, found in advanced colorectal cancers, they are found much less frequently in precursor lesions (Fig. 3.17). *TP53* inactivation is therefore a relatively late event in colorectal tumorigenesis. Carriers of *TP53* mutations, who are affected by LFS, do not have a highly increased risk of colorectal cancer. Collectively, these observations suggest that *TP53* inactivation does not initiate the process of colorectal tumorigenesis, but rather plays a central role in the transition from larger adenomas to invasive cancers.

In many colorectal tumors, early inactivation of *APC* is followed by allelic losses on 18q involving the *SMAD4* locus. Loss of 18q is frequently seen in large (>1 cm),

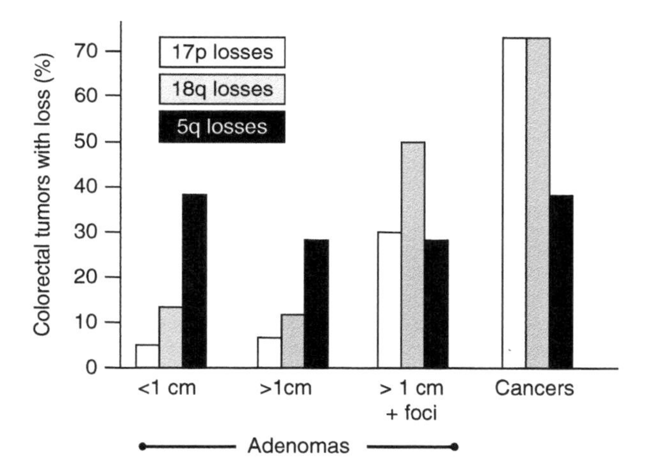

Fig. 3.17 Chromosomal losses during colorectal tumorigenesis. There is a high frequency of LOH involving chromosomes 17p, 18q and 5q in colorectal adenomas and invasive cancers. Allelic losses involving 17p (that contain the *TP53* locus) and 18q (that contain the *SMAD4* locus) tend to occur predominately in larger adenomas with focal regions of carcinomatous transformation, and in invasive cancers. In contrast, allelic losses of chromosome 5q sequences (that contain the *APC* locus) occur at similar frequency in small adenomas, larger adenomas and cancers. These data suggest that 5q loss is an early event, while 17p and 18q losses occur later during tumorigenesis. Note that an evaluation of large allelic losses in the absence of corresponding DNA sequence data from the same tumors can underestimate or overestimate the extent of tumor suppressor gene inactivation. Smaller deletions and point mutations were not assessed by this type of analysis, while large regions of loss can involve multiple tumor suppressor genes. Data from *The Genetic Basis of Human Cancer,* Kinzler and Vogelstein eds, McGraw Hill (2002)

late stage adenomas and in invasive cancers. These alterations are rarely observed in less advanced lesions. Therefore, the inactivation of tumor suppressor loci on 18q typically occurs during intermediate stages of tumor progression, as benign adenomas grow in size. Many cancers with 18q losses also exhibit mutation of *SMAD4*, indicating that *SMAD4* is the relevant gene that is completely inactivated in these cancers.

Colorectal cancer provides a useful model for understanding how cancers arise and progress in step with accumulating genetic alterations (Fig. 3.18). While the genetic principles that have emerged from the systematic analysis of colorectal cancers and their precursors appear to be generally applicable to many other cancers, the specific genes involved and the roles they play varies considerably. As we have seen, many genetic alterations are tumor-specific. *APC* mutations are ubiquitous in colorectal cancers, but generally not observed in tumors that occur outside of the gastrointestinal tract.

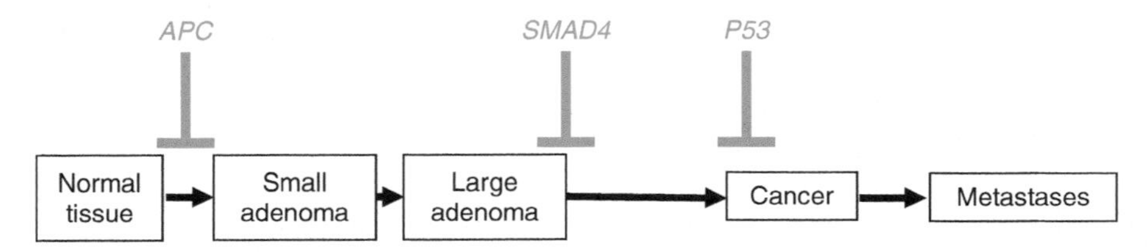

Fig. 3.18 Tumor suppressor genes define rate-limiting steps in the evolution of colorectal neoplasia. The combination of LOH and mutational analyses support defined roles of tumor suppressor genes. *APC* controls the rate-limiting step of initial adenoma formation. Selective pressure favors the loss of *SMAD4* and *TP53* functions later in the process of tumorigenesis, as larger adenomas evolve into invasive cancers

Inherited Tumor Suppressor Gene Mutations: Gatekeepers and Landscapers

In previous sections of this chapter, we have seen how the inheritance of germline tumor suppressor gene mutations leads to an increased risk of cancer. The variable penetrance of different tumor suppressor gene mutations reflects the distinct ways in which these alleles contribute to tumor development. This principle is exemplified by comparing the rates of colorectal cancer associated with germline mutations in *APC* and *SMAD4*.

Inactivated *APC* alleles are highly penetrant while inactivated *SMAD4* alleles are less so. Why do different types of mutations confer different risks for the same disease? The answer to this question lies in the effect of a genetic loss on the characteristics of proliferative cells in the target tissue, and whether this effect directly impacts the growth of cancer progenitor cells. The most potent tumor suppressor genes have demonstrably direct effects on cell growth and survival. Mutations of growth-controlling genes are typically highly penetrant and thus confer the greatest risk of cancer. Inactivation of *APC* directly causes the outgrowth of pre-cancerous polyps. In individual carriers of FAP, every cell has only one functional *APC* allele. Loss of this single allele is sufficient to give rise to a polyp. The large number of polyps that occur in FAP patients is a virtual guarantee that some will eventually develop into cancers. One can readily infer that wild type *APC* must play a critical role in regulating cell growth and preventing neoplasia. In a similar fashion, *RB1* functions as a critical and essential factor for the maintenance of stable growth and tissue homeostasis among the cells of the developing retina. There is not a precursor lesion in retinoblastoma that corresponds to a colonic polyp, but each neoplasm that does arise apparently has a high probability of progressing into a symptomatic tumor.

Classical growth-controlling tumor suppressor genes such as *APC* have been categorized as *gatekeepers*. As this term suggests, gatekeepers directly suppress the first stages of abnormal cell outgrowth. Cells that lose gatekeeper activity are very likely to divide in an uncontrolled manner that perturbs tissue homeostasis, and thereby form neoplasia. Each of the resulting neoplastic lesions has the potential to become a cancer.

As described in an earlier section, the inherited mutations of *SMAD4* affect epithelial cell populations in a less direct manner. Germline *SMAD4* mutations appear to primarily alter the growth of stromal cells, which are not cancer precursors. *SMAD4* inactivation thus alters the tissue structure of the colorectal mucosae, rather than the proliferative cells of the epithelium that have the potential to form cancers. However, the structural changes caused by the inactivation of *SMAD4* create an abnormal microenviroment, providing a fertile landscape for the outgrowth of epithelial neoplasia. Accordingly, mutations in *SMAD4* typify what has been termed a *landscaper* defect. Landscapers like *SMAD4* maintain normal tissue architecture and thereby promote tissue homeostasis.

Maintaining the Genome: Caretakers

A third category of tumor suppressor genes affect cancer precursor cells directly, but not by controlling their growth. Rather, the proteins encoded by these genes function to maintain a stable genome by directly participating in various processes of DNA repair. When DNA repair genes are inactivated, the overall rate of mutation increases. All subsequent generations of cells will have an increased tendency to inactivate additional tumor suppressor genes and to activate oncogenes. The process of tumorigenesis is thus accelerated in these types of developing cancers. The genes that function to maintain genetic stability can be classified as '*caretakers*'. Examples of caretaker genes are *BRCA1* and *BRCA2*, the breast cancer susceptibility genes.

Caretaker defects define a unique category of tumor suppressor gene. As we have seen in the case of familial breast cancers, the penetrance of mutated caretakers varies considerably. Because they function in the repair of DNA lesions, caretakers are an intrinsic component of the cellular response to replicative mutations that occur by chance and those that result of mutagens in the environment. Accordingly, environmental factors have a significant role in determining the penetrance of caretaker gene mutations.

A caretaker defect is the defining characteristic of an inherited colorectal cancer syndrome called hereditary nonpolyposis colorectal cancer (HNPCC). Defects in one of a family of genes involved in a specific DNA repair process cause an overall increase in the rate of somatic mutations. HNPCC illuminates the central role of genetic instability in cancer and will be described in detail in Chap. 4.

Further Reading

1000 Genomes Project Consortium (2010) A map of human genome variation from population-scale sequencing. Nature 467:1061–1073

Allenspach EJ, Maillard I, Aster JC, Pear WS (2002) Notch signaling in cancer. Cancer Biol Ther 1:466–476

Bremmer R (2009) Retinoblastoma, an inside job. Cell 137:992–994

Collins FS (1995) Positional cloning moves from perditional to traditional. Nat Genet 9:347–350 de la Chapelle A (2004) Genetic predisposition to colorectal cancer. Nat Rev Cancer 4:769–780

Evans SC, Lozano G (1997) The Li-Fraumeni syndrome: an inherited susceptibility to cancer. Mol Med Today 3:390–395

Greenblatt MS, Bennett M, Hollstein M, Harris CC (1994) Mutations in the p53 tumor suppressor gene: clues to cancer etiology and molecular pathogenesis. Cancer Res 54:4855–4878

King M-C, Marks JH, Mandell JB et al (2003) Breast and ovarian cancer risks due to inherited mutations in BRCA1 and BRCA2. Science 302:643–646

Kinzler KW, Vogelstein B (1996) Lessons from hereditary colorectal cancer. Cell 87:159–170

Kinzler KW, Vogelstein B (1998) Landscaping the cancer terrain. Science 280:1036–1037

Levine AJ (1993) The tumor suppressor genes. Annu Rev Biochem 62:623–651

Macleod KF, Jacks T (1999) Insights into cancer from transgenic mouse models. J Pathol 187:43–60

Marx SJ (2005) Molecular genetics of multiple endocrine neoplasia types 1 and 2. Nat Rev Cancer 5:367–375

Narod SA, Foulkes WD (2004) BRCA1 and BRCA2: 1994 and beyond. Nat Rev Cancer 4:665–676

Sharpless NE, DePinho RA (1999) The INK4A/ARF locus and its two gene products. Curr Opin Genet Dev 9:22–30

Tan M-H, Mester JL, Ngeow J, Rybicki LA, Orloff MS, Eng C (2015) Lifetime cancer risks in individuals with germline *PTEN* mutations. Clin Cancer Res 18:400

Chapter 4
Genetic Instability and Cancer

What Is Genetic Instability?

When a cell prepares to divide, its genome is first duplicated and then distributed in total to each daughter cell. Every aspect of this fundamental biological process is tightly controlled, ensuring that the information encoded in the genomic DNA is not lost and does not significantly change as it is transmitted from each generation of cells to the next. A full complement of chromosomes is inherited in structurally intact form. The process of DNA replication is similarly characterized by an extraordinarily high degree of fidelity. During the proliferation of normal stem cells, genetic changes arise very rarely. The information content of the genome in the cells that compose normal tissues is therefore highly stable over the lifetime of the individual.

Cancer cells exhibit a variety of defects in genomic DNA repair and chromosome segregation. Not all of these defects are present in every type of cancer cell, but it appears that nearly every type of cancer involves at least one type of molecular defect that impacts genetic stability. Because of these defects, the rate at which genetic alterations occur is consistently higher in cancer cells than in normal proliferating cells. Genetically, the cells of a growing tumor tend to be inherently less stable than those in neighboring normal tissues.

Why is the genetic instability exhibited by tumor cells important? As we have seen in the preceding chapters, tumors are caused by the sequential acquisition of genetic alterations in proliferating cell populations. These genetic alterations do not arise all at once but accumulate over time as clonal cell populations expand. In some cancers, characteristic mutations coincide with each wave of clonal expansion that defines a stage of tumor development. An increase in genetic instability means that the cells of a developing tumor will acquire genetic alterations at a higher rate than would otherwise be expected. The genetic instability that arises during the process of tumorigenesis serves to accelerate the occurrence of all subsequent genetic alterations. Thus, genetic instability increases the pace of clonal evolution.

F. Bunz, *Principles of Cancer Genetics*, DOI 10.1007/978-94-017-7484-0_4

Genetic instability is a heritable cellular phenotype. The genetic instability observed in a cancer cell is the result of an ongoing defect in genome maintenance or chromosome transmission. This is a concept that is of singular importance in cancer genetics. A frequent point of misunderstanding is the relationship between *genetic instability*, which is a defect in a process related to the transmission of genetic material, and *genetic alterations*, which are stochastically-acquired mutations in genomic DNA. Random mutations can and do arise outside of the context of genetic instability. A random mutation does not necessarily indicate, nor cause, genetic instability. But a large number of mutations in a cell clone is a reliable indicator of an underlying genomic instability.

As we have seen in the preceding chapters, mutations that inactivate tumor suppressor genes and activate oncogenes can be found in nearly all cancers, demonstrating that they are not merely incidental occurrences but cardinal features of cancer cells. Similarly, virtually all cancers exhibit some form of genetic instability. The precise type of genetic instability and the mechanisms by which these instabilities cause increased rates of genetic alterations may vary among different cancers.

The Majority of Cancer Cells Are Aneuploid

One of the most readily observable traits of cancer cells is an abnormal number of chromosomes. While normal human somatic cells invariably contain 23 pairs of chromosomes, the cells that compose tumors often deviate significantly from this diploid complement. A cell that has a number of chromosomes that is not a multiple of the haploid number is defined as *aneuploid*. Aneuploid cancer cells most commonly contain an excess number of chromosomes. A chromosome complement of between 60 and 90 chromosomes is frequently observed. This number varies from cell to cell even within a single tumor.

In addition to these numerical abnormalities, the chromosomes in aneuploid cells commonly have structural aberrations that are rarely observed in normal cells. The structural abnormalities associated with aneuploidy include cytogenetically apparent translocations, deletions, inversions and duplications.

Aneuploidy can be visually linked to mitosis, the phase of the cell cycle during which chromosomes condense, are aligned with respect to the division plane and are then pulled to opposing poles of the mitotic spindle. When observed during mitosis, aneuploid cells exhibit mechanical defects in chromosome segregation. The features of aneuploidy in cancer cells were first described by the German pathologist David Paul von Hansemann a decade after the discovery of chromosomes in the late 1870s. Upon microscopic examination of carcinomas, von Hansemann observed several recurring chromosomal abnormalities in mitotic cells. Prominent among these were asymmetrical mitotic figures that appeared to result in 'imbalances' in the chromosome complement of daughter cells (Fig. 4.1). While abnormal mitoses and chromosome complements had been observed in cancer tissues before, the prevailing thinking had held that these features were the result

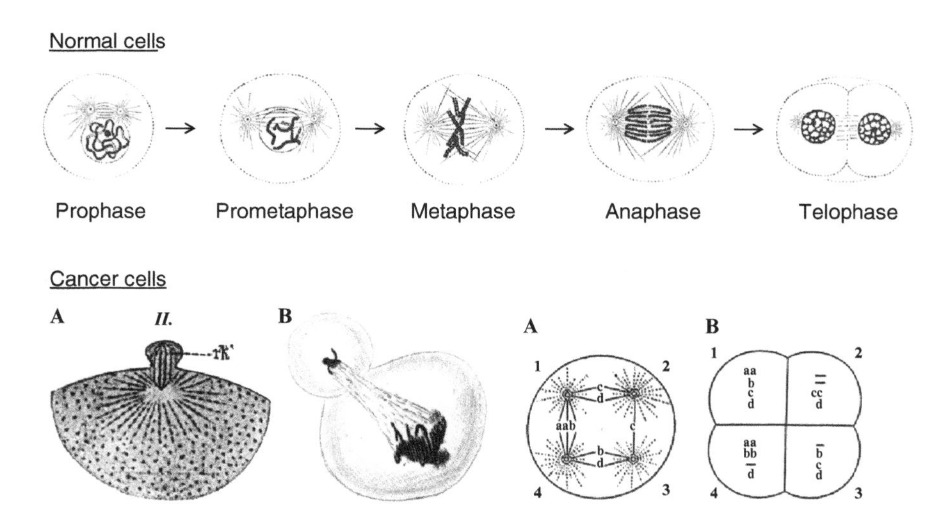

Fig. 4.1 Early observations of aberrant mitoses in cancer cells. In normal cells, mitosis and subsequent cytokinesis result in symmetric daughter cells with an identical chromosome complement. Cancers, in contrast, were found to exhibit symmetrical mitotic figures and tetrapolar mitotic figures. Top panels from Gray (1918) Anatomy of the human body; bottom panels from von Hansemann (1890) Virschows Arch. Pathol. Anat. 119:299–326 and Boveri (1914) Zur Frage der Enstehung maligner Tumoren

of fusions between neighboring tumor cells. Contrary to this idea, von Hansemann proposed that the observed defects in the process that is now known as *chromosome segregation* were an intrinsic defect in cancer cells and a causative factor in tumorigenesis. The hypothesis put forth by von Hansemann was extended and popularized several years later by the German biologist Theodor Boveri, who was among the first to link chromosomes with the functional units of heredity. Boveri noted that mitotic spindles in cancer cells often appeared to be multipolar, and suggested that an underlying mechanical defect that led to abnormal chromosome numbers was a pathological feature of the cancer cell.

Modern cytogenetic techniques vividly reveal both the numerical and structural abnormalities that define aneuploidy (Fig. 4.2). While highly illustrative, karyotypes such as those shown actually underrepresent the full extent of alterations to chromosomes. The reason for this disparity is that cytogenetic techniques allow the visualization of large chromosome regions, but cannot distinguish submicroscopic changes, including the single nucleotide substitutions that predominantly drive tumorigenesis. The genetic consequences of recombination between homologous chromosomes can also be impossible to visualize by cytogenetic methods. As an example, consider a cell that has lost a maternal chromosome 17, but then reduplicated the corresponding paternal chromosome 17. In this scenario, such a cell would have a normal karyotype, but would have lost every unique allele carried on the maternal chromosome 17. Molecular techniques such as SNP analysis or deep DNA sequencing can make this distinction. The use of such molecular techniques has

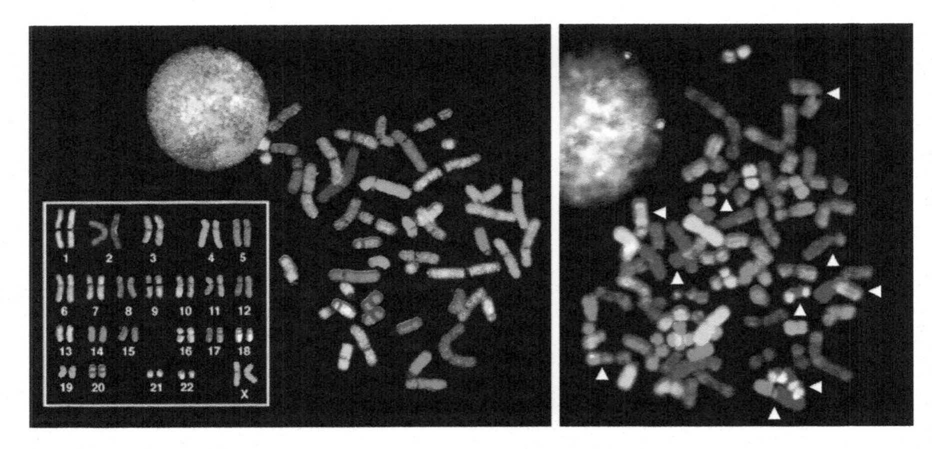

Fig. 4.2 Spectral karyotyping. With the use of chemical inhibitors of mitotic spindle formation, cultured cells can be arrested in metaphase, facilitating the examination of individual, condensed chromosomes. After fixation, these cells are incubated with chromosome-specific DNA probes that are conjugated with fluorophores. The hybridization of these probes with fixed chromosomes effectively results in the painting of each chromosome with an identifiable color. The cell analyzed at *left* has a diploid chromosome complement, with no gross structural abnormalities (image from the NHGRI). In contrast, a spectral karyotype of a cancer cell reveals both numerical and structural abnormalities (*right panel*). Numerous chromosomal rearrangements are indicated by *arrowheads* (Image by Constance Griffin, MD, The Johns Hopkins University)

revealed that in many common cancers, 25 % of alleles are lost. Losses of greater than half of all alleles are not unusual.

What is the meaning of the striking chromosomal abnormalities that are found so frequently in cancer cells? Is aneuploidy causally involved in cancer, or merely a consequence of hyperactive cell division? This point has been a matter of vigorous debate in the century that has elapsed since the observations of von Hansemann and Boveri. The sheer prevalence of aneuploidy in cancer would suggest that it contributes to the process of tumorigenesis, but it has also been proposed that aneuploidy is merely a byproduct of dysregulated cell growth or structural changes that arise during tumorigenesis. Only recently has this issue been definitively resolved. In the sections that follow, we will explore the relationship between aneuploidy and the cancer gene theory.

Aneuploid Cancer Cells Exhibit Chromosome Instability

The descriptions of aneuploidy provided by von Hansemann and Boveri suggested that aneuploidy might be a manifestation of an underlying defect in mitosis. An alternative interpretation is that aneuploidy arises by some other means, and that mitosis is simply more likely to fail in the presence of too many chromosomes. A powerful approach to investigating these two possibilities was devised by Christoph Lengauer, while working with Bert Vogelstein and Kenneth Kinzler in the late

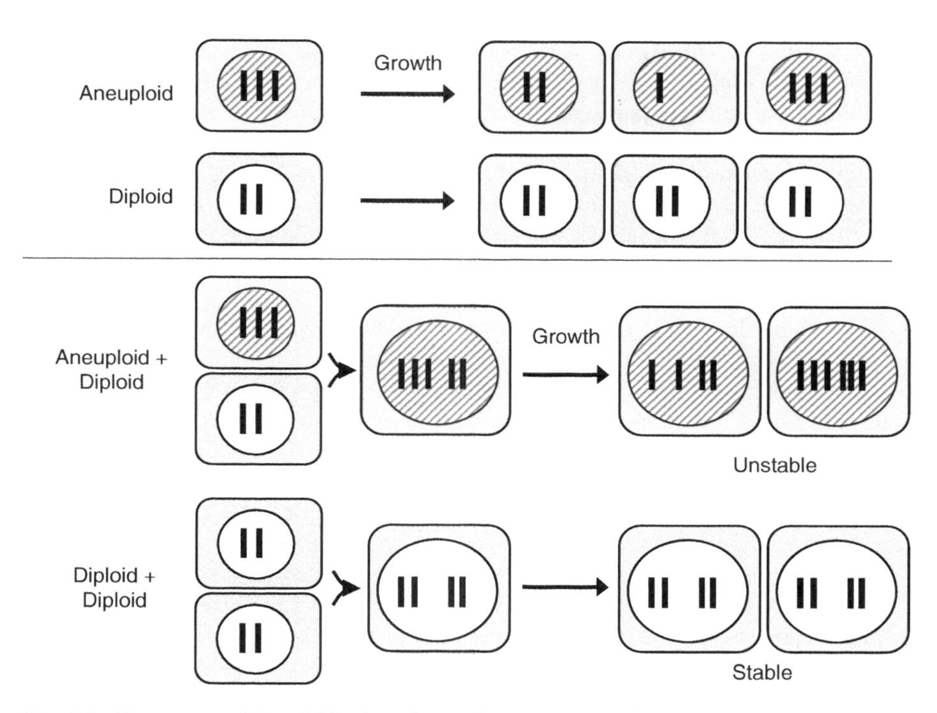

Fig. 4.3 Chromosomal instability in colorectal cancer cells. *In vitro* clonal expansion of an aneuploid cancer cell results in a cell line in which the individual cells have divergent numbers of chromosomes (*upper panel*). This instability defines the CIN phenotype. Diploid cell clones, in contrast, maintain a stable chromosome complement. Fusion of an aneuploid cell and a diploid cell results in a hybrid cell line with a large chromosome complement that exhibits CIN upon expansion (*lower panel*). This result demonstrates that CIN is dominant under these conditions. Fusion of two diploid cells similarly results in a hybrid cell with an abnormal number of chromosomes. Despite this abnormal complement, the progeny of this fused cell maintain numerical stability. This result shows that numerical abnormality does not, in itself, cause CIN

1990s. Using the technique of fluorescence *in situ* hybridization, Lengauer measured the rates at which chromosomes are lost and gained in colorectal cancer cells during long term culture (Fig. 4.3). The results were binary in nature. Diploid cancer cells were observed to maintain a stable chromosome complement when propagated for many generations. In contrast, cancer cells that were aneuploid tended to gain and lose individual chromosomes at the relatively high rate of 0.01 per chromosome per cell division. When clonal populations of these aneuploid cells were propagated for multiple generations, the cells within each expanded clone were found to rapidly diverge from one another with respect to their chromosome complement. The increased rate of chromosome gains and losses in aneuploid cells was termed *chromosomal instability*, often abbreviated as CIN.

Additional insight was gained through cell fusion experiments, similar in design to the seminal experiments of Hill that revealed the recessive nature of tumor suppressor mutations (Chap. 3). Experimental fusions between diploid and aneuploid cells resulted in hybrid cells that were aneuploid. Hybrid cells resulting from the fusion of two diploid cells maintained a constant chromosome number, despite the fact that these cells contained an abnormal chromosome complement. Thus, a cardinal feature of aneuploidy could be experimentally separated from the underlying process that causes CIN. Several conclusions can be drawn from these observations: (1) aneuploidy is a reflection of an ongoing cellular process, (2) aneuploidy does not in and of itself *cause* instability, but rather may *result* from instability and (3) aneuploidy, in the forms examined in this analysis of prototypical colorectal cancer cells, is a dominant phenotype.

The quantification of CIN provides a useful framework for understanding the nature of aneuploidy and its potential role in cancer. Aneuploidy is a state that reflects an ongoing, dynamic process which can be measured as CIN. A significant body of evidence, including the original observations of von Hansemann and Boveri, suggest that the mitotic defects observed in aneuploid cells contribute to CIN. Chromosomes are lost when they fail to segregate equally to daughter cells during the process of mitosis. Chromosome gains occur when chromosomes are unevenly segregated and when they are aberrantly duplicated, suggesting that defects in the regulation of DNA replication might also contribute to CIN.

Aneuploid cancer cells most often have an excess of chromosomes. Cancer cells with a reduced number of chromosomes, which are termed *hypodiploid*, are relatively rare and most often are found in leukemias. The processes that underlie CIN do not appear to be biased; aneuploid cells have been shown to gain and lose chromosomes at equally high frequencies. Why then do aneuploid cancer cells most typically have a chromosome complement that is greater than the diploid number? The answer may be related to cell survival. All human chromosomes, with the exception of the Y chromosome, are essential for cellular viability. Loss of even one chromosome of a homologous pair can have lethal consequences, presumably due to the negative effects of reduced *gene dosage* or the unmasking of non-functional alleles. While CIN can cause the chromosome complement of a given cell to drop below the diploid number of 46, such a cell would be less likely to survive and proliferate. Hypodiploid cell populations are therefore rare. In some cases, the karyotypes of hypodiploid cancer cells reveal an extreme degree of structural rearrangement. Spectral karyotyping of such cells reveals individual chromosomes that contain material originating from multiple chromosomes. These derivative chromosomes can presumably maintain a vital gene dosage in the context of a reduced numerical complement.

Chromosome Instability Arises Early in Colorectal Tumorigenesis

Intriguing clues as to the role of aneuploidy during tumorigenesis have been provided by studies of colorectal tumors. CIN was first characterized in aneuploid cell lines that had been derived from established colorectal carcinomas. Subsequent studies have shown that even the smallest adenomas, less than 2 mm in size, have measurable allelic imbalances. These imbalances are a molecular indication of aneuploidy (which was in the past a cytogenetic observation). Thus, evidence of aneuploidy can be seen in the earliest defined colorectal tumors.

In some very small colorectal adenomas, allelic imbalances are evident in only a subset of the cells. Notably, imbalances involving chromosome 5, which contains the locus for *APC*, are more likely to be present in every cell of a small tumor than are imbalances in other chromosomes. This observation is consistent with the preponderance of evidence that the loss of heterozygosity (described in Chap. 3 and abbreviated LOH) involving the *APC* locus is the event that initiates colorectal tumorigenesis. Although the precise timing of CIN onset remains difficult to ascertain, the available data suggest that CIN occurs very early in the process of tumorigenesis, shortly after the biallelic loss of *APC*.

Does loss of *APC* lead directly to aneuploidy? Aberrant mitotic spindles have been detected in *APC*-null cells from experimental mice, suggesting that *APC* loss may play a direct role in chromosome segregation. However, conclusive evidence for such an affect during human colorectal tumorigenesis remains elusive. It is also important to consider that, while aneuploidy is prevalent in most cancer types, *APC* mutations are mainly restricted to colorectal tumors. Thus, even if *APC* inactivation were to be established as the proximal cause of CIN and in colorectal cancers, the loss of *APC* would clearly not be a general explanation for such a widespread phenomenon.

A general cause of aneuploidy might be expected to be present in many diverse cancer types. Genetic alterations of *TP53* have been proposed to fulfill this criterion. It has been suggested that *TP53*, which is frequently mutated in a wide variety of cancers – including colorectal cancers – might play a critical role in maintaining chromosome stability. Evidence in favor of this hypothesis includes the overall prevalence of *TP53* mutations, and the inevitable association of these mutations with aneuploidy, which is similarly prevalent. Among the tumors that arise in the highly proliferative colorectal epithelia, for example, there is a strong association between *TP53* mutations and aneuploidy. However, there are many examples of chromosomally stable cancers with inactivated *TP53* and, conversely, aneuploid cancers that have retained wild type *TP53* alleles. Furthermore, the experimental mutation of *TP53* alleles in chromosomally stable cancer cells does not generally cause nullizygous to display CIN and aneuploidy at the levels typically observed in aneuploid tumors. An additional consideration is the timing. During colorectal tumorigenesis, aneuploidy is detectable very early in the process in very small lesions. *TP53* inactivation occurs much later, perhaps after decades of benign tumor growth. Indeed, LOH involving the *TP53* locus on chromosome 17, a process accelerated by the forces of CIN, provided the critical insight that led to our understanding of *TP53* as a tumor suppressor gene.

Chromosomal Instability Accelerates Clonal Evolution

The loss of genetic material can be lethal to a cell. There is clearly a lower limit to a chromosome complement, as attested by the relative paucity of hypodiploid cancer cells. There is also an apparent upper limit to how many chromosomes can be contained, maintained and transferred to progeny; few cancer cells have more than ~90 chromosomes. Extreme levels of CIN would therefore be expected to be highly detrimental to the ongoing viability of a cell clone. Consistent with this prediction, the genes that are known to play central roles in mitosis and the mitotic spindle checkpoint have been found to be essential for viability.

A loss of genetic stability can clearly decrease cellular viability. However, an intermediate level of instability, such as that found in highly proliferative cancer cells, can augment clonal evolution and therefore increase the capability of mutable cell populations to adapt to the changing environment of a growing tumor (Fig. 4.4).

Cancer cell clones evolve by the process of genetic mutation followed by successive waves of clonal expansion. How might CIN contribute to clonal evolution? While many aspects of aneuploidy remain mysterious, one consequence of CIN is clear: CIN accelerates the late of allelic loss. As described in Chap. 3, the first step of tumor suppressor gene inactivation is the inactivation of one allele by mutation. The second step is the loss of the remaining wild type allele, known as loss of heterozygosity (LOH). LOH occurs either by an independent mutation, by mitotic

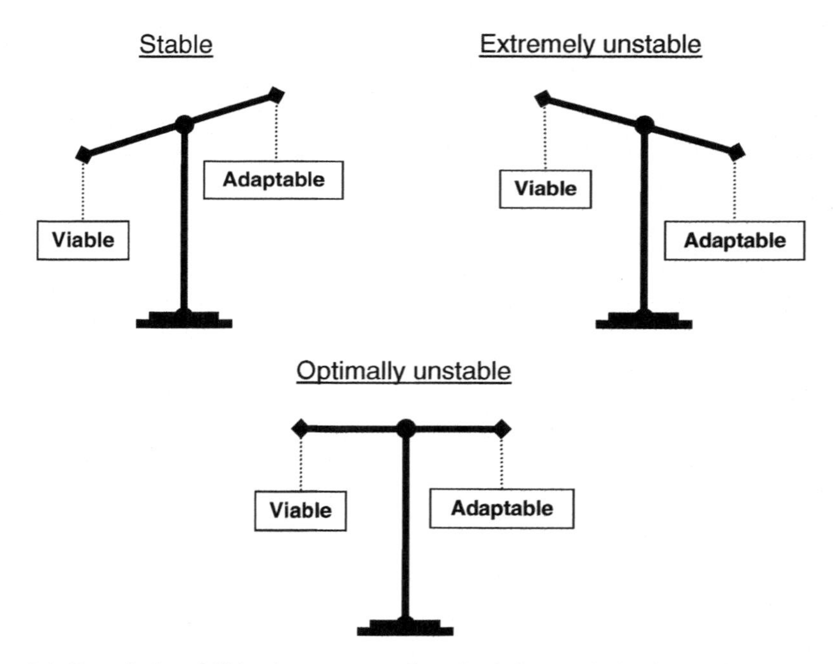

Fig. 4.4 Genetic instabilities in cancers reflect the balance of viability and adaptability. Normal cells with a stable genome are highly viable, but not readily adaptable to changing environments. In contrast, extreme levels of instability would promote adaptability but losses of essential genes would significantly impair viability. The optimal level of instability in cancer cells appears to be high enough to facilitate increased adaptability and promote clonal evolution into expanding microenvironmental niches, but low enough to preserve viability and the capacity for continued proliferation

recombination, or by loss of the chromosome that carries the remaining wild type allele. CIN would be predicted to directly increase the rate of the second step of tumor suppressor gene inactivation by increasing the rate at which whole chromosomes or parts of chromosomes are lost. In most cases, LOH is accompanied by a duplication of the remaining homologous chromosome. The duplication process is also favored in cells with a CIN phenotype, which promotes both numerical gains and losses. Thus, the tendency of CIN cells to gain and lose chromosomes can contribute to two separate components of tumor suppressor gene inactivation: the accelerated loss of the wild type allele and the duplication of the mutant allele.

The clonal evolution of cancer is punctuated by the progressive accumulation of genetic gains and losses. Genetic instability accelerates the rate at which these gains and losses occur, and thereby promotes the progression of clonal evolution. The evolutionary advantage acquired by a cell clone that becomes genetically unstable is finely balanced against the disadvantages of instability. An extreme level of instability would cause the frequent loss of essential genes and other disturbances to cell growth, and would therefore be highly detrimental to cell viability. For example, the mutational loss of genes that contribute to mitosis, which would be predicted to cause an extreme level of CIN, has been shown to be lethal. A more moderate level of CIN, which in many cancers has been measured as a loss or gain of 0.01 chromosomes per cell division, can preserve viability and also accelerate the inactivation of tumor suppressor genes and the activation of oncogenes.

Aneuploidy Can Result from Mutations That Directly Impact Mitosis

The aberrant mitotic figures observed in cancer cell populations suggest that aneuploidy may result from intrinsic defects in the way that cancer cells divide. How might such defects arise? The most obvious potential source of aneuploidy is alteration of the genes that control mitosis. Gene mutations affecting encoded proteins that participate in the machinations of mitosis might be predicted to directly interfere with the ability of cells to maintain a stable number of chromosomes. And in fact several common and deadly cancers harbor recurrent mutations in genes that are required for the efficient and coordinated execution of chromosomal segregation. Experimental manipulation of these genes can cause cells that were formerly diploid to express CIN phenotypes and become aneuploid. Such tumor suppressor genes thus delineate a clear pathway to the phenotypic expression of CIN and aneuploidy.

The segregation of chromosomes during mitosis is monitored by a mechanism known as the *spindle assembly checkpoint*. In normal cells, this checkpoint functions to ensure that mitosis occurs in an orderly and highly coordinated manner. Chromosomes must be properly aligned in metaphase cells and attached to the newly formed mitotic spindle, by a structure called the *kinetochore*, before the separation of sister chromatids can proceed. If one chromosome lags behind or fails to properly attach to the microtubules that compose the mitotic spindle and provide the appropriate level of tension, the spindle assembly checkpoint is activated. The molecular target of the spindle assembly checkpoint is a multi-protein enzyme known as the *anaphase promoting complex*, or APC. (The mitosis factor APC is sometimes referred to as the cyclosome or APC/C. The APC is not to be confused with the unrelated tumor suppressor protein encoded by the *APC* gene.) The inhibition of the APC by signals emanating from the spindle checkpoint transiently blocks the subsequent steps of sister chromatid separation, allowing lagging chromosomes to become properly attached. At this point, the inhibition of the APC by the spindle assembly complex is relieved and anaphase can commence.

Several genes that contribute to the mitotic spindle checkpoint are mutated in a small number of cancers. The first known examples were *BUB1*, which is mutated in less than 10 % of bladder and colorectal cancers, and *BUB1B*, mutated in small numbers of lung and lymphoid cancers. Experimental disruption of these genes has successfully caused diploid cells to express a CIN phenotype.

Germline mutations in *BUB1B* are found in individuals affected by *mosaic variegated aneuploidy*, a rare autosomal recessive disease that causes inherent genetic instability and a significantly elevated risk of cancer. Another gene that is mutated in the germline of some individuals with this disorder is *CEP57*, which encodes a centrosomal protein involved in microtubule attachment. At the cellular level, this disease is characterized by aneuploidies that occur in a *mosaic* pattern, meaning that the karyotypes of cells from the same individual are highly variable. The aneuploid cells of individuals affected by mosaic variegated aneuploidy are predominantly trisomies and monosomies. This rare syndrome of constitutional aneuploidy and cancer predisposition provides evidence that aneuploidy is in fact a contributing factor to developing tumors, rather than a mere byproduct of dysregulated cell division.

STAG2 and the Cohesion of Sister Chromatids

Glioblastoma is a highly lethal type of brain tumor that responds poorly to therapy. In an effort to identify cancer genes that contribute to the evolution of these intractable malignancies, Todd Waldman and David Solomon examined the distribution of known single nucleotide polymorphisms across the chromosomes of these tumor cells, as a means of assessing regions of amplification and deletion. Using this high-resolution scanning method, they identified a focal region of genomic deletion on the X-chromosome that included the locus for the gene *STAG2*.

STAG2 had originally been identified as a protein antigen recognized by antibodies directed against the stromal component of the blood forming organs in mice. Subsequently, STAG2 and the structurally related protein STAG1 were found to be components of a large multi-subunit protein complex known as *cohesin*. The proteins that comprise the cohesin complex assemble into a ring-like structure that encircles sister chromatids and thereby regulates their separation during mitosis.

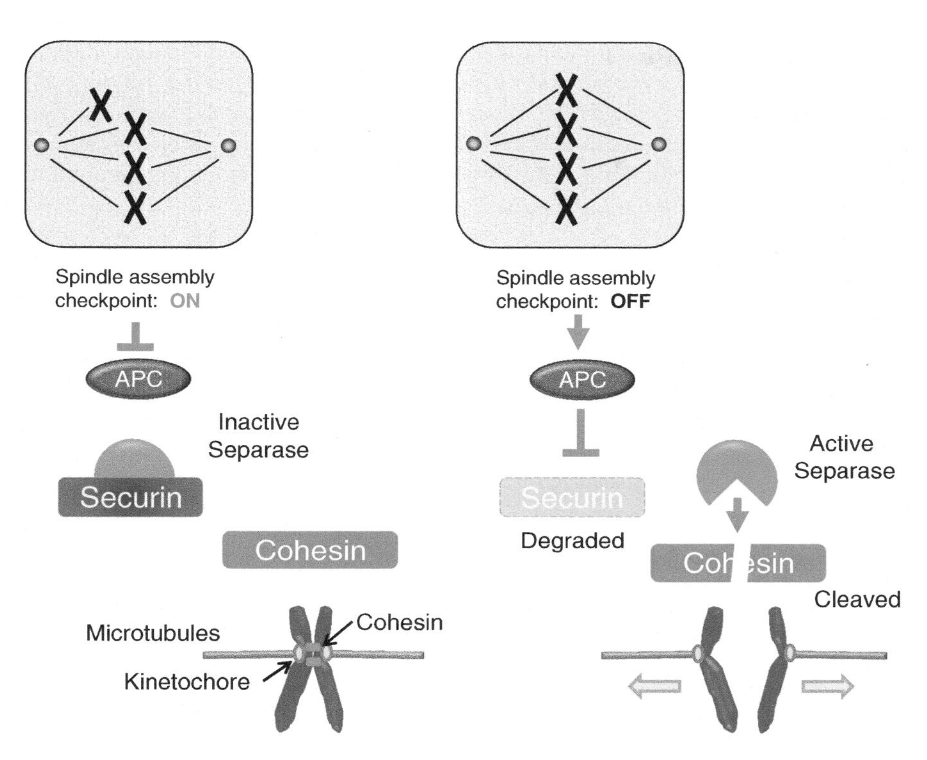

Fig. 4.5 A final wave of sister chromatid separation is orchestrated by the anaphase promoting complex. The spindle assembly checkpoint, activated by an unattached chromatid, prevents the progression of mitosis from metaphase to anaphase by inhibiting the anaphase promoting complex (APC). In this state (spindle checkpoint assembly ON), the cleavage enzyme separase remains largely bound to and thereby inactivated by securin. The proper alignment and attachment of all chromatids to the mitotic spindle results in the deactivation of the spindle assembly checkpoint (OFF) and the activation of the APC. The APC catalyzes the degradation of securin, thus liberating active separase. Separase cleaves the remaining cohesin, the sister chromatid "glue", and thereby facilitates efficient separation of the two sister chromatids to opposite poles of the mitotic spindle. Cancer-associated mutations that affect cohesin function cause dysregulation of sister chromatid separation and thereby promote chromosomal instability and aneuploidy

Cohesin appears to function as a form of molecular glue that binds the two sister chromatids together until it is time for them to be pulled apart during anaphase.

Cumulatively, sister chromatids represent the two complete copies of the genome that are destined to be distributed to both of the daughter cells that arise at the completion of mitosis. The dissociation of sister chromatids defines the onset of anaphase, during which the sister chromatids migrate to opposite poles of the mitotic spindle (Fig. 4.5).

Sister chromatids are primed for separation when cohesin is enzymatically cleaved by a protease called *separase*. This process occurs in several phases as mitosis progresses. Prior to anaphase, separase is largely held in check by its physical association with a protein called *securin*. In the absence of signals from the spindle assembly checkpoint, APC directly targets securin for degradation, and thereby liberates separase activity. Thus, the activation of the APC triggers the final wave of cohesin cleavage and facilitates the separation of sister chromatids. Conversely, the inhibition of the APC by the spindle assembly checkpoint prevents the premature separation of sister chromatids.

The critical role that securin, separase and cohesin play in chromosome segregation has been demonstrated by Prasad Jallepalli and colleagues, who engineered knockouts and knockins in the human genes that encode these proteins and showed that these mutant cells recapitulate some of the features of CIN. Similarly, Waldman and Solomon manipulated the endogenous *STAG2* gene in human cancer cells to demonstrate the role of this cohesin component on the maintenance of a stable chromosome complement. These studies underscore how the precise timing of sister chromatid separation is critical to ensure that all chromatids are faithfully segregated, and demonstrate the direct link between the inactivating *STAG2* mutations found in cancers and aneuploidy.

The *STAG2* locus resides on the X-chromosome and is therefore present as a single functional allele. (In females, one of the X-chromosomes is maintained in a transcriptionally inactive state.) So interestingly, unlike the majority of tumor suppressor genes, *STAG2* requires only one mutational 'hit' to become completely inactivated.

STAG2 is also mutated in about 12 % of bladder cancers. Unexpectedly, *STAG2* mutations correlated poorly with aneuploidy in such tumors, and it has been suggested that the mechanisms by which *STAG2* contributes to tumorigenesis may extend beyond stabilization of the chromosome number. *STAG2* is also mutated in 20 % of Ewing sarcomas, a rare type of pediatric cancer that usually harbors a small number of genetic alterations.

Other Genetic and Epigenetic Causes of Aneuploidy

The genetic basis for CIN in the majority of aneuploid tumors remains largely obscure. This significant gap in our knowledge stems in large part from the incomplete understanding of the many factors that contribute to and regulate mitosis and cell division. Studies in yeast have shown that mutations in over 100 genes can cause a CIN-like phenotype; many of these genes had no previously appreciated link with cell division or chromosome stability. It is possible that many cancer-associated genetic mutations may affect chromosome stability in a manner that is not immediately obvious.

An example of such an unexpected relationship is the effect of alterations in *CCNE* and *CDK4* on chromosome stability. Both of these genes function to regulate the progression of the cell cycle. Amplification of *CCNE*, which encodes cyclin E, and inactivating mutations in *CDK4*, a cyclin-dependent kinase, are both found in cancers at low frequency. Introduction of these alterations in chromosomally stable cancer cells causes these cells to express a CIN phenotype. It had been understood for some time that Cyclin E and Cdk4 proteins function together as part of a multi-protein complex that regulates cell cycle transitions (see Chap. 6). More recently, evidence has emerged that that cyclin E and Cdk4 may regulate the mitotic spindle checkpoint, suggesting that the role of cyclin E and Cdk4 on chromosome stability might be more direct than was previously believed.

Another possible indirect mechanism for CIN involves the control of gene expression. It has been observed that the impairment of the mitotic checkpoint in cancers is frequently associated with changes in the levels of mitotic proteins. As tumor suppressor genes and oncogenes frequently regulate transcription, it is possible that mutations might indirectly affect mitosis by altering the expression of the proteins required for mitosis.

Given the complexities of mitotic regulation and the maintenance of chromosome stability, it is quite possible that frequently mutated tumor suppressor genes and proto-oncogenes might contribute to the development of aneuploidy in many cancers. In depth studies of colorectal tumors underscore the many questions that remain. While aneuploidy has been temporally linked with *APC* inactivation in colorectal cancers, a clear role for *APC* in the stabilization of the chromosome complement has not been established. Similarly, the statistical association of *TP53* inactivation and aneuploidy is compelling, yet experimental manipulation of *TP53* has not supported a direct functional role in the stabilization of the chromosome complement.

Experimental evidence, largely derived from mouse models, suggests that inactivation of tumor suppressor genes involved in DNA recombination and repair might significantly contribute to aneuploidy. Examples of this type of gene include the breast cancer susceptibility genes *BRCA1* and *BRCA2*. Biallelic inactivation of *BRCA1* or *BRCA2* in mice leads to an increased incidence of tumors. These *BRCA1*- and *BRCA2*-null mouse tumors are typically highly aneuploid and exhibit centrosome abnormalities that are strikingly similar to those found in human cancers. It has not been elucidated whether the predisposing event – *BRCA1* or *BRCA2* inactivation – or subsequent alterations that occur during the accelerated process of tumorigenesis are the proximal cause of aneuploidy. It is widely believed that defects in DNA repair might also contribute to the structurally aberrant chromosomes that are strongly associated with aneuploidy.

While studies of mouse tumor models have provided interesting links between known cancer genes and aneuploidy, the mechanism by which aneuploidy arises in the context of these alterations remains incompletely understood. An improved understanding of the molecular mechanisms that underlie cell growth and division as well as new insights into the details of cancer gene function will no doubt contribute to the unraveling of these enduring mysteries.

Given the current paucity of data to firmly support a genetic basis for aneuploidy in many cancers it is worthwhile to consider alternative non-genetic hypotheses. One idea is that epigenetic alterations to the genome (see Chap. 1) might play a central role in the stabilization of chromosomes. In this model, promoters of genes that contribute to the maintenance of genetic stability are silenced by cytosine methylation during tumorigenesis, thereby favoring the CIN phenotype and the development of aneuploidy. There is currently limited evidence to either support or refute this idea. Consequently, a role for epigenetic changes in the CIN phenotype is largely supported as an alternative by a lack of genetic evidence.

An older, but persistent hypothesis holds that aneuploidy is completely independent of genetic mutations or epigenetic changes. Proponents of this view, including the virologist Peter Duesberg, have argued that aneuploidy arises as a random event that precedes genetic alterations. According to this model, the destabilizing effect of aneuploidy is sufficient to promote cellular evolution and ultimately cause all cancer phenotypes. The 'random aneuploidy' theory does not readily account for tumor suppressors, like *STAG2*, that directly control chromosomal segregation, nor does it explain how inherited mutations in genes that control cell ploidy can markedly affect cancer predisposition.

Transition from Tetraploidy to Aneuploidy During Tumorigenesis

The development of CIN during tumorigenesis is one explanation of how cancer cells become aneuploid. The CIN phenotype facilitates gradual changes in the chromosome complement, primarily by the loss or gain of single chromosomes during mitosis. There is a substantial amount of data that suggest that other processes may also contribute to aneuploidy.

Many solid tumors are *polyploid* – they have a chromosome complement that is a multiple of the haploid number. Most often, such cells have twice the diploid chromosome complement and are termed *tetraploid*. Tetraploidy would not be expected to result from gradual losses and gains of individual chromosomes. Instead, tetraploidy represents the aberrant duplication of the entire genome.

There are several lines of evidence that suggest that tetraploidy may represent an intermediate state during the development of some aneuploid cancers. Tetraploid cells are often seen in the lining of the esophagus in individuals prone to esophageal carcinoma. Esophageal carcinoma is known to evolve from a chronic inflammatory condition known as *Barrett's esophagus* by a series of histologically well-characterized steps. During the transition to cancer, the cells of the inflamed epithelium become first tetraploid and then aneuploid.

A high level of tetraploidization has also been observed in the colorectal mucosae of patients with *ulcerative colitis*, an inflammatory disease that strongly predisposes affected individuals to the development of colorectal cancer. Interestingly, the colorectal cancers associated with ulcerative colitis appear to arise from a precursor lesion that is morphologically distinct from a polyp, and which exhibit higher rates of *TP53* inactivation and lower rates of *APC* and *KRAS* mutations. Ulcerative colitis might therefore trigger a distinct sequence of mutations that define an alternative route to colorectal cancer. Interestingly, tetraploidization is seen in the context of ulcerative colitis but is not a common feature of the polyps associated with FAP, nor of sporadic polyps. These data suggest that tetraploidization might contribute to the development of aneuploidy during the evolution of some tumors but not others.

Normal proliferating cells undergo mitosis after a single round of genomic DNA replication. Cells actively monitor this sequence of events. The molecular basis of tetraploidization is incompletely understood, but appears to involve the failure of molecular mechanisms that make the onset of mitosis contingent upon the prior completion of DNA replication.

As in the transition from metaphase to anaphase during mitosis, other cell cycle transitions are negatively regulated by inhibitory mechanisms analogous to the spindle assembly checkpoint. The uncoupling of DNA replication and mitosis by the mutation of stage-specific checkpoint regulators might be expected to increase the number of tetraploid cells. *TP53* is itself a checkpoint regulator that can halt the progression of the cell cycle prior to mitosis, and this activity is therefore frequently absent in cancer cells. There is experimental evidence that loss of *TP53* can lead to an increase in the rate of tetraploidization. While *TP53* inactivation has not been firmly established as a direct cause of aneuploidy, it may contribute to an intermediate stage of numerical aberration, in some cell types. The mechanisms by which cancer genes regulate cell cycle checkpoints will be described in more detail in Chap. 6.

Some mitotic errors can alternatively lead to tetraploidy or aneuploidy. Recent studies have demonstrated that chromosome missegregation during mitosis, which is often observed in aneuploid cells, sometimes leads to mitotic failure resulting in tetraploidization (Fig. 4.6). Detailed studies of evolving breast tumors have suggested that aneuploidy is preceded by tetraploidy, and, furthermore, that tetraploidization is concurrent with the gradual loss and gain of individual chromosomes. These observations suggest that, in some cancers, CIN and tetraploidization together contribute to the development of aneuploidy.

Multiple Forms of Genetic Instability in Cancer

Does genetic instability cause cancer or is it a merely a consequence of dysregulated cell growth? This had been one of the oldest questions in cancer genetics. In the case of aneuploidy, a causal role was initially suggested by its sheer prevalence in cancer and by the potential for CIN to accelerate the process of LOH. The relationship between constitutional aneuploidy and cancer predisposition in the genetic disorder mosaic variegated aneuploidy provides another strong piece of evidence that aneuploidy directly promotes cancer development. Additional evidence that aneuploidy actively participates in the evolution of cancers is provided, perhaps counterintuitively, by cancers that are not aneuploid.

While most solid tumors are composed of aneuploid cancer cells, the smaller proportion of cancers that are not aneuploid often exhibit defects in DNA repair. Every cell contains the machinery to repair DNA sequence errors that arise as a

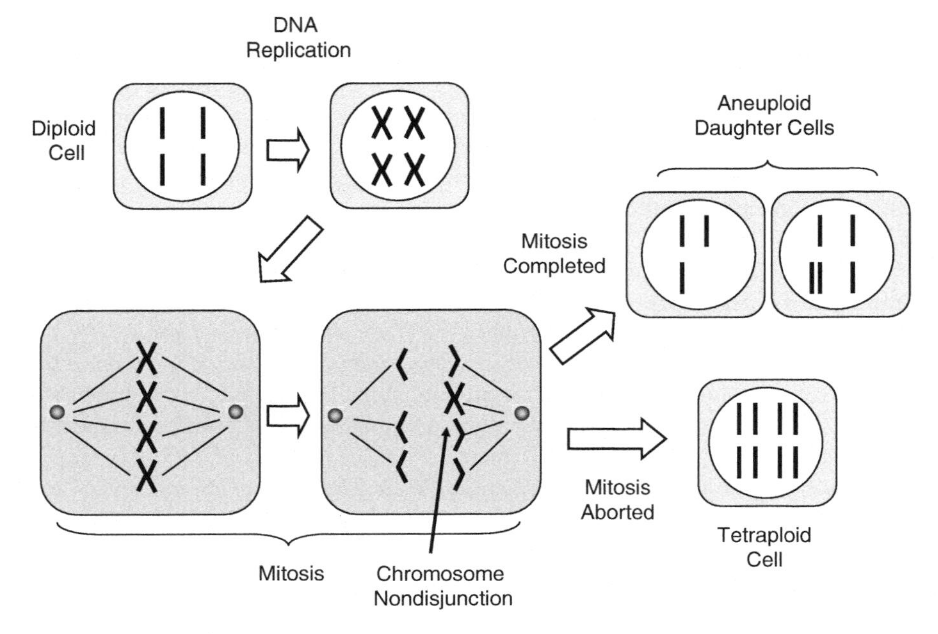

Fig. 4.6 Pathways to aneuploidy and tetraploidy. In this hypothetical model, chromosome nondisjunction can lead to aneuploidy or to tetraploidy. A diploid cell undergoes DNA replication prior to entering mitosis. (For illustrative purposes, only four chromosomes are shown.) Following the breakdown of the nuclear membrane, chromosomes align at the metaphase plate and attach to the mitotic spindle, which is organized by centrosomes. Sister chromatids separate during anaphase and migrate to opposite poles of the mitotic spindle; failure of this process results in chromosome nondisjunction. The activation of the mitotic spindle checkpoint by chromosome nondisjunction will cause mitosis to be delayed or aborted. In the latter case, premature exit from mitosis results in a tetraploid cell. Alternatively, failure of the mitotic spindle checkpoint allows mitosis to be completed in the presence of a lagging chromosome. In this case, chromosome nondisjunction results in aneuploid daughter cells

result of random replicative errors or mutagen exposure. Defects in distinct DNA repair processes have been conclusively shown to significantly accelerate the development of several types of cancer. Summarized here, these repair processes and their inactivation in cancers will be discussed in detail in the sections that follow.

During DNA replication, most misincorporated bases are immediately corrected by the replicative DNA polymerase complex, which has a substantial, intrinsic proofreading capacity. As a result, the error rate of the replicative DNA polymerase complex is estimated to be 1 in 10^8 bases. Repair enzymes revert most of these mutations to the original sequence, and thereby increase the fidelity of DNA replication to 10^{-10} per base pair. This remarkable degree of fidelity implies that, on average, less than one mutation introduced each time the diploid genome is replicated.

The rare misincorporated base that arises during DNA synthesis is processed by the mismatch repair (MMR) system. Approximately 15 % of all colorectal cancers are estimated to have defects in MMR. All DNA repair systems, including MMR, involve the concerted activity of multiple proteins. Germline inactivating mutations in one of several MMR genes are the cause of *hereditary nonpolyposis colorectal cancer* (HNPCC), also known as Lynch syndrome. HNPCC is an autosomal dominant disease that, in addition to a highly elevated risk of colorectal cancer, also predisposes affected individuals to several additional types of epithelial cancers.

Altered bases that result from exposure to many types of environmental mutagens are processed by the nucleotide-excision repair (NER) system. Total inactivation of one of several NER genes causes a disease known as *xeroderma pigmentosum* (XP). XP, an autosomal recessive disease, strongly predisposes affected individuals to skin tumors in areas exposed to sunlight.

Defects in DNA repair processes such as MMR and NER cause genetic instability. Cancer cells with defects in MMR, for example, have a mutation rate that is between two and four orders of magnitude greater than that observed in normal cells with proficient MMR. Cellular defects in NER accelerate the accumulation of UV signature mutations (see Chap. 1).

The changes to the genome that occur at high frequency in MMR- and NER-deficient cells are at the level of the DNA sequence. In contrast, the generation-to-generation changes in genome content associated with aneuploidy involve whole chromosomes or large chromosome segments that are visible upon cytogenetic analysis. Despite these dissimilarities, both aneuploidy and DNA repair defects accelerate the inactivation of tumor suppressor genes and the activation of oncogenes.

Analysis of familial cancers has provided critical insight into virtually every important aspect of cancer genetics. In the case of HNPCC and XP, these disorders once again demonstrate that genetic instability directly promotes tumorigenesis. The cancers that occur in HNPCC and XP patients are clearly the result of the genetic instability caused by the mutational inactivation of repair pathways. It appears that genetic instability in some form, whether aneuploidy or DNA repair deficiency, is a near-universal feature of virtually all cancers, both sporadic and inherited.

Notably, the cancers associated with HNPCC and XP are only rarely aneuploid. In general, aneuploidy and inactivated DNA repair pathways are mutually exclusive. As genetic instability clearly promotes tumorigenesis, it is logical to conclude that aneuploidy is a causal factor in the cancers in which it is observed.

Defects in Mismatch Repair Cause Hereditary Nonpolyposis Colorectal Cancer

The most common inherited form of colorectal cancer, and the most prevalent cancer predisposition syndrome known, is hereditary nonpolyposis colorectal cancer (HNPCC). HNPCC, also known as Lynch syndrome, is an autosomal dominant disorder that is caused by inactivating germline mutations in the genes involved in the mismatch repair (MMR) system. Patients with HNPCC develop cancer at a young age. In the general population, the average age at which colorectal cancer is diagnosed is 64. In contrast, individuals with HNPCC are diagnosed at an average age of 44, and cancers have been reported to arise as early as the teens. Tumors in HNPCC patents occur disproportionately in the proximal segment of the colon. Although larger and less differentiated than the majority of colorectal tumors on average, HNPCC-associated colorectal cancers have a better outcome than stage-matched sporadic tumors. Carriers of germline HNPCC mutations are also susceptible to cancers in epithelial tissues of the uterus, small intestine, ovary, stomach, urinary tract, pancreas, biliary tract and brain.

HNPCC is a relatively common genetic disorder that was recognized as a distinct entity relatively recently. The delayed recognition of this syndrome occurred because colorectal cancer is very common in the general population, and because individuals affected by HNPCC do not have distinguishing traits other than an increased incidence of cancer. These factors contributed to difficulties of ascertainment.

Several families with numerous affected members were originally identified by the University of Michigan pathologist Aldred Warthin in the late nineteenth century. This family came to the attention of Warthin by way of his seamstress, who lamented that many of her relatives had died of cancer and predicted that she would likely die of cancer of the stomach, colon or uterus. This fear was unfortunately realized when she died at a young age from endometrial carcinoma. Clusters of epithelial cancers in this family and others were documented and categorized in the 1960s and 1970s by Henry Lynch, for whom the syndrome was named. It was only in the 1980s that the concept of a familial cancer syndrome became widely accepted and studied.

The initial kindred identified by Warthin and subsequently analyzed by Lynch has exhibited an interesting shift in the types of cancers that develop in affected individuals. In the earlier generations of the family, gastric carcinomas were the predominant cancers that developed. Later generations increasingly developed colorectal carcinomas. This change in cancer incidence mirrors that which occurred in the general population over the same period. Presumably these changes are related to changes in diet.

The search for the molecular basis of HNPCC involved complementary approaches employed by competing teams of researchers. In 1993, the discovery of a new and unusual DNA repair defect in colorectal cancer cells provided the critical clue. A group led by Manuel Perucho, while searching for genomic amplifications and deletions that might point to new oncogenes and tumor suppressor genes, instead found somatic alterations in the lengths of highly repetitive elements known as *microsatellites*. An independent group led by Stephen Thibodeau also came upon these altered microsatellite sequences and found that they were correlated with tumors of the proximal colon. This observation provided a potential connection between microsatellite abnormalities and HNPCC. Concurrently, a collaborative group led by Albert de la Chapelle and Bert Vogelstein was attempting to map the location of a tumor suppressor locus in Lynch kindreds using positional cloning methods. While mapping regions of LOH, the de la Chapelle/Vogelstein group also detected mutations in microsatellite sequences.

Microsatellites are repetitive DNA sequences that are widely distributed throughout the genome. Repeats are typically composed of between 10 and 100 units that are between one and four bases in length. The highly repetitive nature of microsatellites makes them unusually susceptible to mutation by slipped DNA strand mispairing (see Chap. 1). Mononucleotide repeats such as A_n or G_n and dinucleotide repeats such as $(CA/GT)_n$ are the most commonly affected by slippage, which causes either the expansion or the contraction of the number of bases within the repeat. The majority of mispaired bases are repaired by the proofreading mechanisms inherent to the replicative DNA polymerase complex. In normal cells, most of the mispaired bases that escape the proofreading process are subsequently resolved by the MMR system. The relatively high mutability of microsatellites renders them highly *polymorphic* (meaning that they acquire the state of polymorphism). This attribute has made these repeat elements informative markers for a wide range of genetic analysis, including population studies and gene mapping.

Defects in MMR significantly impede the correction of mispaired bases and thereby increase the mutation rate. Microsatellite sequences in MMR-deficient cells are particularly susceptible to this effect and tend to expand and contract from generation to generation. This form of readily-detectable hypermutability is known as *microsatellite instability* (MSI). MSI is a reflection of an increased mutation rate that affects the entire genome (Fig. 4.7). The observation of MSI in colorectal cancer cells illuminated an entirely new mechanism of tumorigenesis. MSI is not restricted to colorectal tumors but can be detected in extracolonic tumors, such as gastic, endometrial, and other cancers that occur in HNPCC patients.

Interestingly, the pivotal insights into the genetic basis for MSI were provided not by studies of cancers, but by studies of model microorganisms. MSI was found

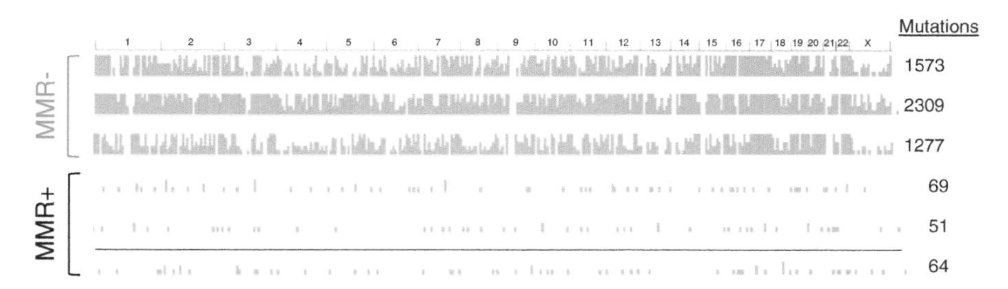

Fig. 4.7 Mismatch repair-deficient colorectal cancers exhibit large numbers of mutations. The mutational load of colorectal cancers is distributed in a bimodal fashion. The majority of these tumors harbor 40–100 mutations. However, colorectal tumors that are mismatch repair-defective (MMR-, *top rows*) accumulate mutations at a greatly accelerated rate, and can therefore harbor thousands of alterations to their genomic DNA. In this figure, mutation numbers are scored in *green* on the *vertical axis*. The *horizontal axis* is a linear representation of the haploid genome, with chromosomes in numerical order. The results shown here are based upon data generated by the TCGA Research Network: http://cancergenome.nih.gov/

Table 4.1 MMR genes involved in HNPCC

E. coli Gene	*H. sapiens* homolog	Chromosomal location	Mutated in HNPCC	Predisposition
MutS	*hMSH2*	2p21-22	40 %	Typical HNPCC
	hMSH6	2p16	10 %	Atypical HNPCC
MutL	*hMLH1*	3p21	50 %	Typical HNPCC
	hPMS1	2q31-33	Rare	Typical HNPCC
	hPMS2	7p22	<2 %	Turcot Syn

to strongly resemble mutation patterns previously found in bacteria and yeast that were defective for MMR. In the bacterium *E. coli*, the MMR system is known as the MutHLS pathway. This system functions to recognize mismatched bases that arise during DNA replication, to excise the mismatched and neighboring bases and to trigger the re-synthesis of a defined region, or "patch", of DNA. This pathway is dependent upon several genes, including *MutS* and *MutL*. Biochemical studies demonstrated that dimeric MutS protein detects the mismatch and recruits a MutL dimer to the repair site.

Eukaryotic homologs of bacterial *MutS*, designated *MutS homolog* or *MSH*, were found in yeast (*yMSH*) and in human cells (*MSH*). In yeast, mutation of *MSH* genes was found to lead to 100- to 700-fold increases in the mutation rate of dinucleotide repeats. The revelation that MSI was related to MMR defects provided a critical clue as to the identities of the HNPCC genes. Shortly following the discovery of MSI in colorectal cancers, groups led by Richard Kolodner and Bert Vogelstein identified a human *MutS* homolog, *MSH2*, on chromosome 2. Germline mutations of *MSH2* were found in a substantial proportion of Lynch kindreds. Additional MMR genes were similarly identified by positional cloning and by virtue of known interspecies protein and DNA sequence homologies.

MMR is a basic biological process that is evolutionarily conserved. Human cells contain at least five *MutS* and four *MutL* homologs. Five of these genes have been shown to play a role in MMR and to cause HNPCC when mutated (Table 4.1). While the first steps of MMR in bacteria involve the activity of MutS and MutL homodimers, the human proteins form heterodimers in various combinations. The different specificities of these complexes allow the recognition of different substrates (Fig. 4.8). MSH2 plays a fundamental role in the recognition and binding of mispaired bases, while MSH3 and MSH6 appear to modify the specificity of this recognition. The MutL homolog MLH1, which is recruited to the repair site by the MutS homologs, functions as molecular matchmaker. As a hetrodimeric complex with PMS2, MLH1 couples mismatch recognition with downstream steps of MMR, which include 'long patch' regional DNA excision, repair synthesis and re-ligation. The role of PMS1 in this process remains to be determined.

Genetic analysis of the human MMR genes revealed that mutations in *MSH2* and the *MutL* homolog *MLH1* account for the majority of documented Lynch syndrome mutations. As has been shown to be the case with other familial cancer syndromes such as familial breast cancer, HNPCC kindreds with different mutations exhibit

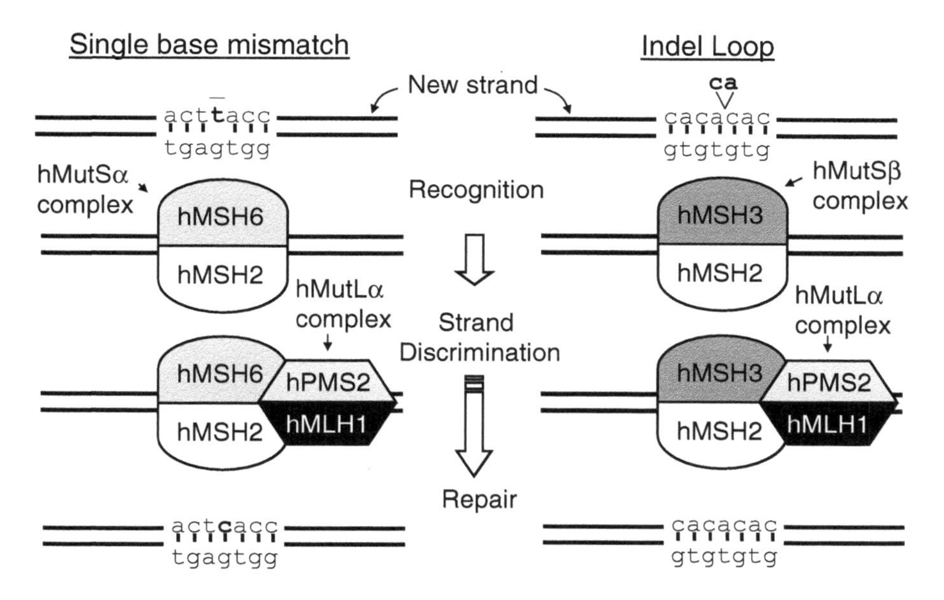

Fig. 4.8 Human DNA mismatch repair. Mispaired bases (shown in *bold*) create a physical deformity in the DNA double helix that is recognized by the MutS homologs. Single base mismatches are recognized by MSH2-MSH6 heterodimers known as the hMutSα complex (*left*). Looped-out bases caused by short insertions and deletions (indels) cause a distinct structure primarily recognized by MSH2-MSH3 dimers, known as the hMutSβ complex (*right*). Note that there is some overlap in the recognition affinities of hMutSα and hMutSβ. The MutLα complex composed of MLH1 and PMS2 is recruited to the repair site and functions to determine which DNA strand contains the error. The MutLα complex communicates this information to downstream repair proteins that excise a region of DNA known as a long patch, resynthesize the damaged strand and ligate the repaired strands

distinct patterns of disease. *MSH2* mutations are more strongly associated with extra-colonic cancers than are mutations in *MLH1*. Mutations in the *MutS* homolog *MSH6* are found in only a small number of kindreds. Germline mutation of *MSH6* is associated with an atypical form of HNPCC, characterized by a somewhat older mean age of cancer diagnosis and a risk of endometrial cancer that is higher than that conferred by mutations in *MSH2* or *MLH1*. A small number of germline mutations have been found in the *MutL* homolog *PMS2*. These mutations are associated with Turcot syndrome, an HNPCC syndrome-related disorder characterized by an increased risk of brain and early-onset colorectal cancers.

While HNPCC was recognized as a disease entity by the identification of large kindreds with multiple affected individuals, many additional carriers of HNPCC gene mutations have been identified by population based genetic screening. Genetic testing has revealed that MMR gene mutations are highly prevalent among individuals with inherited colorectal or endometrial cancers, most of whom are not known members of HNPCC kindreds. Among cancer patients age 50 and younger that have

Table 4.2 Prevalence of MLH1 and MSH2 mutations among cancer patients. Data from Myriad Genetic Laboratories, October 2005

	Family history	
Personal history	No affected relatives (%)	≥1 Relative affected (%)
Colorectal cancer (age < 50)	9.1	22
Colorectal cancer (age ≥ 50)	<5	15
Endometrial cancer (age < 50)	11	23
Other HNPCC-associated cancer	6.5	16

at least one relative with cancer, nearly one quarter have germline mutations in one of the two highly mutated HNPCC genes, *MSH2* or *MLH1* (Table 4.2).

The HNPCC genes are tumor suppressor genes. In terms of their stepwise inactivation, they share the general characteristics of the tumor suppressor genes discussed in Chap. 3. HNPCC genes are present in the germline of cancer-prone families as a single mutated allele. The wild type allele is lost somatically, giving rise to the cellular MMR defect.

Unlike the gatekeeper defects caused by biallelic inactivation of *APC* or *RB1*, the inactivation of HNPCC genes does not directly affect cell proliferation. Rather, HNPCC gene inactivation causes defective DNA repair, a form of genetic instability. Cells with MMR defects have a higher mutation rate than normal cells and thus have an increased probability of acquiring tumor suppressor gene and proto-oncogene mutations. Mutations in HNPCC genes, like those in other tumor suppressor genes that are involved in DNA repair, cause caretaker defects.

The nature of the cellular defect in HNPCC is clearly reflected in the pathogenesis of the disease. HNPCC is readily distinguished from the less common familial adenomatous polyposis (FAP) by tumor number. FAP patients develop an extraordinarily large number of polyps. Although each polyp has only a small chance of developing into an invasive cancer, the cumulative risk caused by the large number of polyps in FAP-affected individuals makes the development of cancer all but inevitable. In contrast, individuals affected by HNPCC do not exhibit polyposis; patients with HNPCC develop polyps at approximately the same rate as the general population. However, the underlying genetic instability greatly increases the chance that a given polyp will progress to a cancer.

The classical tumor suppressor genes, exemplified by *APC*, *RB1* and *TP53*, are mutated in the germline of cancer-prone kindreds, but are also mutated somatically in sporadic cancers. The MMR genes are similarly involved in both inherited and sporadic cancers. In unselected samples, MSI occurs in colorectal cancer at a rate of approximately 13 %. In the majority of MSI-positive cases, germline mutations in MMR genes are not detected in normal tissues from the same patient. Two important conclusions can be drawn from these observations. First, the majority of MSI-positive cancers are not associated with HNPCC, a heritable disorder. Second, a sizable proportion of all sporadic cancers acquire mutations in MMR genes.

Approximately 2–7 % of the 160,000 colorectal cancers diagnosed in the United States each year are attributable to hereditary defects in MMR, which cause

HNPCC. The remaining 10 % of MSI-defective colorectal cancers are caused by somatically-acquired MMR defects.

An understanding of the mutational mechanisms of MMR and the genetic basis of HNPCC are likely to provide direct benefits for cancer-prone individuals. HNPCC is a common genetic disorder that causes a significant number of cancers. Analyzing tumor samples for the presence of MSI can aid the discovery of potential HNPCC kindreds, while searching for germline HNPCC mutations is a strategy for identifying HNPCC-affected individuals before they develop invasive cancers. Given the high incidence of colorectal cancer, the use of genetic analysis to uncover HNPCC promises to have a significant impact on public health. Additionally, recent evidence suggests that MMR-deficient colorectal cancers with high numbers of somatic mutations are more robustly recognized the immune system, and are therefore more responsive to new cancer therapies designed to unleash the immune response against tumors (see Chap. 8).

Mismatch Repair-Deficient Cancers Have a Distinct Spectrum of Mutations

MMR defects cause an increased mutation rate. It can be inferred that mutation of MMR genes leads to increases in the rates at which tumor suppressor genes are inactivated and proto-oncogene are activated. Indeed, the specific mutations found in MSI-positive/MMR-deficient cancers reflect a unique mechanism of mutagenesis.

It appears that the same molecular pathways are disrupted by mutation in MSI-positive/MMR-deficient and MMR-proficient tumors alike. For example, mutations in *APC* initiate the process of colorectal tumorigenesis in both tumor types. However, MSI-positive/MMR-deficient cancers have a higher rate of frameshift mutations at intragenic mononucleotide tracts, most strikingly at A_n (Table 4.3).

The overall prevalence of detectable *APC* mutations is also somewhat lower in MSI-positive/MMR-deficient tumors. In MSI-positive/MMR-deficient colorectal cancers with wild type *APC*, a mutation in the *CTNNB1* gene, which encodes

Table 4.3 Representative inactivating *APC* mutations found in MSI-positive/MMR-deficient colorectal tumors. Insertions and deletions are indicated in bold type. Mutations frequently occur in sequences that contain mononucleotide tracts. Data from Huang et al. *PNAS* 93:9049–9054

Family history	*APC* codon	Nucleotide change	Target sequence
Sporadic	758	1 bp deletion	AAC**a**AAAAGCC
Sporadic	773	2 bp deletion	GAAAC**tt**TTGAC
Sporadic	801	1 bp deletion	TATG**t**TTTTGAC
HNPCC	847	1 bp insertion	TCTG(**A**)AAAAAGAT
HNPCC	907	1 bp deletion	TCT**g**GGTCT
HNPCC	941	1 bp insertion	TCGG(**A**)AAAATTCA
Unknown	975	1 bp deletion	GGT**a**AAAGAGGT

β-catenin, has been found to phenocopy the loss of *APC*. This observation provides one explanation for the lower *APC* mutation rate in MSI-positive/MMR-deficient tumors. A similar situation has been found to affect the pathway mediated by the proto-oncogene *KRAS*. *KRAS* is commonly mutated in MMR-proficient colorectal cancers, but is mutated less often in MSI-positive/MMR-deficient cancers. Such cancers often contain mutations of a gene known as *BRAF*, which encodes a protein that functions downstream of KRAS.

The genetic alteration most frequently associated with MMR-deficiency is mutation of the gene *TGFBR2*, which encodes the transforming growth factor β type II receptor (TGFβ-RII). The coding region of *TGFBR2* contains an A_8 tract that is mutated in 85–90 % of MSI-positive tumors. The TGFβ-RII protein is a cell surface receptor that functions upstream of the tumor suppressor gene *SMAD4*. These two proteins are critical components of a molecular pathway that communicates growth-inhibitory signals from the cell surface to the nucleus, where gene expression is regulated. The *TGFBR2* mutations in MSI-positive cancers have a similar functional result as the *SMAD4* and *SMAD2* mutations that occur in MMR-proficient cancers.

TP53 is mutated at a lower frequency in MSI-positive/MMR-deficient cancers. One possible explanation for this observation is that an alternate gene in the p53 pathway may be preferentially mutated in cells with MMR defects. One candidate is *BAX*, a gene involved in the process of programmed cell death, or apoptosis. The coding region of *BAX* contains a G_8 tract that is mutated in approximately 50 % of MSI-positive/MMR-deficient cancers. *BAX* has been found to be transcriptionally transactivated by p53 in some cell types. It may be possible that mutation of *BAX* in some tissues eliminates the selective advantage of *TP53* mutation. However, it should be noted that experimental *BAX* mutations appear to cause only a small subset of the cellular phenotypes that are associated with *TP53* inactivation.

That a genetically defined pathway can be alternately inactivated by different gene mutations is a central principle of cancer genetics. The basic principles of signal transduction and the roles of proto-oncogenes and tumor suppressor genes in signaling pathways will be discussed in detail in Chap. 6.

Defects in Nucleotide Excision Repair Cause Xeroderma Pigmentosum

Nucleotide-excision repair (NER) is a versatile type of DNA repair required for the processing of a variety of base lesions, many of which are caused by environmental mutagens. The most important mutagen that affects individuals with defects in the NER system is the ultraviolet (UV) component of sunlight. As described in Chap. 1, UV light causes a number of distinctive DNA lesions, including cyclobutane pyrimidine dimers and (6–4) photoproducts. These damaged bases are normally removed from the genome by the process of NER. Bulky pyrimidine and purine adducts formed by psoralen derivatives, the chemotherapeutic drug cisplatin, and the polycyclic carcinogens such as acetylaminofluorene are also processed by the NER system.

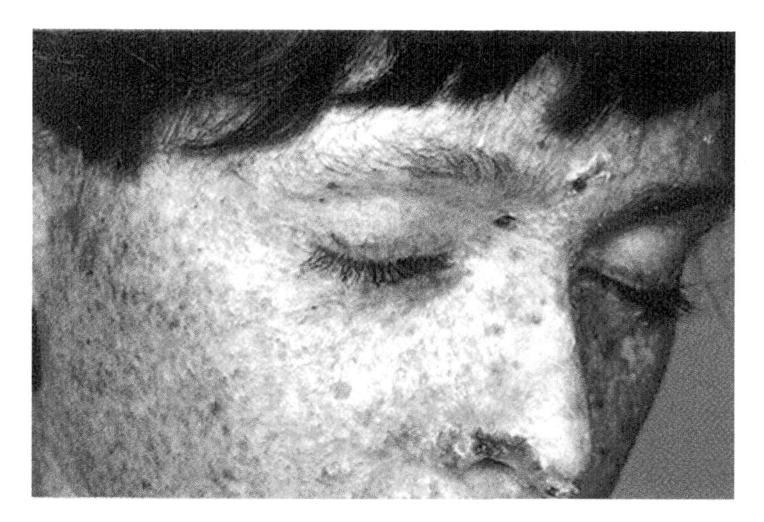

Fig. 4.9 Xeroderma pigmentosum. Individuals affected by this disorder typically have a prematurely aged appearance in sun-exposed areas. Multiple scars and lesions mark sites of treated and developing carcinomas (Reprinted from the Atlas Genet Cytogenet Oncol Haematol, October 2000, Viguie, C. Xeroderma pigmentosum. Courtesy of Daniel Wallach, by permission of the Atlas)

Xeroderma pigmentosum (XP) is a rare disease caused by defective NER. First described by Moriz Kaposi as a skin disorder in 1870, XP was recognized to be often associated with neurological abnormalities by Albert Neisser in 1883. Interestingly, Neisser was also the discoverer of the etiological agent of gonorrhea, the bacterium *Neisseria*.

XP is characterized by an adverse reaction of skin to sunlight, a symptom known as *poikiloderma*, and the development of skin neoplasia. Symptoms most commonly present at the age of 1–2 years, concomitant with the first exposures to sunlight, and include severe sunburns and subsequent freckling. The accumulation of unrepaired DNA lesions results in the progressive degeneration and atrophy of sun-exposed skin and eyes. *Xeroderma* literally refers to the typical parchment-like appearance of exposed skin in affected individuals, while *pigmentosum* describes the pigmentary abnormalities commonly found in these patients (Fig. 4.9). XP patients are prone to cataracts and both benign and malignant ocular tumors. Approximately 20–30 % of XP patients develop a variety of neurologic abnormalities that are often progressive.

XP patients develop an array of benign lesions that arise from various cell types present in the skin. These include the keratinocytes and fibroblasts that are the main structural components of the skin, but also cells of the cutaneous vasculature and adipose tissue. Some, but not all, of these lesions are premalignant and thus have the potential to develop into cancers. XP patients most commonly develop basal and squamous cell carcinomas, but also have a significantly increased risk of developing melanoma, a deadly form of skin cancer that develops from the pigmented melanocytes (see Chap. 7). The onset of cancer in XP patients is strikingly accelerated. Skin cancers occur at a median age of 8 years, which is 50 years earlier than in the general population. The overall risk of skin cancer before the age of 20 is increased more than 1000-fold in XP patients. Many XP patients succumb to cancer before they reach the age of 20.

XP patients also have a moderately increased propensity to develop various solid tumors, most commonly brain cancers. The development of these internal tumors, as well as the neurologic abnormalities that are often detected in XP patients, indicate the complex involvement of NER genes in processes unrelated to the resolution of UV lesions.

XP occurs at a frequency of approximately 1 in 1,000,000 in the US and Europe, 10 to100-fold higher frequencies occur in Japan and North Africa. Unlike the other cancer predisposition syndromes discussed in preceding sections, XP exhibits an autosomal recessive mode of inheritance. Patients are thus homozygous for the primary genetic mutations that underlie the disease. *Consanguinity*, literally blood relation, between patients' parents has been reported in a significant proportion of cases.

Every cell in an XP patient has defective NER. Cellular defects in NER are readily detectable in the laboratory. These two features greatly aided the discovery of the genetic defects that underlie XP. When cultured fibroblasts from normal individuals are exposed to UV light, the damaged DNA triggers DNA synthesis associated with lesion repair, also known as *unscheduled DNA synthesis* (UDS), a term meant to contrast this reparative synthesis with the scheduled type of DNA synthesis that occurs during chromosomal DNA replication. The activation of NER can therefore be directly detected by measuring the uptake of the DNA precursor [^{3}H]-thymidine (Fig. 4.10). Fibroblasts from most XP individuals are defective for NER and therefore usually do not exhibit UDS.

A significant subset of XP patients exhibit normal levels of UDS and thus have no obvious defects in NER. This variant form of XP is nonetheless characterized by an increased rate of mutagenesis upon UV exposure. Designated XP-V, this group is clinically indistinguishable from other XP patients. Further analysis of XP-V cells has suggested that at least some patients in this category have a repair defect that is manifest only during DNA replication. The XP-V patient group exhibits a range of disease severity, with a general lack of neurological abnormalities. The substantial clinical heterogeneity of XP-V suggests that this group might be similarly heterogeneous from a genetic perspective.

Employed in seminal experiments throughout the history of cancer genetics, the technique of cell fusion has been a powerful tool for understanding the nature of cancer cell defects. This strategy proved enormously successful in categorizing the gene mutations that cause XP (Fig. 4.11). Among unrelated XP patients, cells from one patient will functionally complement cells from another patient upon fusion only if the mutated genes in each patient are different. By this technique, XP patients could be categorized into a total of seven distinct complementation groups, designated XP-A through XP-G. (The XP-V group has no UDS defect and cannot, by definition, be complemented.) Each complementation group is defined by a single, distinct mutated gene.

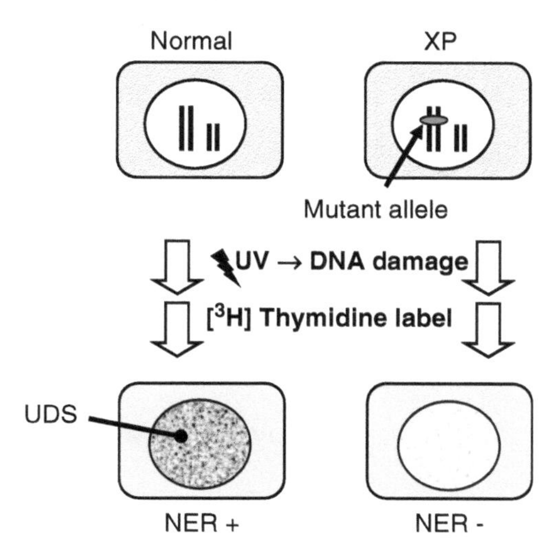

Fig. 4.10 DNA damage triggers unscheduled DNA synthesis. When challenged with UV light, cells harboring normal XP alleles initiate NER processes, which involve the synthesis of new DNA. This phenomenon is known as unscheduled DNA synthesis (UDS). Normal cells will incorporate radio-labeled thymidine at sites of repair, which can then be visualized by autoradiography. Cells from xeroderma pigmentosum patients contain biallelic mutations (shown in *red*) in one of the genes involved in the NER process. XP cells do not exhibit UDS because they are NER negative (NER-). For simplicity, only two homologous pairs of chromosomes are shown

The finding that defective NER can be restored by complementation facilitated the cloning of genes that underlie XP. New reagents were developed for this effort, including mutant rodent cell lines that had defects in DNA repair and were UV-sensitive. Rodent cells could be transformed with either human genomic DNA or with human DNA libraries, allowing the recovery of UV-resistant clones. In a period spanning the mid-1980s and the mid-1990s, groups led by Larry Thompson, Dirk Bootsma and Jan Hoeijmakers cloned human genes that would complement the NER defects of the different rodent cell lines. These genes were designated human *excision repair cross-complementing*, or *ERCC* genes. Several of these were demonstrated to be mutated in XP complementation groups. Randy Legerski and colleagues were able to directly complement a human cell line from an XP-C patient with a gene that was initially designated *XP-C complementing clone*, or *XPCC*. The gene that complements the XP-A group was isolated by a group led by Yoshio Okada. The last complementation group to be genetically characterized, largely by the efforts Stuart Linn and his coworkers, was XP-E. Though there had been some heterogeneity within this group, it appears that the majority of XP-E patients have mutations in *DDB2*, which encodes a DNA damage-specific DNA binding protein. Each gene conclusively demonstrated to be mutated in a specific complementation group has been subsequently so designated (Table 4.4). For example, the gene *ERCC3* has been found to functionally complement the patient group XP-B, and is therefore usually referred to as *XPB*.

The extensive biochemical characterization of XP-V cells conducted independently by the laboratories of Fumio Hanaoka and Louise Prakash revealed a

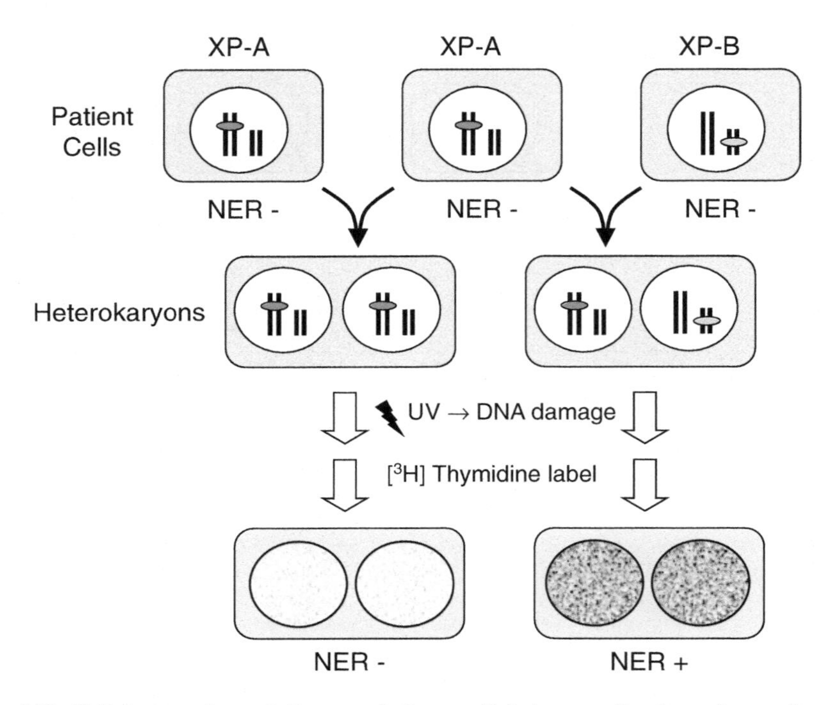

Fig. 4.11 Cellular complementation reveals the genetic heterogeneity of xeroderma pigmentosum. Cells from three individual XP patients are shown (*top*). Pairs of cells are fused to create hybrid cells, known as heterokaryons, that contain nuclei from both patients. The fusion of cells that contain the same mutated gene (shown in *red*) results in heterokaryons that remain NER-negative (NER-), as indicated by the absence of UDS. When cells that contain two different mutations (*red* and *yellow*) fuse, each nucleus contributes complementary wild type genes to the heterokaryon. NER is thus restored in these hybrids (NER+). Such experiments allow the categorization of XP patients into distinct complementation groups, which in this example are denoted XP-A and XP-B. For simplicity, only two homologous pairs of chromosomes are shown

Table 4.4 The XP complementation groups and genes

Comp. group	Relative UDS (%)	Gene	Location	Mutated in XP	Function of encoded protein
XP-A	<2	*XPA*	9q22	25 %	Binds UV-damaged DNA, forms demarcation complex
XP-B	3–7	*XPB*	2q21	Rare	3′ → 5′ DNA helicase, TFIIH subunit
XP-C	10–25	*XPC*	3p25	25 %	Binds UV-damaged DNA, initates GGR
XP-D	25–55	*XPD* *ERCC6*	19q13 10q11	15 %	5′ → 3′ DNA helicase, TFIIH subunit
XP-E	50	*DDB2*	11p12	Rare	Binds UV-damaged DNA during recognition step
XP-F	15–30	*ERCC4*	16p13	6 %	Endonuclease, makes 5′ incision
XP-G	10	*ERCC5*	13q33	6 %	Endonuclease, makes 3′ incision
XP-V	100	*POLH*	6p21	21 %	Translesion DNA synthesis during subsequent S-phase

functional defect in DNA polymerase η. This specialized replicative DNA polymerase, encoded by *POLH*, is involved in translesion DNA synthesis during S-phase. The role of DNA polymerase η in UDS-proficient XP was confirmed by the finding of *POLH* mutations in XP-V patients.

NER is a multistep process that involves the concerted function of numerous protein complexes. There are two distinct modes of NER depending on the whether a lesion is located within an expressed gene. DNA lesions occurring within actively transcribed regions of the genome, which are presumably more detrimental to cellular viability, are repaired by a process known as *transcription-coupled repair* (TCR). In the remainder of the genome, lesions are removed by an NER sub-process known as *global genome repair* (GGR). Some specific types of lesions are more efficiently removed from transcribed regions, via TCR, than they are from the rest of the genome via GGR. In the majority of XP cases, the genetic defect affects both TCR and GGR. The exception is the XP-C group, in which only GGR appears to be affected. That *XPC*-mutant individuals are highly prone to cancer reveals the importance of GGR in tumor suppression.

The first step in NER is the recognition of damaged bases (Fig. 4.12). In TCR, the initial detection of a lesion occurs when the RNA polymerase II holoenzyme complex stalls while transcribing the affected DNA strand. This transcription complex is then rapidly displaced in favor of repair proteins. In GGR, DNA damage recognition is accomplished by a distinct NER protein complex containing the XPC protein. The protein encoded by *XPE* plays a role in DNA damage recognition by both pathways.

Although the mechanism of recognition of damaged bases differs in transcribed genes and untranscribed regions of the genome, the subsequent steps of NER are common to both pathways. Once a site of DNA damage is recognized, the adjoining paired bases are separated by the helicase activities of XPB and XPD, and the site is demarcated by the binding of the XPA protein. Both XPB and XPD are known components of an evolutionarily conserved transcription factor complex known as Transcription Factor II H (TFIIH). TFIIH is a protein complex that controls the initiation of basal gene transcription. The shared requirement of XPB and XPD for these processes reveals the close relationship between NER and the basic mechanisms of gene expression.

The region opened by the TFIIH helicases, spanning about 25 bases, is accessible to the endonucleases XPF and XPG. These enzymes cut the DNA backbone at the junction created by the helicases and thereby excise the bases on the damaged strand. The gap left by the incision process is then filled in by DNA polymerases that specifically function in DNA repair. The newly synthesized DNA strand is covalently joined to the double helix by a DNA ligase.

NER Syndromes: Clinical Heterogeneity and Pleiotropy

XP is a heterogeneous disorder, from both a clinical and a genetic standpoint. Much of this overall heterogeneity is due to the phenotypic differences between the complementation groups. Patients in the XP-C group are affected with what is often

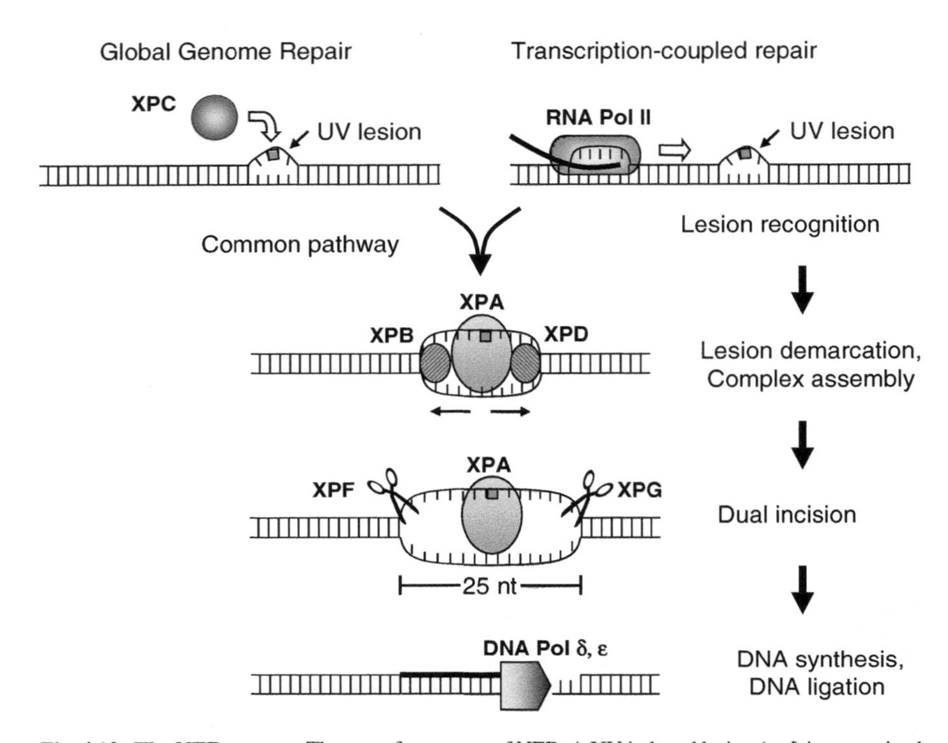

Fig. 4.12 The NER process. There are four stages of NER. A UV-induced lesion (*red*) is recognized either by XPC in global genome repair pathway or by the RNA Pol II complex in the transcription-coupled repair pathway. XPE (not shown) plays a role at the initiation stage of both pathways. The DNA around the damaged region is opened by the TFIIH helicases XPB and XPD, and demarcated by XPA. The damaged strand is then incised by the endonucleases XPF and XPG, allowing the release of the damage-containing oligonucleotide. Finally, the double helix is restored by the sequential activity of DNA polymerases δ and ε, and a DNA ligase. Many additional repair and replication proteins, which are not known to be defective in XP patients, are also involved in NER

termed the 'classic' form of XP. Disease caused by *XPC* mutation is restricted to the skin and eyes, and is dependent on sun exposure. Mutations in *XPA* cause a more severe form of the disease, which is manifest from birth and features progressive neurologic degeneration. A small number of individuals exhibit severe neurological disease along with dwarfism and immature sexual development. This form of XP, generally found within the XP-and D groups, has been termed the *DeSanctis-Cacchione syndrome*.

While there are significant differences between XP-A and XP-C, the presentation of disease *within* each group is fairly uniform. In contrast, several of the XP complementation groups exhibit a significant degree of heterogeneity associated with a single gene. For example, patients in the XP-D group show a widely diverse spectrum of disease severity. Some patients with *XPD* mutations are clinically indistinguishable from those in the XP-A group, while others have a more mild form of the disease resembling classic XP, as seen in the XP-C group. These findings demonstrate that different mutations in the same gene can cause distinct phenotypes. Similarly complex genotype/phenotype relationships are seen in the cancers caused by mutations in other tumor suppressor genes, such as *APC* (see Chap. 3).

Mutations in NER genes can also cause two related syndromes that clinically overlap with XP. Unlike XP, these rare disorders are not typically associated with an increased risk of cancer:

Cockayne Syndrome (CS) Patients with CS typically exhibit sun sensitivity, short stature, severe neurological abnormalities, dental caries, cataracts and a wizened appearance. The average life span of CS patients is 12 years. Cells from CS patients exhibit normal UDS. CS is caused by mutations in either *CSA* or *CSB*, which are involved in TCR. Accordingly, CS cells exhibit defects in TCR, but have normal GGR. A small number of patients with the characteristics of CS have an associated cancer predisposition; this syndrome has been referred to as XP-CS complex and is caused by mutations in *XPB* and *XPD*.

Trichothiodystrophy (TTD) The clinical features of TTD include most of those that define CS. In addition, TTD patients have brittle hair and dystrophic nails that are caused by a reduced content of cysteine-rich, sulfur-containing matrix proteins. TTD is a heterogeneous disorder and at least seven previously described disorders resemble or are identical to TTD. TTD cells exhibit impaired UDS, and are defective in both TCR and GGR. TTD can be caused by some mutations in *XPB* or *XPD*, or by mutations in *TBF5*, which encodes another subunit of the TFIIH transcription complex.

XP, CS and TTD reveal the diverse phenotypic manifestations of NER gene mutation. Mutations in some NER genes are clearly pleiotropic. Distinct mutations in *XPB* and *XPD* have been shown alternatively cause XP or XP-CS or TTD, which collectively encompass a broad range of disease phenotypes. Many of these phenotypes are unrelated to cancer.

The basis of NER gene pleiotropy is thought to be the overlapping activities of the TFIIH complex, which functions in both NER and basal transcription. All of the genes that encode TFIIH are essential for viability, and are therefore never found to be completely inactivated by mutation. The mutations that are found in *XPB* and *XPD* are not inactivating mutations, but rather have subtle effects on TFIIH function. Different mutations in *XPB* and *XPD* can separately affect the two TFIIH-related activities and thus cause distinct diseases. The mutations that underlie CS and TTD are thought to predominantly cause the defective function of the TFIIH complex in basal transcription. The mutations that cause XP, in contrast, affect the role of TFIIH in NER. The mutations that underlie XP-CS appear to affect *both* basal transcription and NER, demonstrating that all of these diverse phenotypes are expressed as part of a continuum.

DNA Repair Defects and Mutagens Define Two Steps Towards Genetic Instability

Although rare, XP and the related NER-associated syndromes illuminate several central principles of cancer genetics. XP-associated cancers, like many types of cancer, can be caused by distinct mutations in different genes that function in a common biochemical pathway. XP gene mutations exhibit pleiotropy. Some germline cancer gene mutations can cause phenotypes entirely unrelated to cancer.

It is revealing that XP carriers, individuals heterozygous for XP gene mutations, are asymptomatic and do not have a measurably increased risk of cancer. By definition, XP genes are tumor suppressor genes because they lose function as a result of mutation. But the tumor suppressor genes that underlie XP are clearly dissimilar from the classical tumor suppressor genes.

The cancer syndromes presented in chapter three are all autosomal dominant. In the more prevalent of these, the inheritance of a single mutated tumor suppressor gene allele confers a significant risk of cancer. In the case of germline *RB1* and *APC* mutations, this risk is close to 100 %. Other tumor suppressor genes, such as the HNPCC genes, are incompletely penetrant, yet still confer cancer susceptibility. In contrast, the penetrance of a single mutated XP allele in the germline is very low.

Classical tumor suppressor alleles become unmasked and exert their phenotypic affects when expanding cell clones lose the remaining wild type allele, a process known as LOH (see Chap. 3). Apparently, LOH at the XP loci is alone insufficient to generate a level of genetic instability that would significantly elevate the overall risk of cancer (Fig. 4.13). Genetic instability in an XP gene-heterozygous cell would be dependent not only on LOH at an XP locus, but also on the mutational effects of UV light.

To understand the rate-limiting role of the environment in XP, it is perhaps useful to compare XP and HNPCC. Although cancers in both diseases arise as a result of defective DNA repair, XP contrasts starkly with HNPCC, an autosomal dominant disorder that causes high rates of cancer in heterozygotes. What is the basis for this difference? NER processes DNA lesions that are largely caused by an interaction with an exogenous environmental mutagen, while MMR processes misincorporated bases that arise endogenously, during normal DNA replication.

In the case of HNPCC, genetic instability occurs immediately and in every proliferating cell that sustains LOH at the affected locus. In XP heterozygotes, loss of the wild type allele would not invariably lead to a higher mutation rate. Rather, genetic instability is manifest in the presence of an environmental mutagen. That the increased occurrence of mutations in NER-deficient cells requires an exogenous component constitutes an extra step towards the acquisition of genetic instability. It appears that this extra step is rate-limiting in XP heterozygotes, which is likely to be the reason that the incidence of cancer in this population is close to normal.

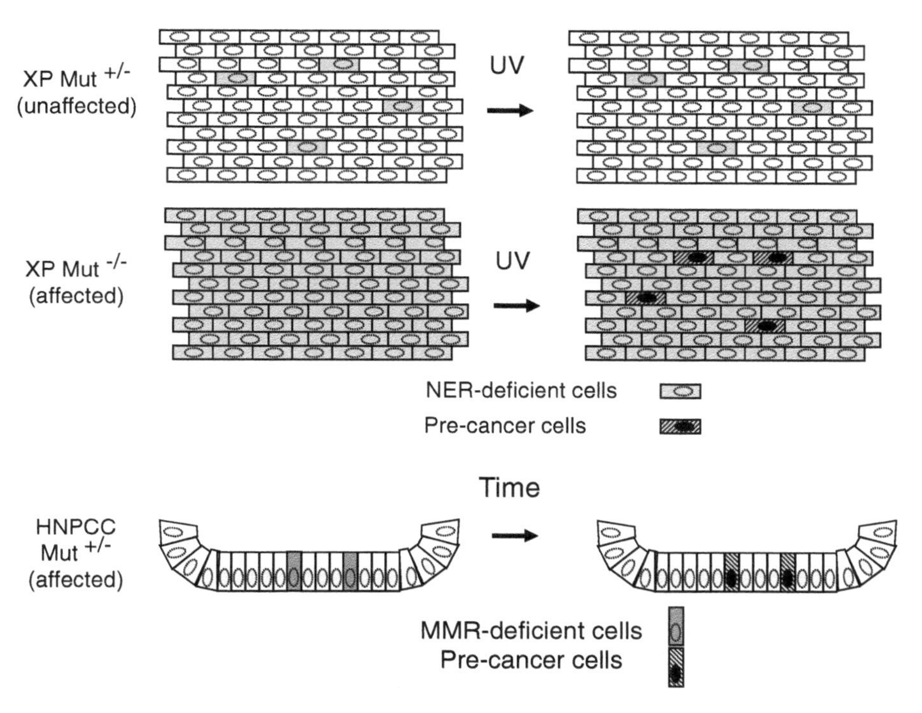

Fig. 4.13 DNA repair defects and environmental mutagens. Patients affected with XP are homozygous for NER gene mutations. Every cell in these patients is therefore NER-deficient (shown in *gray*). Following UV exposure, mutations cause a small but significant minority of proliferating cells in the skin to become cancer precursors (hatched cells). In heterozygous XP carriers, wild type NER genes are presumably lost, via LOH, at a low rate. The total number of NER-deficient cells is therefore very small, and only a small proportion of NER-deficient cells become cancer precursors after UV exposure. Therefore, heterozygous XP carriers do not have a significantly elevated risk of cancer. The situation differs in HNPCC, a disorder with an autosomal dominant mode of inheritance. In individuals heterozygous for HNPCC mutations, LOH in the cells of the colon crypt causes MMR-deficiency (*gray cells*). MMR-defective cells acquire mutations as a byproduct of normal cell proliferation and have significant potential to develop into cancers in later generations

Defects in DNA Crosslink Repair Cause Fanconi Anemia

Fanconi anemia (FA) is a recessive syndrome that features a marked predisposition to bone marrow failure and cancer. Hematological disease appears at a median age of 7 years. FA patients develop both liquid and solid tumors at greatly elevated rates. By age 40, the risk of developing a neoplasm is approximately 30 %. The most prevalent type of cancer associated with FA is acute myelogenous leukemia (AML), which develops at a median age of 14 years. FA patients are also prone to solid tumors, including head and neck and gastrointestinal carcinomas. Solid tumors occur in FA patients at a median age of 26 years. The predisposition of FA patients to solid tumors is particularly striking because of the young age at which they occur, as compared to the general population. FA patients have a markedly reduced life expectancy, with a median survival of 23 years.

Cultured cells from FA patients exhibit elevated levels of spontaneous chromosome breaks and deletions. FA cells are also highly sensitive to agents that cause DNA crosslinks, such as the carcinogen diepoxybutane (DEB) and the chemotherapeutic drug mitomycin C (MMC). It is believed that the failure to normally repair and resolve DNA crosslinks directly leads to double strand DNA breaks. Agents that cause chromosome breaks are known as *clastogens*. The spontaneous chromosome breakage and sensitivity of FA cells to clastogens represents a unique form of genetic instability. It is believed that this form of genetic instability is a direct cause of the cancer seen in these patients, but the specific mechanism of mutagenesis remains incompletely understood.

FA is a highly heterogeneous disorder. FA patients present with diverse clinical features that include congenital abnormalities that can affect any major organ system. First recognized and described by the pediatrician Guido Fanconi in 1927, FA is most commonly characterized by an abnormal reduction in the number of red blood cells, white blood cells and platelets in the blood, a condition known as *pancytopenia*. Other common features include short stature, hyperpigmentation, skeletal malformations, and urogenital abnormalities. Vertebral anomalies, the absence or closure of the anus, fistulae in the esophagus or trachea, limb and skeletal malformations, renal, gastrointestinal and cardiac abnormalities have all been associated with FA. Some patients do not exhibit any congenital abnormalities, or exhibit minor malformations that can be easily overlooked by pediatricians. In such patients, the diagnosis of FA is made after the appearance of hematologic disease. Because the presentation of FA is highly variable, a correct diagnosis may be difficult to make on the basis of clinical manifestations alone. In many cases, FA patients have been identified by virtue of their relatedness to previously diagnosed FA patients. The genetic analysis of FA has been significantly hampered by these inherent difficulties in ascertainment. The assessment of chromosome breakage after treatment with DEB or MMC can serve as a unique and highly useful laboratory test to definitively diagnose FA.

The clinical heterogeneity of FA is partly the result of underlying genetic heterogeneity. Like XP, FA can be subcategorized into complementation groups. The FA complementation groups are defined by their ability to cross-complement the cellular hypersensitivity to the clastogenic effects of DNA crosslinking agents. At least 17 genes, including *FANCA, FANCB, FANCC, FANCD1 (BRCA2), FANCD2, FANCE, FANCF, FANCG, FANCI, FANCJ (BRIP1), FANCL, FANCM, FANCN (PALB2), FANCP (SLX4), FANCS (BRCA1), RAD51C,* and *XPF*, have been identified.

The FA genes were identified by several related strategies that are similar to those used to clone the XP genes. Cells from the FA-C group, for example, were able to be complemented with pooled clones from a human cDNA library that represented most of the protein-coding genes. From these pools, individual clones that could complement the chromosome breakage phenotypes of FA-C cells were identified. The gene corresponding to these complementing cDNAs was designated *FANCC*, and was the first FA gene identified. Analysis of *FANCC* in FA-C patients revealed frameshift, splicing, missense and truncation mutations. Similar approaches, combined with positional cloning, have been used to clone and validate *FANCA*, *FANCB*, *FANCE*, *FANCF* and *FANCG* as the genes corresponding to the FA-A, –B, –E, –F, and –G groups, respectively. The group initially designated FA-D has since been determined to be heterogeneous, with mutations in the genes *FANCD1* and *FANCD2* occurring in subsets of the FA-D group. FA-A represents the largest group of patients, accounting for approximately 65 % of all FA cases.

The molecular cloning of the gene for the FA-D1 complementation group led to the discovery that *FANCD1* is identical to *BRCA2*. Therefore, *BRCA2* mutations can cause two distinct diseases. Germline inheritance of monoallelic *BRCA2* mutations causes familial breast and ovarian cancer susceptibility (an autosomal dominant syndrome), while biallelic germline mutations in *BRCA2* cause FA (an autosomal recessive syndrome).

FA is significantly more common than the NER syndromes. Because carriers appear to be unaffected (with the exception of carriers of mutated *BRCA2*), and because of the difficulties in case ascertainment, the frequency of FA alleles in the general population has been difficult to accurately determine. It has been estimated that as many as 0.5 % of the general population may be heterozygous for an FA gene mutation. The FA allele frequency is about one percent among individuals of South African Afrikaans or Ashkenazi Jewish descent, as a result of founder effects. For example, an A→T splice site mutation in *FANCC*, designated c.711+4A>T, is unique to FA patients of Ashkenazi ancestry. The incidence of FA syndrome is particularly high in ethnic groups in which consanguineous marriages are traditionally common.

The FA gene-encoded proteins are involved in the recognition and repair of DNA damage, particularly covalent DNA crosslinks. The association of FA proteins with sites of DNA damage and repair and the cellular sensitivity of FA cells to crosslinking agents, such as the chemotherapeutic drugs cisplatin and MMC, provide strong evidence that the clinical manifestations of FA result from these DNA repair defects.

FA generally exhibits an autosomal recessive mode of transmission, and accordingly, most FA genes are located on the autosomes. However, the gene mutated in the FA-B group, *FANCB*, was found to be located on the X chromosome. This means that FA-B must exhibit a unique mode of transmission that, interestingly, had not been detected prior to the identification of the underlying genetic defect. Male carriers harbor hemizygous *FANCB* mutations and are therefore invariably affected with the disease. In females, the X-chromosome is randomly inactivated early in development. Normally, females are composed of cells that represent a *mosaic* with respect to the X-chromosome that is inactivated. Female carriers of X-linked *FANCB* mutations would therefore be expected to express the mutant protein in one half of their cells and thus partially express a mutant phenotype. In fact, these individuals appear to be perfectly normal. Cellular and molecular analysis has revealed that

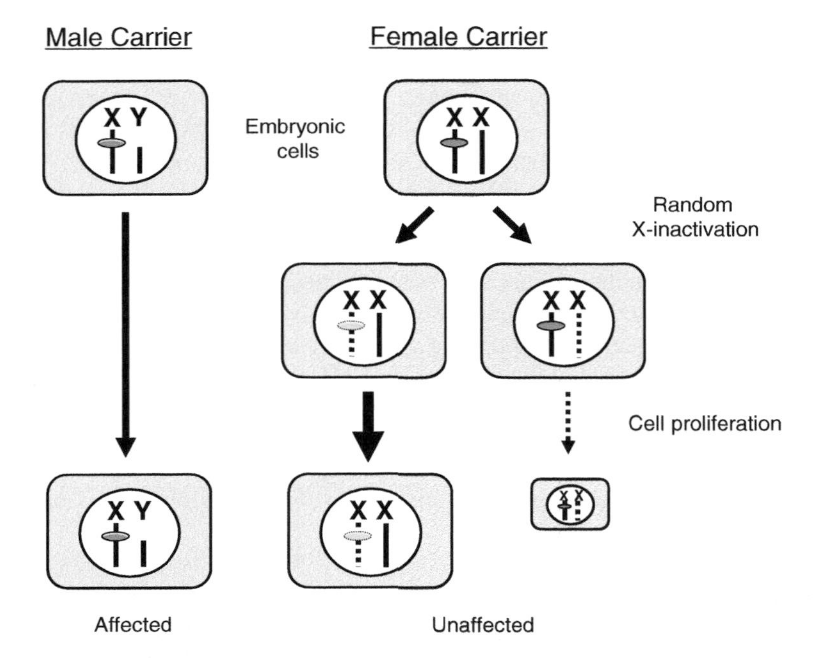

Fig. 4.14 X-linked inheritance of *FANCB* mutations. Male carriers of mutant *FANCB* (shown in *red*) are hemizygous for this recessive allele, and are therefore affected by Fanconi anemia. In females, each X chromosome is subject to random inactivation. However, the cells derived from precursors that had inactivated the wild type *FANCB* allele are apparently at a significant proliferative disadvantage during subsequent phases of development. The large majority of cells in the developed female carrier are derived from the embryonic precursors in which the mutant *FANCB* allele had been inactivated. The female *FANCB* mutant carrier is therefore clinically unaffected

FANCB-mutant female carriers have a markedly reduced level of mosaicism as compared to females that do not carry a *FANCB* mutation. How might this occur? Cells that express mutant FANCB appear to be more prone to spontaneously undergo apoptosis, and are therefore at a significant proliferative disadvantage as compared with wild type cells. Apparently, after X-inactivation occurs, cells that express mutant FANCB are outcompeted by the cells that express wild type FANCB (Fig. 4.14). In the female mutant *FANCB* carrier, the majority of somatic cells are apparently derived from the embryonic precursors in which the copy of the X-chromosome harboring the *FANCB* mutation has been inactivated. This unusual mode of transmission has important implications for the genetic counseling of FA families in which males are exclusively affected.

In contrast to female carriers of *FANCB* mutations, who lose mosaicism during development, about one quarter of FA patients with autosomal mutations have been found to gain mosaicism. In such patients, two distinct populations of blood cells can be detected: one population with a marked chromosome-break phenotype induced by DEB or MMC treatment, and one that is phenotypically normal. In such

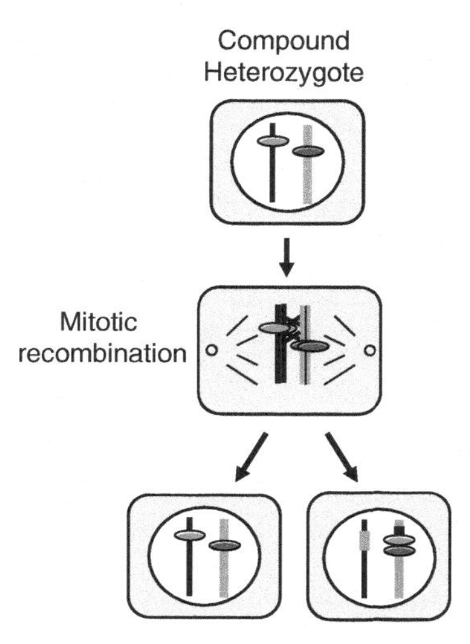

Fig. 4.15 Reversion of FANC phenotypes by intragenic recombination. A Fanconi anemia-affected individual with compound heterozygous FANC mutations (shown in *red* and *blue*) has two inactivated FANC alleles. During mitosis, crossing over leads to an exchange between chromatids on the maternal and paternal chromosomes. A recombination event puts both FANC mutations on the same chromosome, while the other chromosome reverts to wild type. The daughter cell that inherits the revertant allele is phenotypically normal. This patient is said to exhibit mosaicism

mosaic patients, a proportion of blood cells have apparently reverted to a normal phenotype. There are two known mechanisms for reversion. In some cases, reversion is a result of mitotic recombination (Fig. 4.15). Many FA patients are *compound heterozygotes*, in whom two distinct mutations are present in the maternal and paternal FA alleles. Intragenic recombination that occurs during mitosis can result in the transmission of both mutations on the same allele. Another mechanism of reversion is *gene conversion*, which occurs upon introduction of compensatory mutations (Fig. 4.16). It has been demonstrated that frameshift mutations in FA genes can be compensated for by somatically acquired mutations that restore the correct reading frame and thereby revert to wild type function. It is unclear whether reversion of FA mutations in subpopulations of blood cells is sufficient to alter the course of the disease or significantly affect the prognosis.

While the genetic heterogeneity among the FA complementation groups contributes to the overall clinical heterogeneity of the disease, other factors additionally affect the expression of the varying disease phenotypes. Significant phenotypic variation has been reported within families. Even monozygotic twins have been found to be discordant in their expression of congenital abnormalities. These studies conclusively demonstrate that while FA gene mutations are the cause of FA, the specific features of the disease can be shaped by unique genetic and environmental factors.

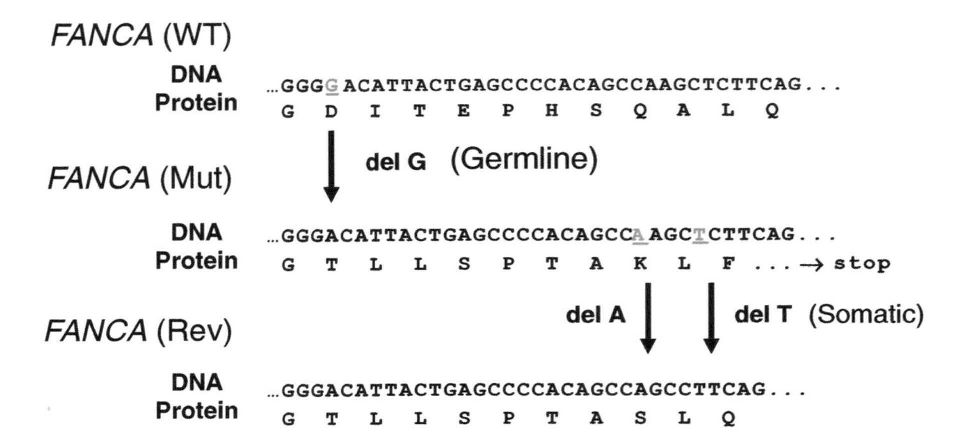

Fig. 4.16 Reversion of FANC mutations by gene conversion. The germline deletion of a single G residue at position 1615 (underlined in *red*) in a Fanconi anemia patient disrupts the open reading frame of *FANCA*. This mutation, *FANCA* (Mut), leads to the premature truncation of the encoded protein. Two somatic deletions occurring downstream of the germline mutation cause a shift back to the wild type reading frame (*FANCA* (Rev)) and restore function of the encoded protein (Example from Waisfisz et al. *Nature Genetics* 22:379–383 (1999))

A Defect in DNA Double Strand Break Responses Causes Ataxia-Telangiectasia

Ataxia-telangiectasia (AT) is an autosomal recessive syndrome characterized by hypersensitivity to ionizing radiation and a predisposition to cancer, most commonly in lymphoid tissues. Major clinical features of this disorder include: (1) a progressively disabling loss of muscle coordination that underlies a gait abnormality known as cerebellar ataxia, (2) an inability to follow an object across the visual fields, a symptom known as oculomotor apraxia, (3) dilated groups of capillaries, known as telangiectasia, which cause elevated dark red blotches on the skin and eyes, and (4) humoral and cellular immunodeficiencies that predispose affected patients to frequent infections. AT patients typically exhibit high levels of a serum protein known as α-fetoprotein, believed to be a suppressor of immune function.

A clue into the cellular basis of AT was provided by the observation that AT patients are highly sensitive to the effects of ionizing radiation, which is often employed as cancer therapy and during diagnostic imaging. Therapeutic doses of radiation are well-tolerated by most cancer patients, but cause serious and often life-threatening complications in AT patients. Ionizing radiation – and drugs that mimic the effects of radiation – imparts several forms of cellular damage, predominant among these are double strand DNA breaks. Double strand DNA breaks present a significant challenge to proliferating cells and are highly lethal when unrepaired.

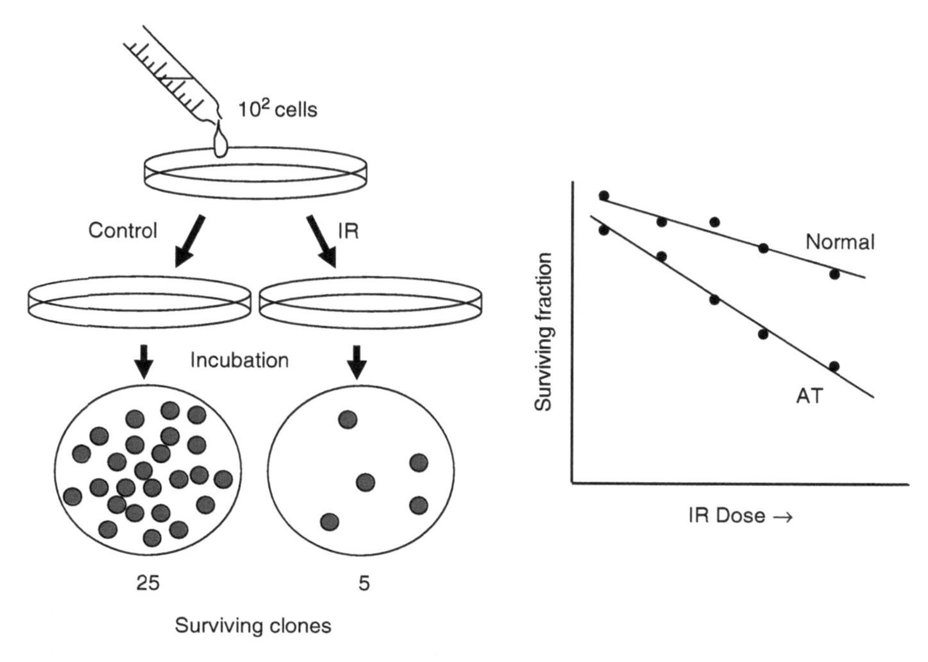

Fig. 4.17 Cells derived from ataxia telangiectasia patients exhibit reduced clonogenic survival following exposure to ionizing radiation. Patient-derived cells – most often fibroblasts – are seeded to culture dishes and exposed to measured doses of ionizing radiation. In this example, 100 cells are plated to multiple plates (*left panel*). Plates are incubated following treatment, allowing the surviving cells to proliferate and form clonal colonies. Only a fraction of cells in the original population are able to generate colonies, such cells said to be *clonogens*. On the untreated (control) plate, 25 colonies (shown in *blue*) are visible after seeding and incubation of 100 cells; the *plating efficiency* of the original cell population is therefore 25 %. The plate treated with IR contains a reduced number of clones compared to the control, reflecting reduced *clonogenic survival*. At this single dose of IR, the *surviving fraction* is 0.2. AT patient-derived cells are more sensitive to ionizing radiation than are cells from normal individuals, across a wide dose range (*right panel*)

Aberrant responses to ionizing radiation can be observed in cultured, AT patient-derived cells. AT-associated radiosensitivity can be observed by measuring the proportional survival of irradiated cells (Fig. 4.17). AT cells also have a characteristic defect in the regulation of DNA replication after irradiation. Normally, cells transiently halt DNA replication that is in progress at the time of radiation exposure. AT cells are defective in this radiation response and thus continue to replicate their genomic DNA without a normal pause. This quantitative cellular trait is known as *radioresistant DNA synthesis* (RDS). RDS can be directly quantified by measuring the uptake of [^{3}H]- thymidine within a timed interval following radiation exposure. It is not clear whether RDS and reduced survival are causally related, but these two *in vitro* responses nonetheless facilitate the quantification of cellular AT phenotypes.

The initial experimental strategies to determine the genetic cause of AT were similar to those employed in the search for the NER genes. It was reported that the RDS phenotype of AT could be complemented by cell fusions. These data were used to categorize patients into a number of distinct complementation groups, similar to the manner in which XP patients were categorized by the complementation of UDS. However, subsequent efforts to clone AT-associated genes by complementation were unsuccessful. The relevance of the originally-defined AT complementation groups remains unclear. Similarly, attempts were made to complement the radiosensitivity phenotype of AT cells by gene transfer. While numerous genes were isolated by this approach, none of these was found to be defective in AT patients. In retrospect, it would appear that the rescue of the RDS and radiosensitivity phenotypes in cultured AT cells did not reflect underlying genetic defect that causes AT but rather were artifacts of the methods employed.

Ultimately, the genetic basis of AT was revealed by linkage to a region on chromosome 11 by Richard Gatti and coworkers. This discovery guided subsequent positional cloning efforts. In 1995, a collaborative group led by Yosef Shiloh identified a single gene on chromosome 11q22-23 that was mutated in the germline of AT patients. This gene was designated *ataxia telangiectasia mutated*, or *ATM*.

ATM is a large gene composed of 69 coding exons. The mutations in *ATM* that cause AT are diverse and distributed throughout the *ATM* coding region. There are only a few relative mutational hotspots; many mutations are unique. The most common types of *ATM* mutations are single base substitutions and short deletions. Of the single base substitutions in *ATM*, more than one third are nonsense mutations. Therefore, the majority of *ATM* mutations result in the truncation of the open reading frame. AT patients are most commonly compound heterozygotes, and thus harbor two different *ATM* mutations.

AT patients have an approximately 37-fold increased lifetime risk of developing any type of cancer. Approximately 85 % of cancers that arise in AT patients are leukemias and lymphomas. The care of AT patients has improved in recent years and resulted in an improvement of the average life span. In the older cohort of AT patients, significant numbers of solid tumors such as breast cancers and melanomas have begun to be observed.

The incidence of AT has been estimated at 1 in 40,000 live births. Almost 1 % of the general population is heterozygous for a mutant *ATM* allele. This implies that there are approximately 2.5 million AT carriers in the US. Cells from heterozygous carriers have been demonstrated to partially exhibit some of the cellular phenotypes of ATM-deficiency. Despite these subtle cellular abnormalities, *ATM* mutation carriers appear to be otherwise phenotypically normal. Population-based studies suggest that carriers may have an increased risk of breast cancer, but the magnitude of this effect seems to be small. Mutant ATM alleles are thus low-penetrance breast cancer genes.

The broad spectrum of disease features suggests that loss of ATM function affects tissues in different ways. For example, the Purkinje cells of the cerebellum degenerate and migrate abnormally in the absence of ATM activity, while the thymus fails to develop beyond the embryonic stage. That the neurological, immunological and neoplastic characteristics of AT are all attributable to a single genetic defect demonstrates an extraordinary degree of *pleiotropy*, or the attribution of two or more phenotypes to a single genotype. The pleiotropy of *ATM* mutations indicates a broad role for DNA break responses in normal human physiology.

ATM encodes a large protein kinase that is rapidly activated at the site of DNA breaks. Activated ATM associates with a multi-protein complex known as the MRN complex, and with the protein encoded by *BRCA1*. The MRN complex binds DNA and has multiple biochemical properties that include the cutting, unwinding and bridging the ends of the damaged double helix. BRCA1 protein is involved in a DNA repair process known as non-homologous DNA end joining. It appears that the MRN complex and the BRCA1 protein are required for the efficient recruitment and possibly the retention of ATM at double strand DNA break sites. The molecular mechanism of DNA break-dependent activation of ATM will be described in Chap. 6.

The MRN complex is so-named because it is composed of three proteins encoded by *M RE11*, *R AD50* and *N BS1*. Germline mutations of each of these genes have been found in individuals with rare autosomal recessive syndromes that clinically overlap with AT. *MRE11* mutations cause the Ataxia Telangiectasia-like disorder (ATLD), mutations in NBS1 cause Nijmegen breakage syndrome (NBS), and mutations in RAD50 have been found in a single individual with an NBS phenotype. While ATLD has not been associated with an increase in cancer risk, individuals with NBS are prone to leukemia, melanoma, and cancer of the prostate, breast and ovary.

The importance of the DNA damage response genes to the suppression of cancer is underscored by the numerous tumor suppressors that are functionally linked to ATM and the DNA damage response. The proteins of the MRN complex are important for ATM activation and the efficient transduction of DNA damage signals to downstream target molecules. Among these molecular targets are the tumor suppressors of the FA complex and p53.

A Unique Form of Genetic Instability Underlies Bloom Syndrome

Among all of the cancer syndromes described in this chapter, perhaps none more emphatically highlights the causal relationship between genetic instability and cancer than does Bloom syndrome (BS). Individuals affected by this very rare genetic disorder exhibit both a readily observable defect in the maintenance of chromosomes and a pronounced predisposition to develop common forms of cancer.

BS patients develop cancer at a higher rate than any other genetically defined group of individuals. The types of cancer and the sites at which they occur are similar to those in the general population. About 30 % of BS patients develop leukemias and lymphomas; a similar proportion develops carcinomas of various types. As is the case with cancer in the general population, the liquid tumors arise in younger

BS patients, whereas the carcinomas develop later in life. Of the BS patients who develop malignant disease, about 10 % have more than one primary cancer. BS patients develop cancers at an early age, with a mean age of onset of 25 years. Other phenotypes associated with BS, include small body size, characteristic facies and voices, sun-sensitivity, immunodeficiency and, in males, infertility. Cancer accounts for a markedly reduced life expectancy for BS patients, the majority of whom succumb before age 30.

Proliferating cells isolated from BS patients exhibit several striking chromosomal abnormalities. Chromosomes from dividing blood lymphocytes exhibit numerous chromatid breaks, gaps, and structural rearrangements. These structural features occur spontaneously, in the absence of any environmental stimulus or clastogen. BS-associated cytological defects are quantitative in nature; similar features can also be seen in cells from normal individuals, but at a much lower frequency. The process that underlies this elevated level of gross chromosomal aberrations is an abnormally elevated rate of recombination between homologous chromosome regions. Recombination can occur between two chromosomes of a homologous pair, between the maternal and paternal chromosome 3, or intra-chromosomally, between the sister chromatids of a single chromosome. These inter- and intra-chromosomal exchanges probably occur during S-phase, when chromosomes are replicated.

Intra-chromosomal exchanges can be visualized by differentially labeling sister chromatids during S phase and examining stained chromosomes during a subsequent metaphase (Fig. 4.18). This type of analysis allows the extent of recombination to be visually observed and quantified. BS cells exhibit a high level of sister chromatid exchanges (SCE). While cells from normal individuals typically exhibit fewer than 10 SCE/metaphase spread, BS-derived cells often exhibit from 60 to 90 SCE/metaphase. This elevated SCE frequency, known as the *high-SCE* phenotype, is highly diagnostic for BS. In addition, BS cells exhibit an elevated frequency of mutations that occur at the submicroscopic level, including point mutations and mutations at repeat sequences. By several criteria, the genome in BS cells is highly unstable.

Interestingly, the cells from some BS patients are found to vary in their phenotypic presentation. While the majority of lymphocytes from a given BS patient exhibit the high-SCE phenotype, a significant proportion might be found to be low-SCE, and thus functionally wild type. These individuals were thus mosaic in respect to expression of the cellular BS phenotype. A similar type of mosaicism is observed in some patients with Fanconi Anemia. The explanation for mosaicism in FA is that compound heterozygotes, individuals who have different mutations on each of the two alleles, can create a normal allele by the process of homologous recombination. As the primary defect in BS is an increased rate of homologous recombination, it appeared probable that such a mechanism would explain the reversion of the BS phenotype observed in mosaic patients. Definitive proof of this hypothesis awaited the identification of the BS gene.

BS is a monogenic disease caused by the mutational inactivation of a tumor suppressor gene. Like many other tumor suppressor genes, the BS gene was cloned by

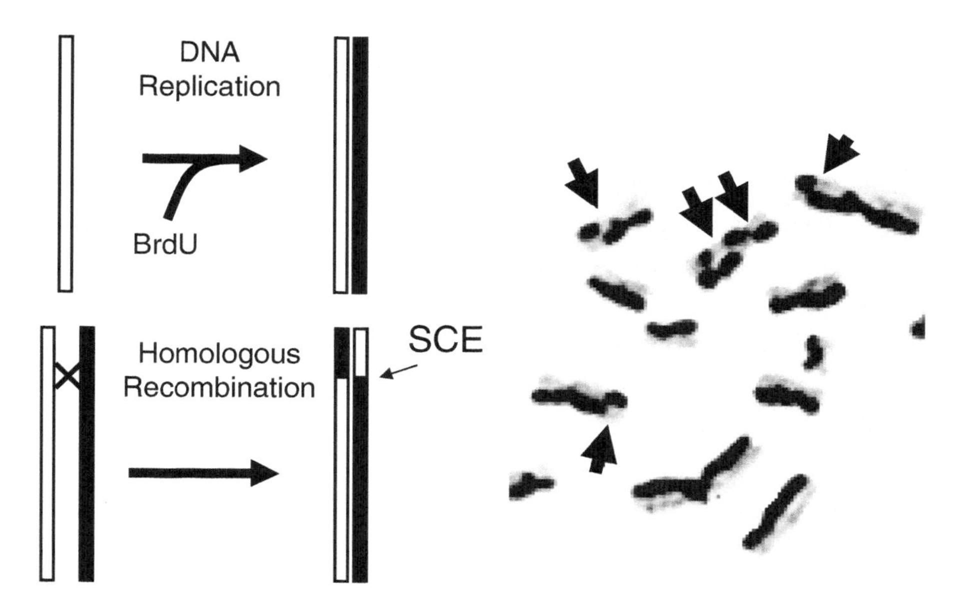

Fig. 4.18 Genetic instability in Bloom syndrome. Sister chromatids can be differentially stained by incubating mitotically active lymphocytes in the presence of the nucleotide analog bromodeoxyuridine (BrdU) for one complete cell cycle. The newly synthesized chromatid contains incorporated BrdU, which can be then photo-bleached and darkly stained (shown in *black*). Sister chromatid exchanges (SCE) resulting from homologous recombination can be visualized as alternating regions of light and dark staining. Bloom syndrome metaphase chromosomes (*right panel*) exhibit numerous SCEs (indicated by *arrows*)

virtue of its chromosomal location. However, the methods employed exploited several unique aspects of BS inheritance as well as the BS-associated cellular phenotype. The overall approach was guided by several unique insights that, in a stepwise fashion, narrowed the search for the gene of interest. The first step in determining the position of the BS gene was the complementation of the high-SCE phenotype by whole chromosome transfer. In 1992, it was demonstrated that the transfer of a normal chromosome 15 could suppress high-SCE in BS-derived cells.

Although extremely rare, BS is significantly more prevalent in the Ashkenazi Jewish population than in other ethnic groups. Among non-Ashkenazi families, the disease arises most frequently as a result of consanguinity. As a result, such affected individuals exhibit many regions of homozygosity. The location of the BS gene on chromosome 15 was localized to 15q26 by using polymorphic markers to determine the extent of homozygosity, a technique that came to be termed 'homozygosity mapping'. In Ashkenazi Jewish families, tight linkage was demonstrated between the BS allele, a gene designated *FES* located at 15q26.1 and several microsatellite repeat sequences.

The precise location of the BS gene was deduced by detailed genetic analysis of the BS-derived cell lines that were low-SCE revertants. In these lines, crossover events had reduced the compound heterozygous BS locus to homozygosity, thereby eliminating the high-SCE phenotype. Loci distal to the BS in these cell lines were homozygous, while proximal loci retained the heterozygosity observed in patients' constitutional DNA. This observation facilitated a third cloning strategy termed 'somatic crossover-point mapping', which involved the identification of the junction between homozygous and heterozygous regions. Because the yet-to-be discovered BS gene had apparently been restored to wild type by recombination, it was expected that the homozygous/heterozygous junction must fall within the locus of interest. Using this strategy, a group led by James German localized the BS gene to a relatively short interval of just 250 kb, and finally cloned the gene in 1995. Thus, the hyper-recombinant phenotype of BS was successfully employed as a tool to pinpoint the disease locus. The BS gene, designated *BLM*, is composed of 22 exons and spans approximately 100 kb on chromosome 15.

The role of *BLM* in BS was confirmed by the presence of mutations that segregate with the disease phenotype. A variety of mutations affect the *BLM* open reading frame, including missense and nonsense mutations, small indels and splice site mutations. Most of the *BLM* mutations found in BS patients result in premature truncation of the open reading frame and predicted inactivation of the protein product. Sequence analysis of *BLM* in the Ashkenazi Jewish population definitively confirmed the existence of a founder effect. The carrier rate in this population is 1 %. Also confirmed by DNA sequencing was the prediction that the individuals exhibiting revertant cell populations were compound heterozygotes.

The *BLM* gene encodes an enzyme that belongs to a previously identified family of highly conserved DNA and RNA helicases. These enzymes catalyze the ATP-dependent unwinding of duplex nucleic acids, a process that is essential for basic cellular processes including DNA replication and repair, RNA transcription and protein translation. The protein encoded by *BLM* most closely resembles a helicase subfamily known as RECQ, named after the prototypic *RECQ* gene in the bacterium *E. coli*. Analysis of RECQ homologs in model organisms has yielded significant clues as to what the specific functions of human RECQ helicases might be. Bacterial *RECQ* is required for recombination during conjugation and also for resistance to UV, which is a potent inhibitor of DNA replication. In the budding yeast *S. cerevisae*, mutants of the *RECQ* homolog *SGS1* feature slow growth, frequent chromosome mis-segregation and chromosome rearrangements, and defects in double strand break repair. In the fruit fly *D. melanogaster*, RECQ mutants confer sensitivity to mutagens as well as a pattern of sterility that resembles that observed in human BS. The sterile phenotype in flies has been attributed to chromosome mis-segregation that occurs prior to meiosis. Experimental disruption of the *BLM* gene in mice and chicken cells results in a high-SCE phenotype that closely resembles the cytological defect in BS.

The cloning of *BLM* and the analysis of homologs in model organisms has revealed a critical role for RECQ helicases in the process of homologous recombination and in the maintenance of genetic stability. The extraordinary risk of cancer borne by BS patients demonstrates in dramatic fashion the role of genetic instability in the development of common types of cancer.

Aging and Cancer: Insights from the Progeroid Syndromes

Cancer is strongly associated with aging. While cancer in its various forms strikes individuals at all stages of life, the overall incidence of the most common solid tumors clearly increases with age.

The relationship between cancer and aging is readily explained by the cancer gene theory. Neoplastic cell clones harboring mutations iteratively expand and accumulate more mutations. The development of these progenitor cells into cancer requires many generations of cell growth. In most tissues this process takes years or even decades. Consequently, cancers tend to disproportionately appear in older individuals. Inborn genetic instability alters the time frame in which tumors develop. Common among HNPCC, XP, FA, AT and BS is the acceleration of the process of tumorigenesis, which causes the greatly increased incidence of cancer at younger ages. By various mechanisms, the genetic mutations that underlie these diseases cause genetic instability that, in turn, accelerates the process of tumorigenesis.

Many of the cardinal signs of aging can also be related to the maintenance of a stable genome. Evidence to support a direct relationship between aging and genetic stability is derived from studies of a category of inherited diseases known as the *progeroid syndromes. Progeria*, or premature aging, can be caused by inborn genetic instability.

The most symptomatically striking progeroid syndrome, and the most intensively studied, is Werner syndrome (WS). WS patients prominently exhibit a prematurely aged appearance that develops during the second and third decades of life. Affected individuals develop normally, but as young adults they develop grey hair, hyperpigmentation and other age-associated skin changes, and a hoarse voice. Individuals with WS appear 20–30 years older than their chronologic age (Fig. 4.19). Many disease states that are strongly associated with aging occur prematurely in WS patients. These typically include arteriosclerosis, cataract formation, osteoporosis and diabetes mellitus. WS patients also have a highly elevated risk of many types of cancer, and cancer is the cause of death in 80 % of cases. The average life span of WS patients is 47 years.

WS patients develop a broad range of cancers, but they are not at uniformly increased risk for all common types of cancer. Rather, WS exhibits a selective increase in some relatively rare cancers. For example, while sarcomas occur infrequently in the general population, they represent approximately one half of the cancers that arise in WS. Conversely, several of the most common cancers in the general population, such as prostate cancer, do not occur at elevated rates in WS patients. WS thus does not exactly recapitulate all of the increases in cancer incidence that are attributable to normal aging. Nor does WS completely recapitulate normal aging, but rather the disease phenotype accelerates segments of the normal aging process. For example, the dermis of WS patients exhibits severe pathology that similar to that seen in normal aging, while the immune system appears to be unaffected. WS appears to mimic individual components, known as *segments*, of aging. To highlight this distinction, WS and the other diseases of premature aging are termed '*segmental progeroid syndromes*'.

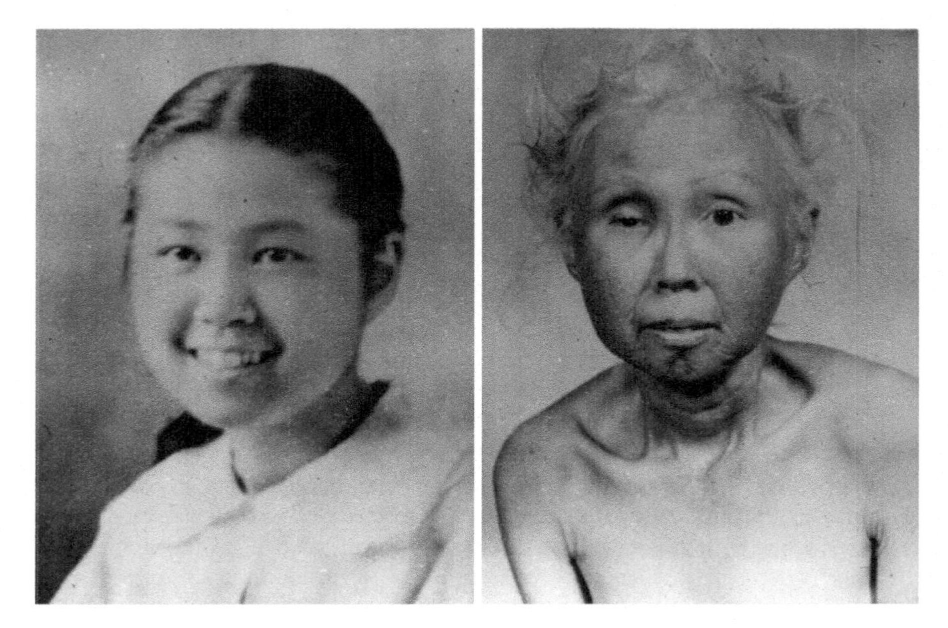

Fig. 4.19 Premature aging in Werner syndrome. A Japanese woman with Werner syndrome photographed at age 15 (*left*) and again at age 48 (*right*). From Epstein CJ, et al. Werner's syndrome: a review of its symptomatology, natural history, pathologic features, genetics and relationship to the natural aging process. *Medicine* 45:177–221 (1966) (Reproduced with permission)

Cells from WS patients show several characteristic cytogenetic phenotypes, including extensive chromosomal deletions, chromosome fusions, elevated rates of homologous recombination, and a prolongation of S-phase of the cell cycle. WS cells are hypersensitive to DNA damaging agents that cause DNA double strand breaks, including ionizing radiation. The degree of radiosensitivity is significantly lower than that seen in cells from AT or NBS patients, suggesting a distinct molecular defect in WS patients. These diverse defects suggest fundamental defects in chromosomal DNA repair and chromosome maintenance.

WS is inherited in an autosomal recessive pattern; affected families often have a high rate of consanguinity. The WS gene was cloned by a positional approach. Localization of the gene was initially guided by homozygosity mapping, similar to the approach employed in the identification of the Bloom syndrome gene, *BLM*. Analysis of linkage to a panel of polymorphic markers narrowed down the location to a 1.2 Mb region on chromosome 8. In a final comprehensive effort, ten genes that lie in this interval were screened for mutations. A previously uncharacterized gene, subsequently designated *WRN,* was found to be mutated in affected individuals and obligate carriers, by a group led by Gerard Schellenberg. *WRN* spans a 140 kb region at 8p11-12 and is composed of 35 exons. The first mutations identified in *WRN* were single base substitutions that created nonsense codons or splice site defects. Thus, the mutations that cause WS lead to the premature truncation of the *WRN*-encoded protein.

Initial characterization of the *WRN* coding region revealed a striking homology to RNA and DNA helicases. Like *BLM*, *WRN* encodes a RECQ-related helicase that unwinds nucleic acids in the $3' \rightarrow 5'$ direction. Unique among the RECQ family members, the WRN protein exhibits an N-terminal $3' \rightarrow 5'$ exonuclease activity that catalyzes the degradation of DNA ends. Biochemical studies have shown that the helicase and exonuclease associated with WRN have specificity to similar types of DNA structures, suggesting that these two domains function coordinately. Such a helicase could conceivably function in a number of cellular processes. The cellular phenotypes of WS suggest that the WRN helicase is likely to participate in some aspect of intra-strand DNA crosslink repair. The precise cellular role of the WRN helicase and the means by which its loss of function causes WS remains to be completely elucidated.

The clinical features of WS would suggest that cancer and aging are part of a common overall process, all inextricably linked to genetic instability. However, a broader examination of the progeroid syndromes shows that the predisposition to cancer and the other various characteristics, or segments, are clearly separable (Table 4.5). Two of the rare nucleotide excision repair syndromes, Cockayne syndrome and trichothiodystrophy prominently feature segmental progeria, but not cancer predisposition. In stark contrast, XP features a 1000-fold increase in the risk of skin cancer, as well as a significantly increased risk of various internal cancers, but is not associated with progeria. Both BS and AT are characterized primarily by can-

Table 4.5 Overlapping and distinct phenotypes related to inborn genetic instability

Disease	Gene(s)	Cellular defect: encoded enzyme activity	Cancer	Progeria
Xeroderma pigmentosum	*XPA- XPF*	NER: various DNA binding proteins, DNA helicases, endonucleases	+++	–
XFE progeroid syndrome	*XPF*	NER: Endonuclease	Unknown	+++
Trichothiodystrophy	*XPB XPD*	NER: DNA helicases	–	++
Cockayne syndrome	*CSA CSB*	Transcription-coupled repair: coupling factors	–	++
XP-CS complex	*XPB XPD*	NER: DNA helicases	+++	++
Ataxia telangiectasia	*ATM*	Double strand DNA break recognition: Ser/Thr kinase	+	+
Bloom syndrome	*BLM*	DNA repair: RECQ helicase (exo-)	+++	++
Rothmund-Thomson syndrome	*RECQL4*	DNA repair: RECQ helicase (exo-)	++	++
Werner syndrome	*WRN*	DNA repair: RECQ helicase (exo+)	+++	+++

cer predisposition, but also feature mild phenotypes related to segmental premature aging.

Genetic defects that affect nucleotide excision repair can variably cause cancer predisposition, segmental aging, both or neither. In the interesting case of the *XPD* gene, different point mutations cause XP (cancer predisposition only), trichothiodystrophy (progeria only), or the XP-CS complex (cancer predisposition and progeria). Similarly, distinct mutations in *XPF* cause xeroderma pigmentosum or XFE progeroid syndrome, a phenotypically profound disease first described in 2006 and based on the discovery of a single affected individual. Rothmund-Thomson syndrome, a heritable disease that exhibits significant clinical overlap with WS, is caused by mutations in another RECQ family member, *RECQL4*. Rothmund-Thomson syndrome patients are at a greatly increased risk of developing osteosarcoma. Interestingly, different mutations in the *RECQL4* gene have been shown to cause two other rare, autosomal recessive disease syndromes, neither of which appear to feature an increased cancer risk nor segmental progeria. As clearly exemplified by *XPD* and *RECQL4*, different alleles of the same gene can lead to dramatically distinct diseases.

Instability at the End: Telomeres and Telomerase

A critical aspect of chromosome stability is the proper maintenance of the DNA-protein structures called *telomeres* that define chromosome ends. Telomeres are composed of unique repetitive DNA sequences and DNA-binding proteins that shield these termini from nucleases and other enzymes that could otherwise recognize and process them as DNA strand breaks. Functional telomeres thus suppress the growth suppressive signals that would be triggered by the exposed ends of chromosomes. At the cytogenetic level, intact telomeres prevent end-to-end fusions that result from DNA repair.

The molecular machines that faithfully replicate chromosomal DNA during S-phase are enzymatically incapable of fully completing the synthesis of the lagging strand and therefore leave a small terminal region incompletely replicated. Because of this limitation, each round of cell division would theoretically result in a small loss of DNA from the end of every chromosome. In addition, telomeric DNA is particularly susceptible to damage by the highly reactive free radicals that are generated as a metabolic byproduct of continuous cell growth. Many proliferating cells counter these chronic losses of telomeric DNA by expressing the enzyme *telomerase*. Telomerase is a multi-component enzyme complex that catalyzes the addition of telomeric DNA repeats, and thus reverses the attrition of chromosome ends.

The function – and dysfunction – of telomeres is intimately involved with both normal aging and the process of tumorigenesis. As normal stem cell populations age and reach the end of their finite replicative potential, their telomeres erode. This unique form of chromosomal DNA damage triggers intracellular signals that impede the progression of the cell cycle and thereby slow further proliferation. Accordingly, young individuals have, on average, longer telomeres (ie. more telomeric repeats) than their elders. Interestingly, cells derived from WS patients with progeria exhibit short telomeres, suggesting a constitutional defect in telomere maintenance.

Telomere-deficient cells are prone to a unique form of chromosomal instability that was first suggested by the American geneticist Barbara McClintock. When a chromosome that has a critically short telomere is replicated, the two sister chromatids that arise each share the same telomere defect that renders them, in effect, sticky. In the absence of a protective telomeric structure, the two sister chromatids fuse at their sticky ends. During the subsequent anaphase, the sister chromatids are pulled into opposing poles of the mitotic spindle, but remain covalently attached at the site of the telomeric fusion. The traction of the spindle eventually causes the two chromatids to break apart, but this break does not necessarily occur at the original site of fusion. The resulting daughter cells will each contain a chromosome with a broken end, and so the same sequence of events, known as the *breakage-fusion-bridge cycle*, will be repeated during in each subsequent round of cell division (Fig. 4.20).

Cancer cells acquire the capacity to proliferate indefinitely, a property known as *immortality*. During their development, most cancer cells activate the expression of telomerase, which greatly increases their proliferative potential. Despite this mea-

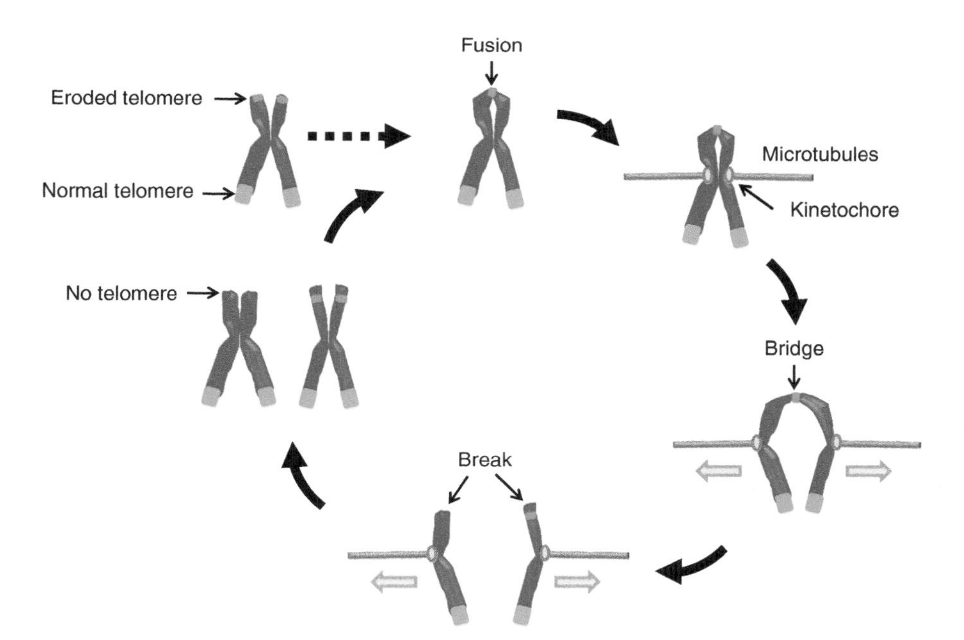

Fig. 4.20 The breakage-fusion-bridge cycle. Critically eroded telomeres (shown in *red*) trigger a repair process that creates a fusion between sister chromatids. This telomere-to-telomere fusion creates a dicentric chromosome that, during anaphase, forms a bridge spanning the two nascent daughter cells. The traction generated by the microtubules attached to the kinetochore causes the fused chromosome to break. This breakpoint can be distinct from the telomere repeat region (*red*) that defines the point of fusion. Each daughter cell thus acquires a chromosome with no telomere, which is replicated with all of the other chromosomes at the subsequent S-phase. This breakage-fusion-bridge cycle accompanies each subsequent cell cycle

sure, cancer cells typically have shortened telomeres with limited functionality. The short, partially defective telomeres harbored by many cancer cells appear to contribute to chromosomal loss and the formation of non-reciprocal translocations.

A significant fraction of cancers do not activate telomerase expression, but instead utilize a mechanism known as the *alternative lengthening of telomeres* (ALT). The ALT pathway in a non-enzymatic mode of telomere regeneration involves the homologous recombination-mediated transfer of telomere repeats between sister chromatids.

A number of genetic disorders have been attributed to defects in telomere maintenance, the most prominent of which is *dyskeratosis congenita* (DKC). DKC is an extremely rare syndrome that is clinically defined by varying degrees of abnormal skin pigmentation, nail malformation, and white patches on the oral mucosa. Affected individuals exhibit many characteristics of progeria and have an increased risk of malignancy, particularly in the oral cavity and at other mucous membranes. At the cellular level, DKC is characterized by short telomeres. The telomere defect that underlies DKC is caused by a variety of mutations that directly or indirectly alter an RNA encoded by the *TERC* gene, a core component of the telomerase enzyme complex.

DKC illustrates the complex relationship between telomerase activity, telomere length and cancer. In most cancers, the activation of telomerase allows continued proliferation but apparently this induced enzymatic activity is insufficient to fully maintain telomeric integrity. In the case of DKC, telomerase is mutationally inactivated, leading to short, dysfunctional telomeres, and ultimately to chromosomal instability. It would therefore appear that telomeric dysfunction, rather than telomerase activation *per se*, provides the selective advantage that promotes neoplastic growth.

Overview: Genes and Genetic Stability

Autosomal recessive diseases of cancer predisposition such as Bloom syndrome, Werner syndrome and dyskeratosis congenita are rare diseases that have minimal impact on the overall health of the human population. While certainly devastating to the affected individuals and their families, the respective germline cancer genes have a low frequency in the general population and such diseases are fortunately rare. With the exception of *ATM*, these genes are not frequently mutated in any type of sporadic cancer. Nonetheless, the study of diseases caused by homozygous mutations of DNA repair genes diseases has led to key insights into the relationship between DNA repair, chromosomal maintenance, aging and the growth and development of neoplasia. Unraveling the molecular underpinnings of these unusual cancer syndromes has provided a unique view into the types of cellular processes that, when either partially or totally disabled, can lead to cancer. The identification of specific genes has directed vigorous research activity into how the information content of the genome is stably maintained.

Not all of the mutations that cause genetic instability are rare. Hereditary nonpolyposis colorectal cancer accounts for a small but significant proportion of the nearly 50,000 deaths from colorectal cancer that occur in the United States every year, and contributes to the incidence of several other types of cancer as well (see Chap. 7). Both Fanconi anemia and ataxia telangiectasia are caused by cancer genes that are present in up to 1 % of the general population. As the consequences of carrier status remains to be conclusively determined, it remains a possibility that germline mutations in the Fanconi anemia and ataxia telangiectasia genes could measurably increase the risk of cancer in the many individuals that harbor mutant alleles.

The genes that ensure the maintenance of a stable genome are, by definition, tumor suppressor genes and fall into the subcategory known as caretakers. As described in detail in Chap. 3, the mutation of caretaker genes does not directly increase the proliferation of cell clones. Instead, caretaker genes prevent aberrant cell proliferation indirectly, by preventing the accumulation of mutations in other tumor suppressor genes and proto-oncogenes that modulate growth control.

Intriguingly, the most common form of genetic instability observed in cancer, aneuploidy, remains in many respects the most mysterious. A central goal of ongoing research is to systematically identify the many genetic and epigenetic changes to the cancer cell genome and to understand how these functionally interact to cause cancer cell phenotypes. This effort promises to provide new insight into how cancer cells become aneuploid, and how aneuploidy shapes the responses of cancer cells to therapy.

Further Reading

Ahmed M, Rahman N (2006) ATM and breast cancer susceptibility. Oncogene 25:5906–5911

Andressoo JO, Hoeijmakers JH, Mitchell JR (2006) Nucleotide excision repair disorders and the balance between cancer and aging. Cell Cycle 5:2886–2888

Cahill DP, Kinzler KW, Vogelstein B, Lengauer C (1999) Genetic instability and darwinian selection in tumours. Trends Cell Biol 9:M57–M60

Cleaver JE (2005) Cancer in xeroderma pigmentosum and related disorders of DNA repair. Nat Rev Cancer 5:564–573

de Laat WL, Jaspers NG, Hoeijmakers JH (1999) Molecular mechanism of nucleotide excision repair. Genes Dev 13:768–785

Duesberg P (2005) Does aneuploidy or mutation start cancer? Science 307:41

Ellis NA (1996) Mutation-causing mutations. Nature 381:110–111

Ellis NA, German J (1996) Molecular genetics of Bloom's syndrome. Hum Mol Genet 5:1457–1463

Fearon ER (1997) Human cancer syndromes: clues to the origin and nature of cancer. Science 278:1043–1050

Gatti RA (2001) The inherited basis of human radiosensitivity. Acta Oncol 40:702–711

Gurtan AM, D'Andrea AD (2006) Dedicated to the core: understanding the Fanconi anemia complex. DNA Repair 5:1119–1125

Joenje H, Patel KJ (2001) The emerging genetic and molecular basis of Fanconi anaemia. Nat Rev Genet 2:446–457

Kastan MB, Lim DS (2000) The many substrates and functions of ATM. Nat Rev Mol Cell Biol 1:179–186

Kipling D, Davis T, Ostler EL, Faragher RG (2004) What can progeroid syndromes tell us about human aging? Science 305:1426–1431

Lengauer C, Kinzler KW, Vogelstein B (1998) Genetic instabilities in human cancers. Nature 396:643–669

Margolis RL (2005) Tetraploidy and tumor development. Cancer Cell 8:353–354

Michor F, Iwasa Y, Vogelstein B, Lengauer C, Nowak MA (2005) Can chromosomal instability initiate tumorigenesis? Semin Cancer Biol 15:43–49

Modrich P (1994) Mismatch repair, genetic stability, and cancer. Science 266:1959–1960

Mohaghegh P, Hickson ID (2001) DNA helicase deficiencies associated with cancer predisposition and premature ageing disorders. Hum Mol Genet 10:741–746

Negrini S, Gorgoulis VG, Halazonetis TD (2010) Genomic instability – an evolving hallmark of cancer. Nat Rev Mol Cell Biol 11:220–228

Rajagopalan H, Lengauer C (2004) Aneuploidy and cancer. Nature 432:338–341

Rajagopalan H, Nowak MA, Vogelstein B, Lengauer C (2003) The significance of unstable chromosomes in colorectal cancer. Nat Rev Cancer 3:695–701

Shiloh Y (2006) The ATM-mediated DNA-damage response: taking shape. Trends Biochem Sci 31:402–410

Siegel JJ, Amon A (2012) New insights into the troubles of aneuploidy. Annu Rev Cell Dev Biol 28:189–214

Tomlinson I, Bodmer W (1999) Selection, the mutation rate and cancer: ensuring that the tail does not wag the dog. Nat Med 5:11–12

Vijg J, Suh Y (2013) Genome instability and aging. Annu Rev Physiol 75:645–668

Chapter 5
Cancer Genomes

Discovering the Genetic Basis of Cancer: From Genes to Genomes

Our efforts to fully understand cancer have always been shaped by the methods and technologies that can be applied to the study of genes. Emerging recombinant DNA technologies allowed Bishop and Varmus to build on the prior observations of Rous to identify the first oncogene—and in the process, to bring the study of cancer into the molecular age. Subsequent developments, from PCR to increasingly powerful methods for DNA sequencing, have allowed scientists to delve ever more broadly and deeply into the genome of the cancer cell.

The previous chapters have summarized many of the early efforts to identify and characterize the genetic elements of cancer. At each stage of discovery, technical innovations facilitated new and powerful experimental approaches. Critical advances in molecular cloning, gene transfer and cell culture allowed the isolation of oncogenes that could confer new cell growth characteristics. The hunt for tumor suppressor genes within discrete chromosomal loci was unleashed by new methods to probe, map and sequence what at the time were uncharted regions of the human genome. While these approaches were amazingly successful, they were also inherently piecemeal. For the first three decades of molecular cancer research, the genetic basis of cancer was uncovered one gene at a time.

A rough draft covering the DNA sequence of about 80 % of a prototypical human genome was released in 2000. Most of the remaining gaps were filled in over the following several years, marking the culmination of the Human Genome Sequencing Project. The mapping of the human genome at the ultimate level of resolution was a watershed for all fields of human biology and genetics, including oncology. With the sequence of the prototypical human in hand, scientists were now empowered to consider not just individual genes, but entire genomes. This chapter will highlight and summarize what we have learned about the genome of the cancer cell.

F. Bunz, *Principles of Cancer Genetics*, DOI 10.1007/978-94-017-7484-0_5

What Types of Genetic Alterations Are Found in Tumor Cells?

The comprehensive genomic analysis of a cancer involves the enumeration of all single nucleotide substitutions, insertions and deletions, inversions, translocations and other more structurally complex rearrangements, as well as an assessment of the overall chromosome complement. As described in Chap. 4, aneuploidy is prevalent in cancers, occurring in 90 % of all solid tumors and 85 % of hematologic malignancies (the so-called "liquid" tumors). The chromosomal imbalances caused by the processes that underlie aneuploidy result in changes to the number of alleles of each gene, a factor also known as *gene dosage*. Most importantly, cells with chromosomal instability have an increased tendency to lose functional tumor suppressor alleles.

Most of the genetic alterations that cause cancer are subtle mutations that can be detected by DNA sequencing. About 95 % of the of the subtle DNA sequence alterations found in cancers are single nucleotide substitutions (also known as point mutations). The rest are small deletions or combined insertion/deletions (indels). Among the single-base substitutions detected, approximately 91 % result in missense mutations, nearly 8 % result in nonsense mutations, and fewer than 2 % affect sites involved in splicing or translation.

Efforts to identify single nucleotide substitutions, small deletions and indels typically focus on the exons of all genes that express mature RNAs. These informative genetic elements are collectively referred to as the *exome*. The exome represents just 1.5 % of the total genome, but the in-depth analysis of this component captures the majority of the somatic alterations that underlie the process of tumorigenesis. Whole exome sequencing of cancer cells and corresponding normal cells from the same individual allows somatically acquired mutations to be distinguished from single nucleotide polymorphisms that are present in the germline. In this way, the mutations that arise in cancer can be detected against the background of human genetic diversity.

How Many Genes Are Mutated in the Various Types of Cancer?

Whole exome sequence analysis applied to the most common and deadly solid tumors from the colon, breast, brain and pancreas has revealed an average of 30–70 base changes per tumor that would be predicted to alter an encoded protein (Fig. 5.1). However, many types of tumors harbor average numbers of mutations that are significantly outside this range. These outliers clearly illustrate several basic principles of cancer genetics.

Lung tumors in smokers and melanomas of the skin each harbor relatively large numbers of mutations that are attributable to the highly mutagenic effects of tobacco

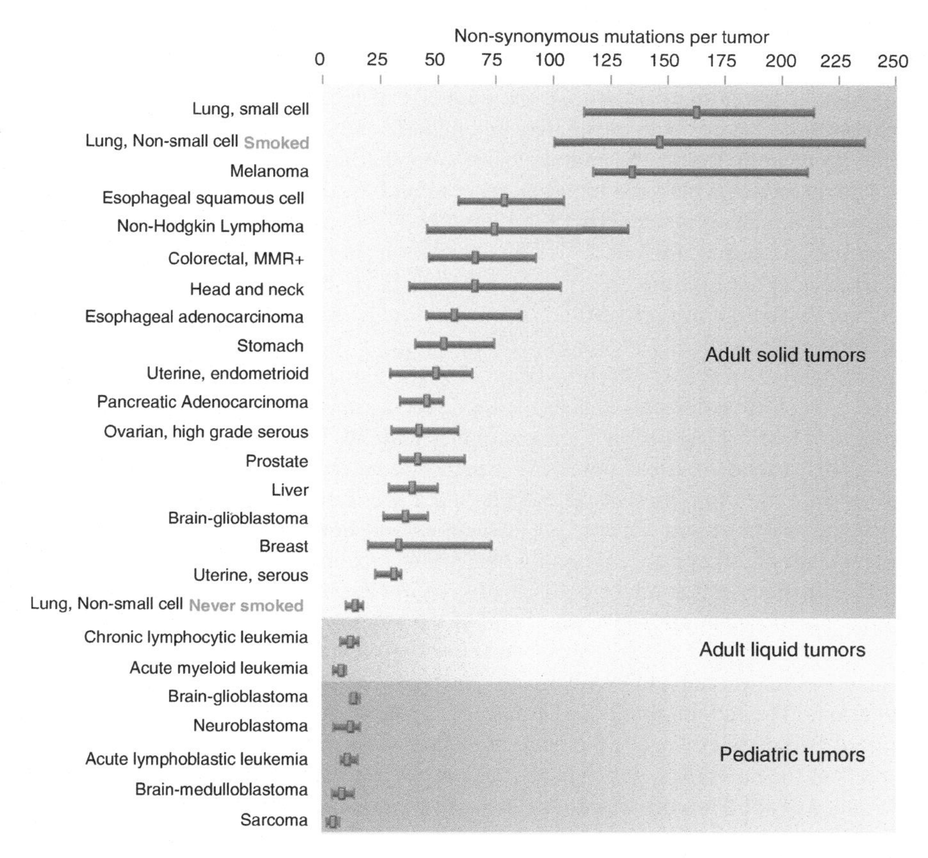

Fig. 5.1 The number of mutations per tumor in various types of cancer. *Red markers* indicate the median number of non-synonymous mutations per tumor; the *blue bar* spans the first and third quartiles. Colorectal-MMR+, mismatch repair-proficient colorectal adenocarcinoma; mismatch repair-deficient colorectal cancers, which often exhibit thousands of mutations, are not shown. This figure is based on an illustration in Vogelstein et al. *Science* **339**, 1546–1558 (2013)

smoke and ultraviolet radiation, respectively. Even in the absence of known mutagens, the common adult tumors harbor more mutations than the tumors that tend to arise in children. This observation reflects the chronological component of tumorigenesis; mutations occur in evolving neoplasms over time as a function of cell division. Tumors that manifest as solid cancers in the elderly most often arise in highly proliferative tissues and develop over decades. The large number of cell divisions that occur over an extended period of time leads to the accumulation of a relatively large number of mutations. In contrast, the solid cancers observed primarily in children tend to arise in tissues that are inherently less proliferative throughout life, such as brain tissue. Such tumors are relatively rare, but when they do arise, tend to develop in a much shorter time period, suggesting that they require fewer mutations to grow. Leukemias arise in both pediatric and adult populations, and in either case typically harbor relatively small numbers of mutations. This is because the bone marrow compartments in which leukemia develops are less proliferative (ie. contain fewer stem cells) than the epithelia of the liver or colon. At the other extreme are cancers with mismatch repair deficiency. Such tumors, which most often occur in the colon and endometrium, often harbor thousands of mutations.

The relationship between mutation number and the timing and incidence of various types of cancer is supported by a large body of epidemiological evidence. As described in Chap. 1, there is a striking correlation between the number of stem cell divisions and the lifetime risk of cancer across all tissues. The most common cancers are those that primarily afflict older individuals. Accordingly, the incidence of carcinomas dramatically increases with age, with a 100-fold increase in incidence occurring over an average lifetime (Fig. 5.2). The clonal evolution of common solid tumors, such as colorectal cancer, occurs over a time frame that is measured in decades. The final expansion of cancer clones with 30–70 subtle mutations is manifest as disease late in life. Conversely, cancer occurs much less often in young people, and the rare tumors that do arise harbor fewer mutations. The most common malignancies in young patients are leukemias and brain cancers. These pediatric cancers harbor, on average, 10 single nucleotide substitutions.

The distinct mutational requirements of different cancers are reflected in mutagen-exposed cohorts. The survivors of the atomic bombings of Hiroshima and Nagasaki during World War II have been closely followed over long periods of time. Ionizing radiation causes DNA damage. The repair of these lesions can leave behind mutations. The radiation-exposed cohort of Japanese atomic bomb survivors experienced two distinct waves of cancer incidence. Leukemias began to appear within 3 years of the bombings, with a peak incidence 7 years after exposure. An increased incidence of solid tumors was not evident until more than 10 years after exposure, a

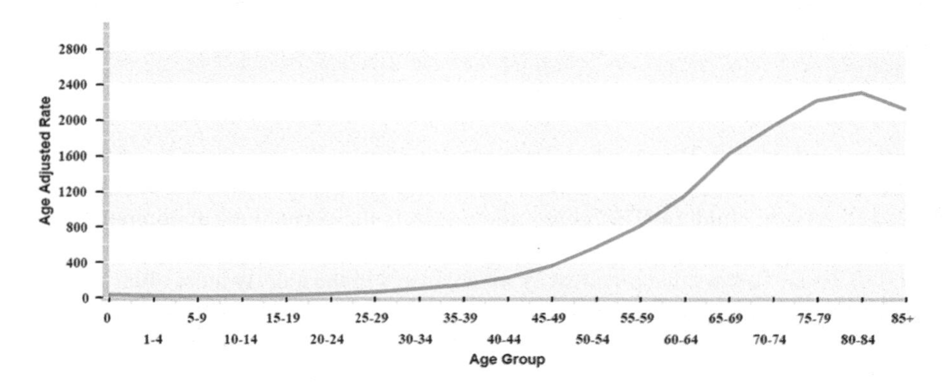

Fig. 5.2 Cancer incidence, by age group. The overall incidence of cancer at all sites rises with increasing age and peaks around age 80. Incidence rates include both sexes and all races, are per 100,000 and are from surveys dating from 1975 to 2012, age-adjusted to the 2000 US population. Primary data are from the Surveillance, Epidemiology and End results program (SEER), of the National Cancer Institute

period that allowed the requisite number of cell divisions, and additional mutations, to accumulate.

What Is the Significance of the Mutations That Are Found in Cancers?

As described in Chap. 1, there are two major types of mutations: passengers and drivers. Driver mutations impart a selective growth advantage and are therefore required for tumor development. Driver mutations affect proto-oncogenes and tumor suppressor genes. The cancer-associated alleles of these genes are sometimes accordingly referred to as *driver genes* or *mut-driver genes*.[1] In contrast to driver mutations, passenger mutations do not impart any growth advantage and do not directly participate in tumorigenesis. Many passenger mutations occur in the vast regions of the genome that do not encode proteins; such mutations are not detected in studies that rely on whole exome sequencing.

Passenger and driver mutations are defined by their effects on growth, not by the genes in which they occur. Passenger mutations can and do occur in tumor suppressor genes, proto-oncogenes and their cancer associated alleles. The extent to which this occurs is simply related to gene size. Larger genes represent larger targets for the stochastic processes that result in mutagenesis. With 18 exons spanning 138 kb on chromosome 5, *APC* is an example of a large cancer gene that frequently accumulates passenger mutations. Importantly, only the mutations that cause truncation of the open reading frame within the first 1600 codons appear to promote tumorigenesis. Most of the other mutations that arise in *APC* are passengers. By definition, passenger mutations do not confer a selective advantage and therefore do not contribute to tumorigenesis, even when they occur in a known driver gene.

In common cancers that harbor many mutations, passengers far outnumber drivers. In many cases, prior functional studies can be used to distinguish one category of mutation from another. A mutation that occurs in a functionally defined and frequently mutated cancer gene such as *TP53* or *KRAS* is generally most straightforward to categorize. Driver mutations in *TP53* tend to occur in the exons that encode the DNA binding domain and result in the loss of transcriptional transactivation; driver mutations in *KRAS* recurrently affect amino acid residues in a regulatory domain and result in constitutive activation.

In the lexicon of tumor genome topography (Fig. 5.3), frequently mutated cancer genes such as *TP53* and *KRAS* are referred to as mutational *mountains*. Many other cancer genes are mutated recurrently, but in relatively small numbers of tumors. Such mutant alleles represent relative mutational *hills* in the cancer genome land-

[1] 'Driver gene' and 'mut-driver gene' are synonyms for the more generic term 'cancer gene' that is used throughout this book. The term mut-driver gene was coined by Kinzler and Vogelstein to distinguish such genes from *epi-driver* genes, which are cancer genes that are functionally altered by epigenetic mechanisms.

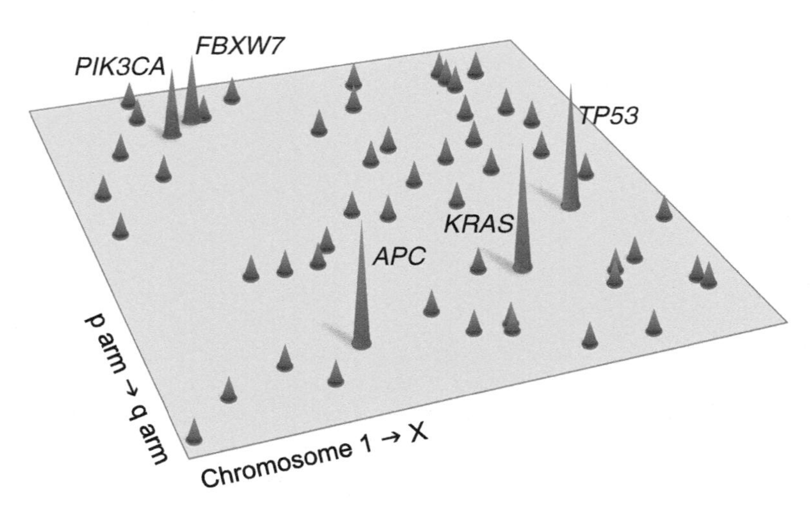

Fig. 5.3 The landscape of the cancer genome: mountains, hills and flatlands. A two-dimensional map of the colorectal cancer genome landscape shows the cancer genes positioned according to their chromosomal locations. Five gene 'mountains' are mutated in a large proportion of tumors, the remaining 'hills' represent genes that are mutated less frequently. This map indicates the frequency of mutations in many samples; any given two tumors will have a different combination of mutations. The landscapes of other types of cancer are similarly defined by mountains, hills and intervening 'flatlands', which can be defined as regions of the genome that harbor only passenger mutations. This figure is based on an illustration in Wood et al. *Science* 318, 1108–1113 (2007)

scape. In the case of these less frequently mutated genes, informative functional data is typically lacking. Distinguishing such driver mutations from more numerous passenger mutations can be a challenge.

Which of the less frequent mutations represent real driver genes? Statistical tools and structure-based algorithms have been devised to identify probable driver mutations and thereby define driver genes. For example, the absolute mutation frequency in the coding sequences of a given gene, normalized to the total size of all of the exons and corrected for the predicted functional impact of the specific mutations observed, can provide some indication of whether a gene might represent a driver. In practice, methods based solely on mutation frequency have proved to be unreliable. An alternative method for driver gene evaluation, proposed by Vogelstein, Kinzler and their colleagues, relies not on the number of mutations that occur in a gene, but on the patterns and characteristics of these mutations. Mutations in validated oncogenes tend to be missense mutations at recurrent positions. If more than 20 % of identified mutations in a given gene are at positions that are recurrently altered in that type of cancer, that gene is probably an oncogene. In the case of validated tumor suppressor genes, more than 20 % of the mutations cause functional inactivation or loss of the encoded protein. This method of ratiometric analysis is known as the *20/20 rule*. All well-documented cancer genes easily meet these lenient criteria. If the patterns of mutation fail to fulfill these criteria – for example in the case of a prospective proto-oncogene that harbors few recurrent mutations or a prospective tumor suppressor gene that is only rarely inactivated – then the gene in question is unlikely to be a true cancer gene.

When Do Cancer-Associated Mutations Occur?

The complete analysis of a cancer genome represents, in essence, a historical record of the alterations that accumulated in the normal precursor cells and in their progeny over many generations. The majority of cancer-associated mutations are passengers that did not directly contribute to tumor growth. Although they do not actively participate in tumorigenesis, passenger mutations can provide information about the history of a given neoplasm. Because mutations arise spontaneously at a constant and measurable rate, the absolute number of mutations in a tumor provides, in essence, a clock that can indicate how long a tumor cell population has been growing and dividing.

Linear regression analysis of the relationship between mutational burden and the age of the patient suggest that more than half of all somatic mutations occur prior to the onset of neoplastic growth in self-renewing tissues. Indeed, passenger mutations are known to be present in proliferative tissues that are phenotypically normal. Therefore, many mutations predate tumors, and arise during the course of normal cell proliferation. Stem cells in older people have undergone more generations of growth than stem cells in younger people and therefore harbor more mutations. This explains why a tumor found in an elderly patient will probably have more mutations than the same type of tumor that develops in a younger individual.

Interestingly, driver mutations can also be found in some tissues that appear normal under the microscope. In skin, driver mutations in genes such as *NOTCH1* have been found in heavily sun-exposed sites, prior to the onset of any histologically apparent neoplastic growth. Such mutations appear in as many as 20 % of cells, indicating that they were harbored in clones that expanded as a result of positive selective pressure. Studies of tissues chronically exposed to environmental mutagens provide insight into the evolutionary processes that can occur, even as these tissues that retain their normal architecture prior to the onset of tumor growth.

In the colon, the ultimate rate limiting step for tumor growth is mutational inactivation of the tumor suppressor *APC* in epithelial cells. Accordingly known as a gatekeeper mutation, the loss of *APC* defines the point at which normal proliferative cells first acquire the functional capability to expand beyond their normal bounds and form a histologically definable lesion. In understanding the molecular evolution of a hypothetical colorectal cancer, it is important to understand that the truncation of the *APC* open reading frame was probably not the first mutation to be acquired by that initial tumor cell. All of the mutations present in the initial cell that lost *APC* will be present in the small neoplasm that results, as well as in the large tumor that becomes clinically apparent decades later. Older individuals will have accumulated a larger number of mutations in their normal precursors, and will thus have more mutations in their eventual tumors.

How Many Different Cancer Genes Are There?

Each of the 20,000 protein-encoding genes in the human genome has been sequenced in thousands of individual tumors from many different patients. While hundreds of genes have been associated with the growth of cancer cells – whether by sequencing, chromosome analysis, functional assay or by RNA and protein expression analysis – a surprisingly small number of these genes have been conclusively shown to provide a selective advantage when altered in the genome of evolving cancer clones. In 2013, Kinzler and Vogelstein used the 20/20 rule to define a set of high probability cancer genes from the many more genes that had been less stringently associated with cancers. They concluded that a total of 125 mut-driver genes are created by subtle genetic alterations. Of the cancer genes created by single nucleotide substitutions or small indels, 71 are tumor suppressor genes and 54 are oncogenes. An additional set of 10 oncogenes that are recurrently amplified and three tumor suppressor genes that are frequently lost from the cancer genome within regions of homozygous deletion was also defined. According to this incisive analysis, the vast majority of all human cancers can be attributed to 138 genes.[2] This calculation implies that about 0.7 % of human protein-coding genes are cancer genes.

All of the cancer genomes that have been evaluated to date represent a small fraction of the annual cancer incidence in the US. How completely does the existing data reflect the total contribution of human genes to cancer? How many cancer genes remain to be discovered? While there are statistical approaches to answering these related questions, an inspection of recent cancer exome sequencing results readily provides a simple answer. With rapidly increasing regularity, assessments of new cancer genomes reveal only those cancer genes that have already been described. As a result, the rate of discovery of new cancer genes appears to be rapidly reaching a plateau. It is highly unlikely that new genetic mountains remain to be discovered in the genomic landscapes of the most common kinds of cancer.

The high-throughput, high-depth sequencing technologies that have enabled the complete, rapid and cost-effective analysis of the cancer genome have transformed the field of molecular oncology. However, it is worth noting that of the 125 cancer genes validated by the 20/20 rule and the 13 genes recurrently found in amplicons or deletions, over 70 % had been previously identified by the diverse – and dauntingly laborious and time-consuming – experimental approaches that predated the era of unbiased exome and genome sequencing. Most oncogenes were discovered on the basis of their ability to confer unusual growth properties to cultured cells (Chap. 2); most tumor suppressors were identified by iterative mapping and candidate gene sequencing and subsequent functional characterization (Chap. 3). That these indirect or low resolution approaches uncovered the majority of all cancer genes is a testament to the ingenuity, creativity and tenacity of the individuals and teams who pioneered molecular cancer research.

[2] Several additional high-probability cancer genes have been described since this 2013 study.

How Many Cancer Genes Are Required for the Development of Cancer?

About 30–70 mutations can be found in the protein-coding genes of the most common types of cancer. Some types of cancer have more mutations than this average number, some have fewer. Only a small proportion of these are drivers. How many driver mutations are required for the full evolution of a deadly cancer?

This fundamental question predates our understanding of molecular genetics. Classic epidemiologic studies focused on the readily apparent relationship between age and cancer incidence and mortality. In the early 1950s, Nordling and then Armitage and Doll examined age-specific mortality rates for diverse types of cancer. These seminal population-based studies suggested that cancers ultimately result from the successive accumulation of five to eight cellular changes, which we now understand to be genetic alterations. Later estimates derived from molecular studies of individual genes in highly mutated cancers, which we now know to be atypical, were much higher – in some cases by many orders of magnitude.

Modern genetic analysis has confirmed the early epidemiologic predictions, for the most part. Common adult tumors of the pancreas, colon, breast and brain most often are observed to have three to six mutational variants of the 138 cancer genes that have been identified to date; most of these observed mutations in cancer genes are thought to represent true driver mutations. Epidemiologic data can now be analyzed in tandem with genome sequence data. Based on this dual approach, some of the early population-based estimates have been refined and revised. Cristian Tomasetti and Bert Vogelstein have recently calculated that only three driver mutations are required for common lung and colorectal cancers.

No two tumors are genetically identical, but tumors that occur in the same tissue often share common cancer genes. For example, colorectal cancers frequently harbor mutations in *APC*, *TP53*, *KRAS*, *PIK3CA* and *FBXW7*, which accordingly represent the five 'mountains' in the colorectal tumor landscape (Fig. 5.3). The majority of colorectal cancers (about 90 %) harbor a truncating mutation in *APC*. *TP53* and *KRAS* are also very commonly mutated in colorectal tumors, while mutations in *PIK3CA* and *FBXW7* are found less frequently, and thus represent smaller mountains in the colorectal cancer landscape. Standing in the shadows of these looming mountains are the many hills that represent genes that are less frequently altered in the colorectal cancer genome. Based on current estimates, a combination of three driver mutations corresponding to mountains or hills provides a sufficient selective advantage for the eventual development of a small neoplasm into a colorectal cancer.

Cancer Genetics Shapes Our Understanding of Metastasis

A metastasis is a cancer that has spread from its original site to another site in the body. The process of metastasis causes the transformation of a cancer from a highly localized illness to a more systemic one. Once a cancer has metastasized to multiple sites, it is in most cases incurable. Most cancer mortality is attributable to metastatic disease.

If cancer is considered as a step-wise progression of disease states, metastasis is the final step. In the colorectal epithelia, the steps of neoplastic tumor growth have been clearly defined by discrete precursor lesions that harbor specific cancer gene mutations. The smallest detectable lesions typically harbor inactivating *APC* mutations, while subsequent adenomas often activate the proto-oncogene *KRAS*. Mutational loss of *TP53* frequently accompanies the critical transition from a benign adenoma to an invasive cancer. Based on this highly enlightening model, originally proposed by Fearon and Vogelstein, it would seem reasonable to expect that a similar rate-limiting genetic alteration, or series of alterations, might facilitate metastasis. For many years, researchers have diligently sought cancer genes that are distinctly required for metastasis. Cancer gene mutations mark cellular pathways and processes that underlie newly acquired cellular phenotypes, and therefore represent prospective targets for new therapies. The identification of stage-specific genetic mutations that confer distinct metastatic phenotypes could suggest new avenues to treat highly lethal, late-stage tumors. The search for these metastasis genes has been accordingly driven by a sense of urgency. But the question remains: do such genes exist?

Cancers most commonly metastasize to the bone, brain, liver and lung via the bloodstream and lymphatic vessels. As they spread to these anatomically distant sites, metastatic cancer cells typically retain the general morphology, molecular marker profile and karyotype of the cells in the corresponding primary tumor. Phenotypically, metastatic cells resemble the cells in the large tumors from which they arose. It has therefore remained unclear if metastasis is a distinct stage that represents the acquisition of new cellular phenotypes, or whether metastasis is simply the inevitable result of an ever-expanding cell population with aggressive growth characteristics.

One would expect a metastasis gene to be exclusively and recurrently mutated in metastatic tumors, while the normal germline sequence would be retained in the corresponding primary tumors as well as in tumors that have not yet metastasized. Despite intensive study, such mutations have not been conclusively identified. It therefore seems possible that there are no cancer genes that specifically promote metastasis.

Large, late stage tumors constantly release many cells into the blood. Most of these circulating tumor cells die, but a very small fraction survive to proliferate and found colonies in distant tissues. The development of a detectable metastatic tumor could thus be the result of stochastic process, rather than a discrete genetic event. If this is true, then the overall probability that a given tumor will metastasize would be a function of the total number of cells in circulation and the very low probability that any one of them will lodge at a site that provides the minimal requirements for continued proliferation.

Tumors Are Genetically Heterogenous

Mutations arise as a byproduct of cell division. As a result, any population of proliferating cells will become progressively more genetically diverse with each successive generation. In advanced cancers, there is typically a very large population of proliferating cells that are many generations removed from the original founder cell. Such tumors will exhibit an accordingly high level of *intratumoral genetic heterogeneity*. A sample taken from one portion of a large tumor will harbor some unique mutations that are not present in a sample taken from another part of the tumor. Cells from sites within a tumor that are spatially distant will exhibit a larger number of genetic differences than cells that are closer together, simply because cells become increasingly separated as they become further removed from a common ancestor. This concept can be illustrated as an evolutionary tree, with branch points that correspond to new somatic mutations (Fig. 5.4).

Most of the mutations that are found within a tumor will be present in all cells. Many of these mutations were therefore present in the founder cell, while others could have arisen at an early point in the clonal evolution process. As the majority of mutations in most cancers are passengers, the largest proportion of intratumoral heterogeneity involves passenger mutations that vary from cell to cell. In contrast, driver genes are much more likely to be present in most or all cells, because they contributed the early rate-limiting stages of tumor growth.

Secondary tumors that arise at anatomically distant sites during the late stages of disease exhibit a large degree of *intermetastatic genetic heterogeneity*. This is because each metastasis is founded by a single cell that escaped from an advanced primary tumor. Each metastasis in a patient is therefore a descendant of a distinct region of a heterogeneous primary tumor, and is therefore unique. Again, in the majority of cases, the mutations that differ from one metastatic tumor to another in the same patient are mostly passenger mutations. In common cancers, a single metastatic lesion may have 20 mutations in every cell that are not shared by other metastases in the same patient.

As the cells in metastatic tumors continue to proliferate, additional mutations continue to accumulate, and each tumor will successively become more heterogeneous as it becomes larger. This level of heterogeneity, known as *intrametastatic genetic heterogeneity*, arises by the same simple process that dictates intratumoral genetic heterogeneity.

The high degree of genetic heterogeneity that exists in late stage and often widely disseminated cancers often poses a significant obstacle to effective therapy. Tumor heterogeneity largely reflects the distribution by expanding subclones of newly arising passenger mutations. These mutations by definition do not provide a selective advantage during tumorigenesis, but they are not necessarily functionally inert. Some passenger mtuations can have phenotypic effects, even if they are not directly relevant to tumor growth at that time of their occurence. Together, all of the passenger mutations in a late stage tumor represent a reserve pool of phenotypic heterogeneity. Individual mutations could become relevant to continued cell growth if the tumor experiences a new environmental challenge.

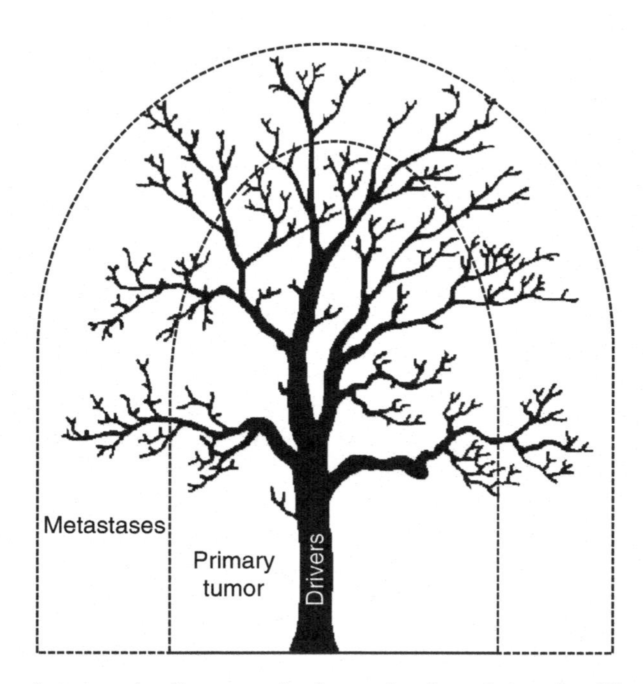

Fig. 5.4 Tumor heterogeneity. Cancers evolve from a clonal population of proliferative cells that becomes increasingly more genetically heterogeneous with each successive generation. The evolution of somatic mutations in cancer can be illustrated in the form of a tree. The original driver mutations present in the first cells of a tumor are represented by the trunk. These drivers feed the growth of every part of the tree. The branches are somatic mutations that arise later, as a product of cell division, and come to define distinct subpopulations within the tumor. The majority of these mutations are passengers. Metastases develop from founder cells that differ substantially from one another, and therefore exhibit a large degree of intermetastatic genetic heterogeneity

Metastatic tumors are most often non-resectable, and must therefore be treated with a systemic chemotherapeutic agent or a combination of agents. If a therapeutic regimen creates an altered local environment that favors new phenotypic traits, some passenger mutations may provide a new selective advantage to the distinct cell subpopulations that harbor them. Thus, rare passenger mutations present in small numbers of tumor cells may increase drug resistance. These populations will be more likely to survive the therapeutic insult and continue to grow as other subclones are killed. These passengers can, in effect, become drivers under a new set of environmental conditions. Larger tumors have more passenger mutations and are composed of more subclones that can potentially survive therapy. Accordingly, tumor heterogeneity has been found to correlate with disease recurrence after therapy.

Beyond the Exome: The 'Dark Matter' of the Cancer Genome

According to the cancer gene theory, cancer in all of its forms is a genetic disease, shaped by mutations. It may therefore be surprising that some types of cancers, particularly pediatric cancers, are characterized by a very low number of driver gene mutations. Indeed, there are examples of unusual tumors in which no driver gene mutations have been detected. How could such tumors possibly arise? One simple possibility is that current sequencing methods are systematically failing to detect driver mutations.

Modern cancer genome analysis has thus far been primarily focused on the genes that encode and express proteins, the exome. For practical reasons, investigators willfully ignore 98.5 % of the genome. Experience has shown that the exome will harbor the majority of the mutations that provide positive selection during tumorigenesis, whereas sequence analysis of the whole genome remains more technically challenging and accordingly more expensive. DNA sequencing is remarkably facile and efficient, but some mutations are not routinely captured by current methods and approaches. Kinzler and Vogelstein have appropriated the cosmological term *'dark matter'* to refer to those regions of the cancer genome that are currently unseen.

What might constitute genomic dark matter? One possibility is the portion of the genome that is involved in the regulation of protein-encoding genes. Regulatory elements such as promoters and enhancers control levels of RNA and protein expression and thereby have a large influence on gene function. An example of a cancer-associated mutation that affects a regulatory element was discovered upon expanded genomic analysis of melanomas. In these tumors, functional mutations involve the promoter region of the gene *TERT*, which encodes the catalytic subunit of the enzyme telomerase. As described in Chap. 4, telomerase is required for telomere maintenance and this activity is upregulated in most cancers. The *TERT* promoter mutations found in melanomas increased the transcription of *TERT*-encoded RNAs, and therefore caused increased telomerase activity.

Other possibilities abound. The prevailing view of what exactly constitutes a functional genetic unit has expanded substantially. Large-scale analyses of expressed RNAs have revealed the human genome to be much more extensively transcribed and functionally regulated than was previously appreciated. Overall, experimental evidence suggests a higher level of biochemical activity than would be predicted if only protein coding regions of the genome were functionally significant. The Encyclopedia of DNA Elements (ENCODE) project completed in 2012 determined that over 80 % of the genome is functional in some quantifiable respect; 62 % of genomic DNA is actively transcribed into RNA.

What is the function of all this RNA? Are these transcripts somehow involved in cancer? These questions are important, but they remain incompletely answered. At least 50 % of the genome is composed of mobile DNA elements that are retroviral in origin and may be parasitic in nature, functional in the biochemical sense, but not necessarily contributing to the cellular phenotypes most relevant to cancer. However, the sheer mass of RNA produced, and the energy required to produce it, suggests that there are physiological roles for many regions of the genome outside the protein-encoding genes that have been most extensively studied. It is therefore possible that some of the 'missing' mutations that provide positive selection for tumor growth might be located in these vast and underexplored regions of the genome.

Another potential source of dark matter, as defined by Kinzler and Vogelstein, is not genetic in essence, but epigenetic. Chromosomes are not a merely a static repository of DNA sequences. Chromosomes are made of chromatin, a highly dynamic store of information both in the form of ordered DNA bases and in the covalent modifications to both DNA and to the proteins that are tightly associated with them. Understanding which among these myriad heritable protein and DNA modifications contribute to the positive selection of cancer cell clones – and which may thus represent *epi-driver* alterations – remains an important challenge for the future.

A Summary: The Genome of a Cancer Cell

DNA sequencing studies have provided a wealth of information about the genome of a typical cancer cell. Here is a brief synopsis of what we know:

Most mutations that cause cancer are subtle, with the notable exception of the chromosomal rearrangements that are predominantly involved in mesenchymal and liquid tumors. Common solid tumors have 30–70 mutations, on average. Most of these mutations are passengers that do not contribute to the process of tumorigenesis. The total number of mutations in a given type of tumor correlates with the age of the patient. Many of the mutations present in a cancer were originally present in the normal precursor cell. There are about 140 different cancer genes that provide a selective advantage to expanding cell clones, and thus drive tumorigenesis. Therefore, about 0.7 % of protein encoding genes in the human genome are cancer genes that can be altered by driver mutations. Between two and seven driver mutations are required for the evolution of most tumors; just three are thought to be required for common tumors in the lung and colon. Metastatic lesions do not appear to have distinct cancer genes compared to the preceding primary tumors. Genetic heterogeneity in primary and secondary tumors can affect the response to systemic therapies.

Further Reading

Armitage T, Doll R (1954) The age distribution of cancer and a multi-stage theory of carcinogenesis. Br J Cancer 8:1–12

ENCODE project consortium (2012) An integrated encyclopedia of DNA elements in the human genome. Nature 489:57–74

Garraway LA, Lander ES (2013) Lessons from the cancer genome. Cell 153:17–37

Martincorena I, Roshan A, Gerstung M, Ellis P, Van Loo P, McLaren S et al (2015) Tumor evolution. High burden and pervasive positive selection of somatic mutations in normal human skin. Science 348:880–886

Meyerson M, Gabriel S, Getz G (2010) Advances in understanding cancer genomes through second-generation sequencing. Nat Rev Genet 11:685–696

Nordling CO (1953) A new theory on cancer inducing mechanism. Br J Cancer 7:68–72

Stratton MR, Campbell PJ, Futreal PA (2009) The cancer genome. Nature 458:719–724

Tomasetti C, Vogelstein B, Parmigiani G (2013) Half or more of the somatic mutations in cancers of self-renewing tissues originate prior to tumor initiation. Proc Natl Acad Sci U S A 110:1999–2004

Tomasetti C, Marchionni L, Nowak MA, Parmigiani G, Vogelstein B (2015) Only three driver gene mutations are required for the development of lung and colorectal cancers. Proc Natl Acad Sci U S A 112:118–123

Vogelstein B, Papadopoulos N, Velculescu VE, Zhou S, Diaz LA Jr, Kinzler KW (2013) Cancer genome landscapes. Science 339:1546–1558

Chapter 6
Cancer Gene Pathways

What Are Cancer Gene Pathways?

The previous chapters have described what cancer genes *are* and how they are acquired. But what do cancer genes *do*? How does the inactivation of tumor suppressor genes and activation of proto-oncogenes cause proliferating cells to evolve into cancers? The answer to this question has been revealed by the functional analysis of the proteins encoded by cancer genes and their wild type counterparts.

Individual proteins do not typically perform their functions in isolation, but rather operate in functional units composed of groups or complexes of proteins that work together towards a common purpose. Multi-protein units often catalyze a sequence of biochemical reactions that occur serially, and these reactions can span several compartments within the cell. Because of the linearity and directionality of these reactions, the multi-protein units that carry them out are often referred to as pathways.

Cancer genes populate the cellular pathways that control three fundamental cellular processes: (1) the determination of *cell fate*, (2) the optimization of *cell survival*, and (3) *genome maintenance*. Cell fate refers to the processes by which stem cells are instructed to stop proliferating and to differentiate into the highly specialized cells that populate mature tissues. Cell fates are physiologically determined during embryonic development and in the regenerative tissues of the adult. The survival of proliferating cells is determined by their programmed responses to local conditions. When normal cells encounter microenvironmental conditions that are sensed as suboptimal or stressful, they arrest their growth, or, in some cases they undergo a form of controlled cell death known as *apoptosis*. Genome maintenance refers to the mechanisms that cells employ to sense and repair damaged DNA.

Some cellular pathways appear to be exclusively dedicated to one of these core processes. Other pathways are able to influence more than one process. For example, the gene that is mutated in the greatest proportion of cancers, *TP53*, defines a multifunctional pathway that can influence cell fate, cell survival, and impact genome maintenance.

F. Bunz, *Principles of Cancer Genetics*, DOI 10.1007/978-94-017-7484-0_6

To understand the roles that *TP53* and other cancer genes play in the evolution of cancer cell clones, it is helpful to appreciate the extent to which normal cells interact with, and are controlled by, their microenvironment. In normal regenerative tissues, cells grow and divide in response to myriad cues, or signals. The outer membrane of most cells is in direct contact with the extracellular matrix, with extracellular fluid and with neighboring cells. Various molecules traverse these routes carrying information. Diverse signals instruct cells to grow or to stop growing, to differentiate and mature or – in some cases – to die. Cells in the proliferative compartments of the human body are literally bathed in signals.

Signals arise from many extracellular sources and are transmitted by several types of molecules. The diversity of cell signaling pathways can be exemplified by three types of signaling molecules: cytokines, free radicals and hormones. Local signals are produced by activated inflammatory cells in the form of small water-soluble proteins known as *cytokines*. Cytokines typically bind specific receptors on the cell surface and are potent stimulators of cell growth as well as triggers of cell death. The free-radical *nitric oxide* (NO) is a small signaling molecule that has the ability to cross numerous anatomical boundaries and affect virtually every cellular function. NO is highly unstable in nature, and its levels can therefore rapidly change to provide highly dynamic signals. *Hormones* secreted by the endocrine system are potent signals that affect the function of distant cells. For example, insulin secreted by the islet cells of the pancreas stimulates the uptake of glucose by hepatocytes in the liver, and the growth of adipocytes that compose fatty tissues. Cytokines, free radicals, and hormones are examples of signaling molecules that facilitate communication between one cell type and another.

Regulatory signals also arise from intracellular sources. The cell growth and division cycle is highly regulated and closely monitored. The sequential stages of the cell cycle, particularly the entry into S-phase and mitosis, are exquisitely sensitive to damaged chromosomes and to stalled DNA replication forks. Interruption of cell cycle progression triggers vigorous cellular responses that strongly affect proliferation and survival.

Cellular pathways are the conduits by which these diverse signals affect proliferating cells. Mutations in cancer genes and the pathways they control alter the cell's ability to appropriately respond to the signals that would otherwise determine its fate, decrease its survival potential in adverse conditions and allow it to properly maintain its chromosomes. These genetic alterations cause the phenotypes that we can recognize as growth and invasion, which eventually lead to cancer morbidity. The fundamental phenotypic traits of cancer cells are listed below. Each cancer ultimately acquires at least one of these traits.

- Loss of the ability to transition from a proliferative, undifferentiated state to a terminally differentiated state, in which the cell has exited the cell cycle. An undifferentiated cancer cell keeps growing at a point where a normal cell would stop dividing and become a functionally defined adult cell.

- Gain of the ability to survive in adverse environments. A cancer cell lives and continues to proliferate in inhospitable sites where a normal cell would become quiescent or die.
- Loss of the ability to maintain a stable genome. A cancer cell continues to proliferate with damaged DNA so that its progeny accumulate mutations, whereas a normal cell would initiate a coordinated response to DNA damage and initiate DNA repair.

Cellular Pathways Are Defined by Protein-Protein Interactions

Biochemical reactions within proliferating cells regulate their growth, maturation and death. Upstream pathways monitor both intracellular and extracellular environments, and create downstream signals that allow cells to adapt to changing physiologic states. Cellular signaling pathways transmit information between these upstream sensors and downstream effectors. The resultant flow of information within the cell allows it to respond to a dynamic environment.

The pathways that dictate cellular physiology are numerous and complex. Consider an electronic microprocessor that contains integrated circuits. Microprocessors receive many inputs in the form of electrical currents. Some of these currents are amplified, others are quenched or transformed. The circuitry of the microprocessor integrates many inputs and generates an organized output. Like microprocessors, the signaling pathways of the cell are highly integrative and interconnected circuits that act as conduits of information (Fig. 6.1).

Proteins are the primary nodes of the cellular pathways that are defective in cancer. Proteins communicate with one another through direct, physical interactions. As a result of these types of interactions, one protein can be structurally and functionally altered by another.

The majority of proteins involved in cancer gene pathways are enzymes that catalyze the covalent modification of other proteins on specific amino acid residues. A covalent modification to an existing protein is known as a *post-translational modification*. There are many ways in which proteins can be post-translationally modified; several of the most impactful types of modifications are listed on Table 6.1.

The common covalent protein modifications are reversible. In each of these cases, the covalent attachment of the modification to a specific amino acid residue is catalyzed by one enzyme, and the reverse reaction is catalyzed by a second, distinct enzyme. Covalent posttranslational modifications can thus define two distinct states (Fig. 6.2). Because the enzymes that add and remove modifications (depicted as ON and OFF enzymes respectively, in Fig. 6.2) are distinct, one state is usually strongly favored over the other, depending on which modifying enzyme is most active. The transition from one state to another can have several interrelated effects:

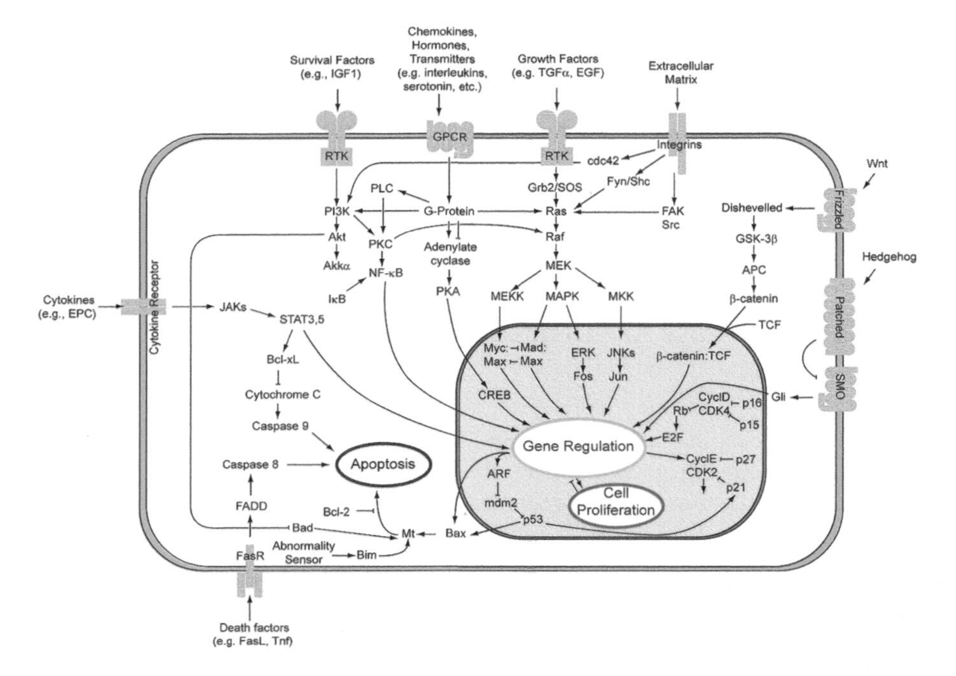

Fig. 6.1 Overview of cell signaling pathways. Human cells have highly integrated signaling pathways that sense changes in the external and internal environments. These signaling pathways allow cells to maintain a stable genome, control their developmental fate and adjust their potential for survival. Many of these pathways are recurrently altered by mutations during tumorigenesis (From Wikimedia Commons, uploaded by user Roadnottaken)

Structural effects. Many modifications cause a change in either the tertiary structure (the three dimensional protein conformation) of a protein, or in the quaternary structure of a multiprotein complex.

Functional effects. The structure and function of any protein are inextricably interrelated. Modifications that change protein structure therefore usually alter change protein function. In the case of proteins that are enzymes, modifications can change the activity of the catalytic domain, often by altering the ability of the substrate to bind. Modifications can either increase catalytic activity or decrease catalytic activity, depending on the protein, the location of the modification and the modifying group.

Localization. Modifications can affect the trafficking of a protein within the cell, and thereby affect its localization. Altered localization can affect access to interacting proteins, or in the case of modifying enzymes, to substrates.

Stabilization. Modifications can dramatically alter the half-life of a protein. Proteins can be either stabilized or destabilized as a result of modifications.

Table 6.1 Reversible protein modifications

Molecule	Size	Target	"ON" enzyme	"OFF" enzyme
Phosphate group **$-PO_3$**	79 Da	Ser, Thr, Tyr	Protein kinase	Protein phosphatase
Methyl group – **CH_3**	15 Da	Arg, Lys	Protein methyltransferase	Protein demethylase
Acetyl group-**$COCH_3$**	43 Da	Lys	Protein acetylase	Protein deacetylase
Ubiquitin-**polypeptide**	8.5 kDa	Lys	Multiple sequential enzymes	De-ubiquitinase
Small Ubiquitin-related modifier (SUMO) **-polypeptide**	10–11 kDa	Lys	Multiple sequential enzymes	SUMO isopeptidases

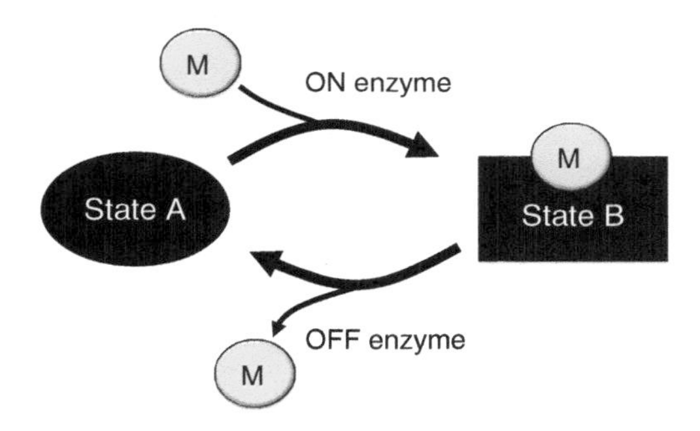

Fig. 6.2 The covalent modification of a protein reversibly alters its functional state. A hypothetical protein exists in two states, A and B. The transition from state A to B is mediated by the addition of a modifying group (M, shown in *yellow*) to an amino acid residue. This reaction is catalyzed by a hypothetical "ON" enzyme. The reverse reaction, resulting in the removal of the modification and the transition from state B to state A, is catalyzed by a distinct "OFF" enzyme. Either state A or state B can be the activated state, depending on the protein and the modifying molecule. (Note that "ON" and "OFF" states depicted here simply refer to the presence or absence of a hypothetical post-translational modification; a pathway that includes such a protein might be upregulated or downregulated by the presence of the covalent modification)

Individual Biochemical Reactions, Multistep Pathways, and Networks

The covalent modification of an individual protein is a single step in the series of biochemical reactions that define a pathway. Most pathways have several steps that involve multiple proteins and modifying molecules (Fig. 6.3). When compared with a single biochemical reaction, a complex series of reactions has several added functional attributes. First, a higher order of organization significantly increases the extent to which a response to a stimulus can be controlled. Second, the multistep nature of most pathways allows a greater range of signal strength – known as the amplitude of the signal – than could be transmitted by a single reaction. Third, a

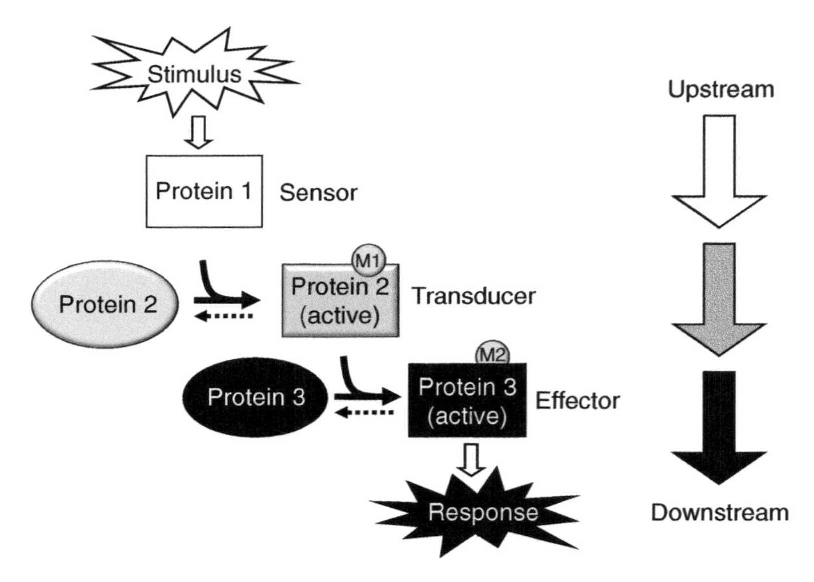

Fig. 6.3 A generic pathway. Several features that are common to many cellular pathways are shown. All pathways are characterized by directionality; signals are said to be transduced from an upstream stimulus to a downstream response. This hypothetical pathway is activated by a stimulus that activates a sensor (Protein 1). This sensor protein then adds a modification (M1, shown in *yellow*) to a second protein (Protein 2), causing it to become catalytically active. Once activated, Protein 2 serves as a transducer of the signal to a downstream effector (Protein 3) by catalyzing the addition of a modifying group (M2). Protein 3 then directly catalyzes a response. In many pathways, the intermediate transducer proteins can amplify upstream signals. The removal of a modifying group at any stage (*dotted arrows*) can result in the deactivation of the entire pathway. The hypothetical pathway shown has a single sensor, transducer and effector. Actual pathways can have multiple upstream and downstream proteins

multistep pathway allows a signal from a single location to have effects in multiple locations within the cell that may be physically distant. Some of the most extensively characterized pathways involved in cancer transduce signals from the cell surface to the nucleus, where genes are regulated.

Some pathways serve the purpose of amplifying a faint stimulus to produce a profound biochemical response. A notable example of this type of amplification is programmed cell death, also known as apoptosis. The interaction of two protein complexes on the cell surface is sufficient to generate a signal that is sequentially amplified and ultimately results in the proteolytic destruction of the cell. Pathways that sequentially amplify signals are in some cases referred to as *enzyme cascades*.

Multiple pathways can converge on a single protein (Fig. 6.4). In such cases, the protein common to different pathways functions as a *node*. Pathways can be either stimulatory or inhibitory. Because the nodes of a pathway integrate several types of proximal, or *upstream* signals, they represent critical regulatory elements.

Other, more subtle interactions can also occur between pathways that, upon initial analysis, may appear to be unconnected. In such cases, two pathways will have distinct stimuli and distinct responses (Fig. 6.5). Although such pathways are paral-

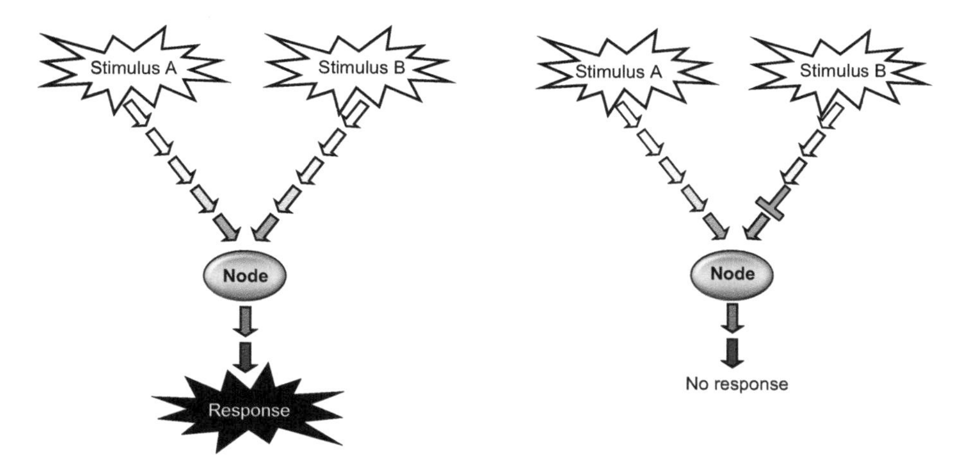

Fig. 6.4 Convergent pathways. Distinct upstream signals can lead to a common response. On the left, two pathways, triggered by stimulus A and stimulus B, converge at a single point and join a common downstream pathway. Points at which pathways intersect are sometimes referred to as nodes. Some pathways can trigger reactions (shown in *red*) that inhibit downstream signaling events. In the example on the *right*, the response that would be triggered by stimulus A is attenuated by the pathways activated by stimulus B

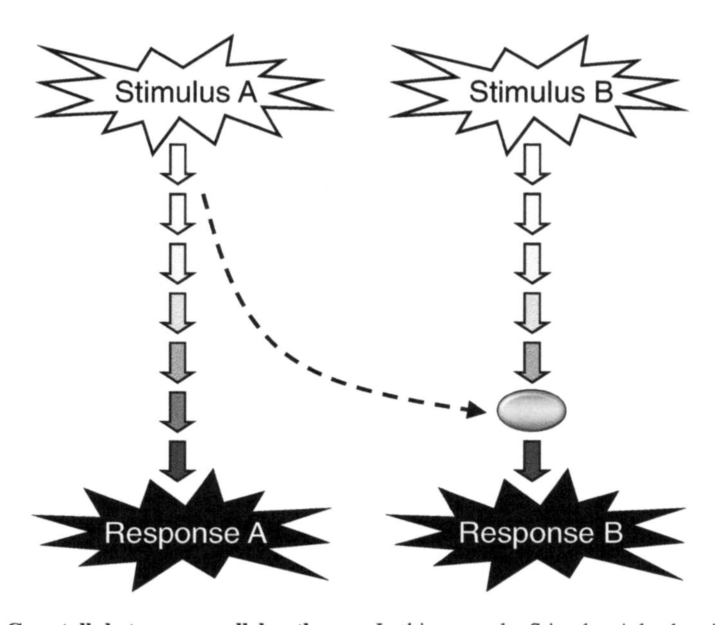

Fig. 6.5 Crosstalk between parallel pathways. In this example, Stimulus A leads primarily to Response A. Stimulus B leads to Response B via a distinct pathway. The "A" pathway is interconnected (*dotted line*) with the "B" pathway at a node. Stimulus A can thus affect Response B to some degree. Crosstalk can increase or decrease the signals transduced by pathways that are otherwise parallel in structure

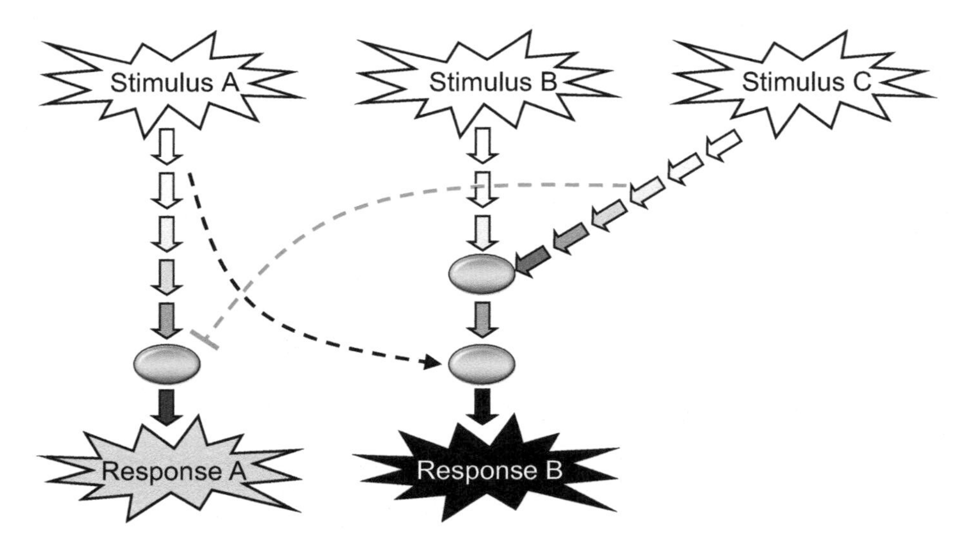

Fig. 6.6 Interconnected pathways form signaling networks. Multiple upstream signals affect multiple downstream responses. The activation of pathways that are influenced by crosstalk provides highly modulated signals that can create nuanced responses. Shown is a simple multi-nodal network in which responses are stimulated by three activating pathways that are influenced by both stimulatory (*black dashed line*) and inhibitory (*red dashed line*) crosstalk. Responses A and B can thus be modulated with high precision

lel in structure, the activation of one can sometimes, and under some conditions, positively or negatively affect the activation of the other. This type of regulation is often referred to as *crosstalk.*

In effect, nodes link multiple individual pathways into functional signaling networks (Fig. 6.6). The integration of multiple stimulatory and inhibitory pathways that are modulated by crosstalk creates a highly sensitive system with a large dynamic range. The extraordinary degree of connectivity that defines a network facilitates the finely tuned cellular responses to complex environmental stimuli.

As will be described in a later section, the p53 protein is a node of several critical pathways that regulate cell growth and survival. This extraordinary degree of interconnection is probably why the *TP53* gene is so frequently mutated in so many types of cancer.

Protein Phosphorylation Is a Common Regulatory Mechanism

One versatile form of protein modification is phosphorylation. The phosphorylation and dephosphorylation of proteins are catalyzed by protein kinases and protein phosphatases, respectively. Kinases catalyze the transfer of the $\gamma-$phosphate group from adenosine triphosphate (ATP) to protein residues, while phosphatases catalyze the removal of this phosphate group. As many as 30 % of the proteins encoded by

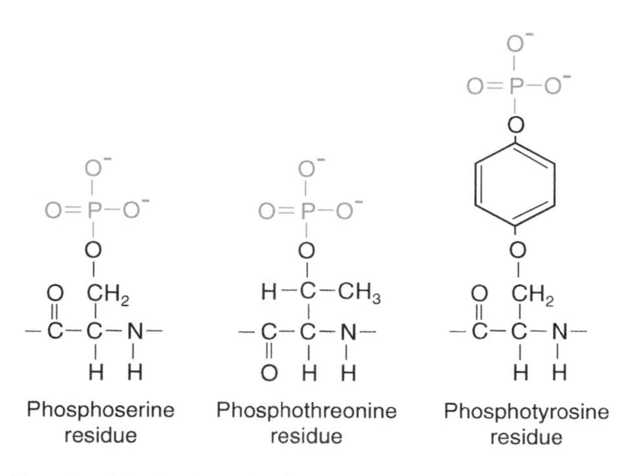

Fig. 6.7 Phosphorylated derivatives of serine, threonine and tyrosine. The addition of a phosphate group (*red*) adds a negatively charged moiety to a protein, altering its hydrophobicity and structure

the human genome are modified by covalently-bound phosphate at least some of the time. The human genome encodes approximately 1000 kinases and 500 phosphatases that mediate these transactions. The reversible phosphorylation of proteins affects many cellular activities and functions.

Until the 1970s, protein phosphorylation was viewed primarily as a specialized mechanism for the control of the pathways involving carbohydrate metabolism. The broader importance of protein phosphorylation only became apparent during the late 1970s and early 1980s, when roles of phosphorylation in diverse cell signaling pathways were discovered. Also appreciated at that time was that not all phosphorylated proteins are enzymes. Proteins that lend structure, organization and motility to cells are also targets of kinases and phosphatases. The reversibility and versatility of phosphorylation probably explains its evolutionary selection as a general mechanism of regulation.

A role for phosphorylation in cancer gene pathways was first discovered in 1978 by Ray Erikson, who demonstrated that the transforming protein encoded by the Rous sarcoma virus *V-SRC* gene encodes a protein kinase. Shortly thereafter, Tony Hunter demonstrated that the V-SRC protein catalyzes the addition of phosphate moieties to tyrosine residues, the first time such a catalytic activity had been observed. Abnormalities involving protein phosphorylation are now known to be among the most common defects found in cancer cells.

In addition to tyrosine, proteins can also be phosphorylated on serine and threonine residues (Fig. 6.7). The addition of a phosphate group increases the molecular weight and the overall space occupied by an amino acid residue. Most importantly, phosphorylation changes the ionic charge of a residue so modified. Serine, threonine and tyrosine residues are neutrally charged; upon phosphorylation they become negatively charged.

The conformation of a protein is largely determined by interactions with neighboring water molecules. *Hydrophilic* regions of a protein tend to be in greater contact with water, while *hydrophobic* regions tend to associate more closely with one another. The covalent addition or removal of negatively charged moieties lowers the hydrophobicity of the protein at that position, and thereby alters protein conformation.

The addition or removal of a phosphate moiety is a chemically simple modification that can have many functional consequences. Phosphorylation states can affect protein conformation and thereby increase or decrease biochemical activity. Phosphorylation and dephosphorylation can also control protein localization, protein stability and the direct interactions of proteins with other biomolecules.

Proteins that are regulated by phosphorylation/dephosphorylation are typically modified not at just one residue, but at several. Proteins can be phosphorylated at multiple sites by the same upstream kinase, or by kinases that belong to two different pathways. The phosphorylation of a single protein at multiple sites increases the extent to which is activity can be regulated by upstream signals. Additionally, multisite phosphoryation allows two different aspects of protein function, such as catalytic activity and half-life, to be separately regulated. The phosphorylation of a protein at one site can facilitate the phosphorylation or dephosphorylation of another site. In such cases, phosphorylation states are said to exhibit *cooperativity*.

In some cancer gene pathways, protein phosphorylation/dephosphorylation functions essentially as a molecular on/off switch. Some of the key cell surface receptor proteins that control growth function in such a binary manner. In other pathways, phosphorylation functions as an extremely fine-tuned mechanism for regulating and coordinating the activity, timing and location of biochemical reactions. In the case of p53 activation, the phosphorylation of numerous residues, and other posttranslational modifications, allow p53 to integrate numerous types of upstream signals and serve to regulate many aspects of p53 activity.

Signals from the Cell Surface: Protein Tyrosine Kinases

Many signals that stimulate cell growth, cell division and cell death arise from the local microenvironment. Cells can sense the presence of both soluble and cell-associated signaling molecules known as *ligands*. Ligands, such as cytokines and hormones, represent extracellular signals that can be sensed and interpreted by receptors at the cell membrane. As a result of ligand-receptor interactions, signals from the cell surface are transmitted into the cells, and thereafter transduced throughout the cytoplasm and into the cell nucleus. Many cell surface receptors function as protein tyrosine kinases. These signaling molecules process extracellular signals and, in response, activate intracellular cancer gene pathways. In many cases, protein tyrosine kinases are themselves encoded by cancer genes.

While protein phosphorylation is a very common posttranslational modification, only about 0.05 % of all phosphorylated proteins are phosphorylated on tyrosine residues. Nonetheless, protein-tyrosine kinases are critical components of the signaling pathways that regulate cell proliferation. Several important proto-oncogenes encode protein tyrosine kinases, and the oncogenic forms of these genes contribute to many cancers.

There are two broad categories of protein tyrosine kinases. *Receptor tyrosine kinases* (RTKs) are transmembrane proteins that span the cell membrane and channel signals from the outside of the cell to the cytoplasm. *Cytoplasmic protein tyrosine kinases* (CTKs) are intracellular enzymes that transduce signals throughout the cytoplasm and into the nucleus. Many CTKs are associated with the interior surface of the cell membrane, but do not span the lipid bilayer.

Of the roughly 100 protein tyrosine kinases that are encoded by the human genome, 58 are transmembrane proteins that function as receptors. On the basis of their structure, these RTK can be grouped into 20 distinct families. The RTKs are highly specialized molecules that have evolved to mediate cell-to-cell communications and are particularly important during development. Accordingly RTKs are found exclusively in metazoans.

RTKs have a typical structure that defines their function (Fig. 6.8). An extracellular domain is involved in ligand binding. A hydrophobic transmembrane domain

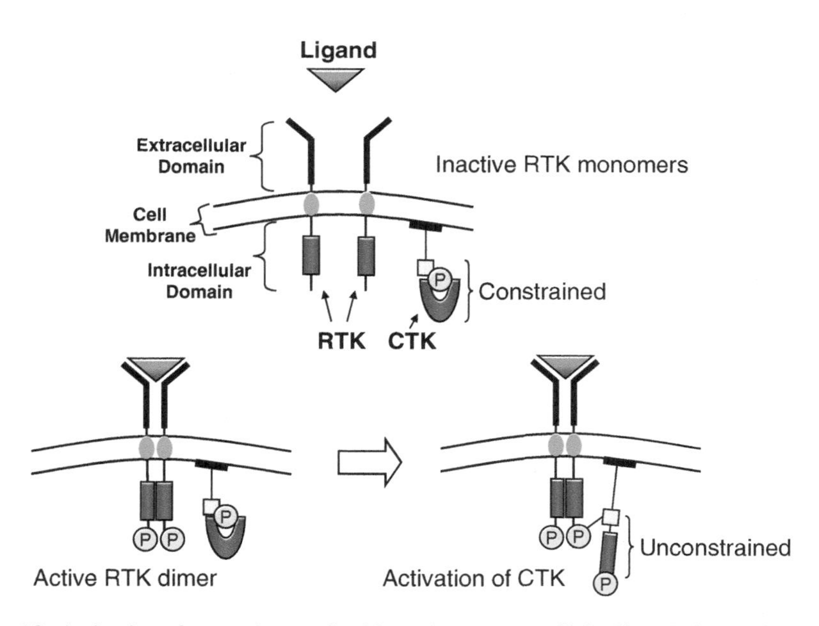

Fig. 6.8 Activation of a protein tyrosine kinase by an extracellular ligand. A generic receptor protein tyrosine kinase (RTK) is composed of an extracellular domain (*black*) that directly interacts with ligands (*red*), a transmembrane domain (*green*) and an intracellular domain that contains a conserved catalytic region (*blue*). A membrane-associated cytoplasmic tyrosine kinase (CTK), is maintained in inactive form by intramolecular constraints that inhibit its catalytic domain. Upon ligand binding, the RTK molecules form dimers, and activate their catalytic domains by autophosphorylation. The intramolecular constraints that keep the CTK inactive are relieved when the SRC-homology domain (*gray*) preferentially associates with the phosphorylated form of the RTK dimer. Thus activated, RTK and CTK can turn on downstream pathways

spans the lipid bilayer that composes the cell membrane. An evolutionarily conserved catalytic domain, which contains protein tyrosine kinase activity, resides in the intracellular portion of the molecule. The binding of ligands to RTKs causes the formation of dimers or higher-order oligomers. Concomitant with this oligomerization is the activation of protein tyrosine kinase activity and autophosphorylation of each receptor molecule on specific tyrosine residues. The oligomeric, phosphorylated RTK complex can then function to recruit cytoplasmic protein tyrosine kinases.

There are many variations in the generic mode of RTK function. Some receptors can recognize several related ligands, others are highly specific. Some types of RTKs, such as those in the epidermal growth factor (EGF) receptor family, are activated by the binding of a single ligand molecule. Others, such as the fibroblast growth factor (FGF) family require the simultaneous binding of two different ligands for activation of kinase activity. The ERBB2 protein apparently requires no ligand at all, but rather interacts with other EGF family members. Within the cytoplasm, some types of RTKs such as those in the FGF receptor family assemble highly ordered complexes of docking proteins that provide an additional level of control.

Several RTK genes are mutated at high frequency in diverse types of cancer. Among the most frequently mutated are *EGFR* and *ERBB2* (Table 6.2), which are members of the EGF receptor gene subfamily.

By several mechanisms, cancer-associated genetic alterations result in the dysregulation of RTK catalytic activity. The most common genetic alterations that affect RTK genes are point mutations and amplification of the entire gene. Single nucleotide substitutions affecting the extracellular or transmembrane domains can promote receptor dimerization in the absence of ligand (Fig. 6.9). Alternatively, single nucleotide substitutions can affect a motif within the catalytic domain known as the *activation loop* and cause an increase in basal kinase activity. A third type of genetic alteration that can dysregulate RTK activity is translocation. In cases wherein the translocated protein domain is normally involved in protein-protein interactions, the mutant receptors dimerize. Translocations are often found in leukemias and lymphomas. In other cancers, amplification of RTK genes can cause receptor overexpression and overactive signaling (Fig. 6.10).

Once activated, RTKs recruit and activate various signaling molecules in the cytoplasm, including CTKs. CTKs are sometimes referred to as *nonreceptor tyrosine kinases*. CTKs are typically associated with the plasma membrane via an N-terminal posttranslational modification, but they are not transmembrane proteins.

The prototype CTK is SRC, encoded by the first identified cancer gene. As described in Chap. 2, the SRC protein is normally phosphorylated on a c-terminal tyrosine residue. An N-terminal domain has a high affinity for the phosphorylated c-terminus. SRC is thus maintained in a constrained, inactive form. Following an upstream stimulus, the intracellular domains of neighboring RTK molecules become phosphorylated on multiple tyrosine residues (Fig. 6.8). The N-terminal domain of SRC has a greater affinity for the newly phosphorylated RTKs than for its own C-terminus. As a result, SRC undergoes a conformational change that results in activation of its kinase domain.

Table 6.2 RTK genes commonly altered in cancers

Proto-oncogene	Ligand	Oncogenic alteration	Cancers
EGFR (ERBB1)	Epidermal growth factor (EGF), Transforming growth factor β (TGFβ)	Point mutation, deletion	Lung, Colorectal, and Breast Carcinoma
		Amplification	Glioblastoma
ERBB2 (HER2/neu)	None	Amplification	Breast, ovarian, gastric, cervical, and lung carcinoma
		Point mutation	Neuroblastoma
FLT3	FLT3L (cytokine)	Tandem duplication	Acute myelogenous leukemia (AML)
MET	Hepatocyte growth factor	Amplification	Medulloblastoma, Esophageal and Gastric carcinoma
		Point mutation	Hereditary papillary renal cell carcinoma
RET	Glial-derived neurotropic factor	Complex rearrangement	Thyroid carcinoma
		Point mutation	Multiple Endocrine Neoplasia syndromes 2A & 2B
KIT	Stem cell factor	Point mutation	Acute myeloid leukemia, germ cell tumors
		Amplification	Glioblastoma
FGFR1	Fibroblast growth factor	Point mutation	Glioblastoma
		Translocation	Acute myelogenous leukemia, lymphoma

Several oncogene products function in a manner similar to SRC and are considered members of a protein family. Proteins in the SRC family exhibit significant amino acid sequence homology. Several regions are critical to their function in signaling, and are known as SRC homology domains SH1, SH2 and SH3. SH1 contains the protein kinase domain. SH2 is required for the binding of the C-terminal phosphotyrosine residue, and SH3 is required for additional protein-protein interactions.

Mutations in *SRC* are found at a relatively low frequency in several cancers including colorectal carcinomas. While activated *SRC* is not a prevalent oncogene, *SRC* and closely related proteins are central components of cancer gene pathways that involve RTKs. It is most likely this important attribute that led *SRC* to be appropriated by the Rous sarcoma virus.

The tyrosine kinase encoded by the *ABL* proto-oncogene represents a distinct CTK family. Unlike other CTKs, *ABL* is located in both the cytoplasm and the nucleus. The translocation that generates the *BCR-ABL* fusion gene in chronic myeloid leukemia has three effects on ABL signaling. First, because the *BCR* gene promoter is highly active, *BCR-ABL* is overexpressed relative to the level that *ABL*

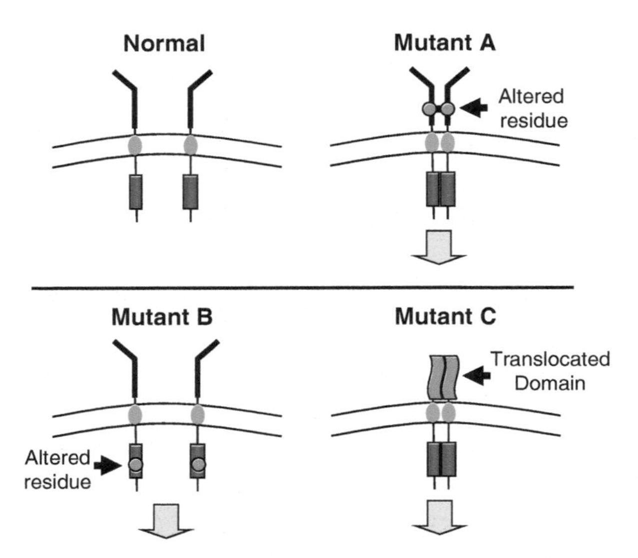

Fig. 6.9 Point mutations can result in RTK dysregulation. Mutant A contains an amino acid substitution (shown in red) in the extracellular domain that causes RTK molecules to have an increased affinity for one another and to dimerize. Mutations in the transmembrane domain can have a similar effect (not shown). Mutant B carries an amino acid substitution mutation in the activation loop of the catalytic domain, increasing the basal kinase activity of RTK monomers. Mutant C is a fusion protein in which the extracellular domain derived from an unrelated protein that is normally 'sticky' and therefore participates in protein-protein interactions. In each case, signaling is ligand-independent

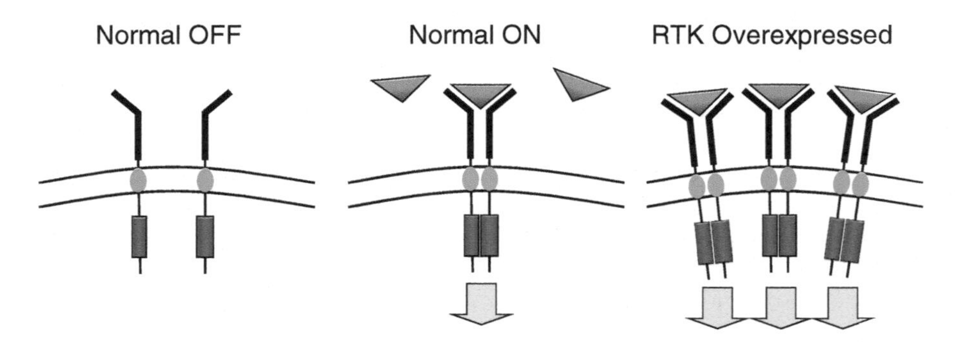

Fig. 6.10 Amplification of RTK genes can cause cells to become hypersensitive to ligand. RTK proteins encoded by wild type genes normally trigger downstream responses (*yellow arrow*) that depend upon the presence of ligand (*red*). Amplification of RTK genes leads to overexpression of RTK receptors, and their increased numbers at the cell surface. Although each receptor is normal in structure and function, cells are hypersensitive to ligand

would normally be expressed. Second, the BCR domain of the fusion protein facilitates the formation of oligomeric complexes, which result in the constitutive activation of ABL tyrosine kinase activity. Third, the BCR-ABL fusion protein is excluded from the nucleus, which restricts access to a subset of the substrates normally phosphorylated by ABL.

The proto-oncogene *FLT3* encodes a receptor tyrosine kinase that is recurrently activated by mutations in acute myeloid leukemia. In bone marrow progenitors, *FLT3* is commonly amplified by a mechanism that involves the generation of internal tandem duplications. The resulting overexpression of FLT3 is a negative prognostic marker, which means that it portends an unfavorable outcome. Signaling through FLT3 engages multiple downstream pathways that control cell survival, proliferation and differentiation.

Membrane-Associated GTPases: The RAS Pathway

A distinct mechanism by which signals at the cell membrane are processed and disseminated involves the binding and hydrolysis of guanosine triphosphate (GTP). Membrane-associated enzymes known as GTPases are activated when GTP is noncovalently bound and inactivated when GTP is hydrolyzed to guanosine diphosphate (GDP). The role of GTPases in cancer cell signaling was revealed by the discovery of the RAS family of oncogenes. RAS-encoded proteins are membrane-bound GTPases that, when present in mutant form, play an important role in the aberrant growth properties of cancer cells.

The three human RAS genes (*HRAS*, *NRAS* and *KRAS*) encode highly related 21-kDa proteins that are localized to the interior surface of the cell membrane. These proteins essentially function as molecular switches that can be turned on and off by the binding and subsequent hydrolysis of GTP, respectively. This binary mode of signaling is highly regulated by additional proteins that regulate a *GDP/GTP cycle* (Fig. 6.11).

RAS proteins exist in equilibrium between GTP bound (active) and unbound (inactive) states. RAS proteins have intrinsically low levels of GTP binding and hydrolytic activities. GDP/GTP cycling by RAS is modulated by two types of regulatory proteins. *Guanine nucleotide exchange factors* (GEFs) promote formation of the active, GTP-bound state. Two examples of GEFs are the SOS proteins SOS1 and SOS2, named for the *Drosophila* genes *Sons of Sevenless*, with which they share significant homology. SOS proteins directly interact with RAS and stimulate the exchange of GDP for GTP. The hydrolysis of GTP is facilitated by the interactions of RAS with *GTPase activating proteins* (GAPs). These include the GTPase activating protein known as p120 GAP, and neurofibromin, which is encoded by the *NF1* tumor suppressor gene (see Chap. 3). The GEFs and GAPs control RAS signaling by influencing the balance of GTP-bound and unbound forms.

Membrane association is a requirement for RAS activity. At this location, RAS is activated in response to upstream signals by nearby RTKs (Fig. 6.12). An impor-

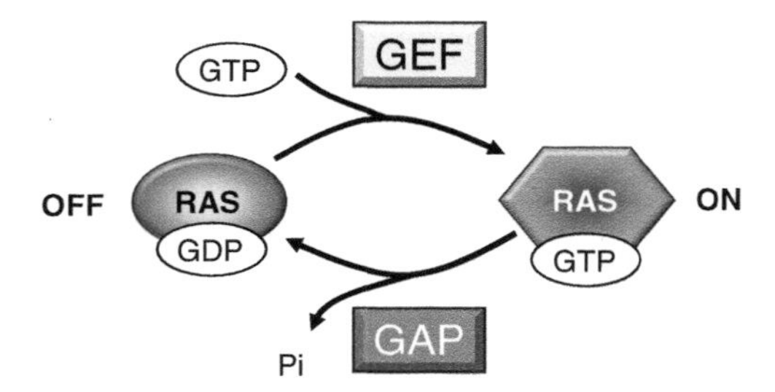

Fig. 6.11 Regulation of RAS-mediated GTP binding and hydrolysis. RAS proteins have low intrinsic GTP binding activity, which can be greatly stimulated by physical association with a guanine nucleotide exchange factor (GEF). Similarly, the hydrolysis of GTP by RAS is stimulated by a GTPase activating protein (GAP). The binary mode (ON and OFF) of signaling by RAS is highly regulated by these interactions

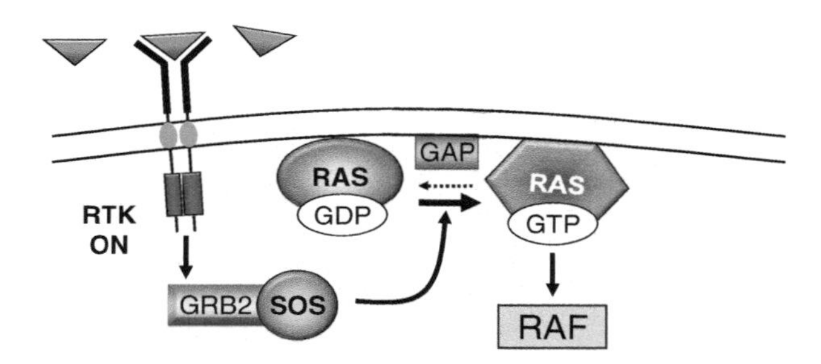

Fig. 6.12 RAS proteins are activated by RTKs. A transmembrane RTK such as EGFR is activated by ligand (*red*) binding and recruits GRB2 and SOS proteins. SOS is a GEF that triggers the exchange of GDP for GTP and thereby results in a change in RAS conformation. This activated form of RAS can interact with downstream molecules, including the RAF serine/threonine kinases. The GAP proteins, which stimulate GTP hydrolysis, can also be recruited to the cell membrane and attenuate downstream responses

tant RTK-RAS relationship involves the epidermal growth factor receptor (EGFR), a proto-oncogene that is frequently amplified in malignant gliomas and mutated in lung adenocarcinomas. Activated by the presence of ligand, the EGFR receptor phosphorylates its own cytoplasmic domain on specific tyrosine residues. An adaptor protein known as GRB2 associates with the activated EGFR complex via an SH2 domain. GRB2 recruits an SOS protein, and thus brings it into the proximity of RAS. SOS stimulates the exchange of GDP for GTP by RAS, triggering a conformational change. Thus activated, RAS can productively interact with downstream molecules. The GAP proteins that function to deactivate RAS also contain a SH2 domain that allows them to be recruited to the membrane.

An Intracellular Kinase Cascade: The MAPK Pathway

The conformational change that accompanies the binding of RAS with GTP allows RAS proteins to activate downstream signaling molecules. Prominent among these regulators is the RAF family of serine/threonine kinases. In a complex, multi-step process, the three RAF kinases are activated upon their recruitment to the cell membrane by activated RAS. Once activated, RAF proteins phosphorylate and activate two signaling molecules belonging to the mitogen activated protein kinase kinase (MAPKK, alternatively known as MAP2K), family alternatively known as the MEK family. The MEKs are unusual protein kinases that have dual specificity; they can phosphorylate proteins on serine/threonine and on tyrosine residues. Activated MEKs translocate to the nucleus and phosphorylate several downstream targets. Among these are two mitogen-activated protein kinases (MAPKs), alternatively known as extracellular signal regulated kinases (ERKs). Activated ERKs are able to translocate across the nuclear membrane. Thus, via sequential activation of the MEKs and the ERKs, RAF proteins trigger a cascade of protein kinase signaling that spans the cytoplasm and reaches effectors in the nucleus (Fig. 6.13).

In human cells, the ERKs are the primary effector of numerous types of proliferative signals. Via phosphorylation, ERKs can directly activate transcription factors and thus affect gene expression. Other important substrates of the ERKs include the ribosomal protein S6 kinases (RSKs), that are regulators of protein synthesis, and the Rho-like GTPases, which have been shown to stimulate changes in cell shape and motility.

The RAS pathway affects many aspects of cell survival that are aberrant in cancer cells; MEKs and the ERKs as the major downstream effectors of these critical responses. Inhibition of the RAF, MEK or ERK proteins by the overexpression of dominant inhibitory mutants has been shown to impair the ability of RAS to transform primary cells. Conversely, experimental overexpression of RAF or MEK genes can phenocopy the transformation and tumorigenic properties of RAS mutants.

Genetic Alterations of the RAS Pathway in Cancer

Activation of the RAS and MAPK pathways occurs very frequently in many types of cancer. There are several types of genetic alterations that affect RAS signaling. By far the most prevalent are mutations of RAS genes themselves. The most frequently mutated RAS family member is *KRAS*. The majority of tumor-associated mutations in *KRAS* affect codons 12, 13, 59 or 61. These codons are in the proximity of the guanine nucleotide binding sites. In cancers, mutant RAS proteins fail to respond to the stimulatory effects of GAP. As a result, mutant RAS proteins remain in the GTP-bound state and are constitutively active.

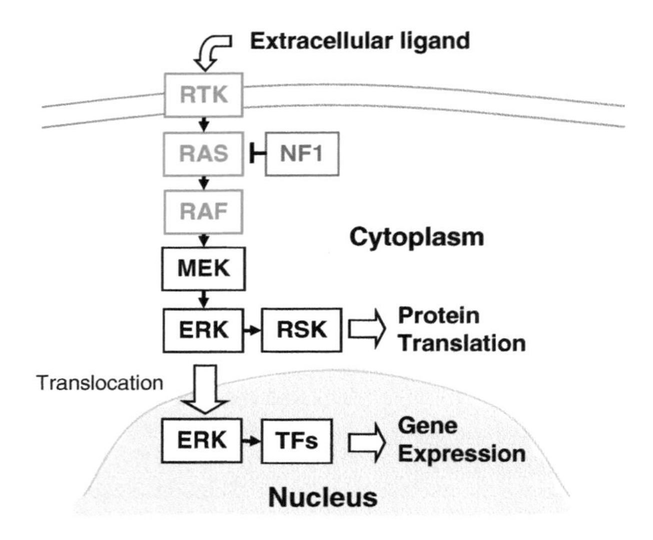

Fig. 6.13 RAS signaling connects RTKs with kinase cascades that alter gene expression and protein translation. RAS represents a node at which upstream and downstream pathways converge. In response to RTK signaling, RAS proteins activate RAF family members. RAS can be deactivated by the GAP proteins, which include the product of the *NF1* gene. RAF proteins phosphorylate and activate the MEKs, which in turn phosphorylate and activate the ERKs. The ERK proteins can activate the ribosome-associated RSK proteins, thereby affecting protein synthesis. ERKs can also translocate into the nucleus and regulate numerous transcription factors (TFs). Thus, RAS signals are transmitted throughout the cell. Proteins that can be constitutively activated via oncogenic mutations are shown in *red*. NF1 is the product of a tumor suppressor gene and is shown in *blue*

The tumor suppressor *NF1* encodes a GAP protein. In cells with biallelically inactivated *NF1*, RAS is maintained in its constitutively active, GTP-bound form. Thus, inactivating mutations in *NF1* have a similar effect on overall RAS activity as activating mutations in RAS genes. As described in Chap. 3, *NF1* mutations are found in both sporadic tumors and in the germline of patients with neurofibromatosis type 1, a syndrome that predisposes affected individuals to cancer (Chap. 3).

More widespread than inactivating *NF1* mutations are activating mutations in the RAF family member *BRAF*. The most common *BRAF* mutation is a T→A transversion that changes the normal valine at codon 599 to a glutamic acid residue (V599E). This mutation is located in a highly conserved protein kinase motif involved in ATP binding. The V599E mutation causes a ten-fold increase in basal BRAF kinase activity. Thus, single nucleotide substitutions in *BRAF* can cause constitutive activation of the RAS pathway.

BRAF mutations have been found in more than 60 % of melanomas and thyroid cancers, about 10 % of colorectal cancers and lung adenocarcinomas. In melanomas, the mutations in *BRAF* are notably distinct from the UV signature mutations that are frequently associated with skin cancers.

In colorectal cancers, the pattern of *BRAF* mutations notably reflects the mechanism of genetic instability present in individual tumors. *BRAF* mutations occur in the modest proportion of tumors with mismatch repair deficiency, while *KRAS* mutations are found in the majority of colorectal tumors that are mismatch repair proficient (see Chap. 4). Notably, *KRAS* and *BRAF* mutations do not occur together in individual tumors. This observation strongly suggests that *KRAS* mutations and *BRAF* mutations are equivalent in their downstream effects on cell survival.

Mutations in the RAS pathway illustrate key principles of cancer genetics. While RAS-activating mutations are neither sufficient nor required for the development of tumors, *KRAS* and downstream components of its signaling pathway are activated in diverse cancers. In some tissues, there is evidently a significant amount of selective pressure to inactivate the RAS signaling pathway. This selective effect is apparent in colorectal cancers. In the mucosae of the colon and rectum, the constitutive activation of RAS signaling occurs as tumors progress from small to intermediately sized adenomas (Chap. 2). About one half of all colorectal tumors accumulate an activating mutation in *KRAS*. However, mismatch repair-deficient colorectal tumors frequently harbor a mutated *BRAF* allele, which similarly activates the pathway. Once the RAS pathway is constitutively switched on by either one of these genetic alterations, there is apparently no selective pressure to inactivate additional genes that populate the pathway.

Membrane-Associated Lipid Phosphorylation: The PI3K/AKT Pathway

In response to mitogenic ligands, receptor tyrosine kinases (RTKs) can activate several downstream pathways that promote cell survival. One pathway that is particularly important in cancer cells involves the phosphatidylinositol 3-kinases (PI3Ks). This unique class of enzymes is phosphorylated and thus activated by RTKs at the plasma membrane, and then catalyzes the phosphorylation of inositol-containing lipids. The resulting phospholipids act as second messengers that stimulate downstream signaling and effector molecules. Several RTKs are known to trigger PI3K dependent signaling, including the EGF receptor (EGFR) and receptors that respond to the growth stimulatory effects of insulin.

PI3K was first discovered in the 1980s as a novel enzymatic activity associated with partially purified viral oncoproteins, including SRC. Further purification and analysis revealed that this activity could be attributed to a two-subunit enzyme complex. An 85 kDa protein (p85) associates with RTK proteins and serves a regulatory function. Catalytic activity of PI3K heterodimers is contained in a separate 110 kDa protein (p110). The isolation of the genes that encode the catalytic and regulatory domains of PI3K revealed a large and complex family of proteins. The PI3K proteins known to be involved in cancer belong to a subcategory known as Class 1A.

Phosphatidylinositol phosphates contain a fatty acid moiety that is associated with the inner surface of the cell membrane. A glycerol backbone links the fatty acid moiety to an inositol head group that is the target of both lipid kinases and lipid

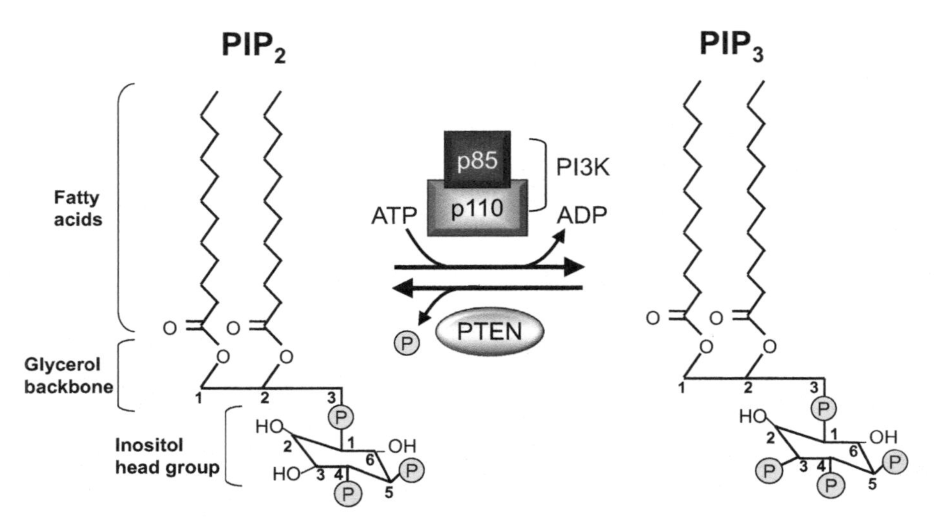

Fig. 6.14 Regulation of the PIP_2-PIP_3 cycle by PI-3 K and PTEN. The heterodimeric PI3K complex catalyzes the ATP-dependent phosphorylation of phosphatidylinositol (4,5)-bisphosphate (PIP_2) at the D3 position of the inositol moiety to generate phosphatidylinositol (3,4,5)-triphosphate (PIP_3). The reverse reaction is catalyzed by the lipid phosphatase encoded by the *PTEN* tumor suppressor gene. Relevant phosphate groups are shown in *yellow*

phosphatases (Fig. 6.14). Class 1A PI3Ks catalyze the phosphorylation of phosphatidylinositol (4,5)-bisphosphate (called PIP_2) to produce phosphatidylinositol (3,4,5)-triphosphate (called PIP_3). The catalytic and the regulatory domains of the Class 1A PI3Ks are each encoded by a family of three distinct but evolutionarily related genes. The activating subunits contain SH2 and SH3 domains that interact with RTKs. The catalytic subunits contain protein domains that are critical for kinase activity, membrane anchoring and interactions with the regulatory subunit.

Normal cells that are unstimulated by mitogenic ligands have very low levels of PIP_3. Following ligand-dependent RTK activation and autophosphorylation, a PI3K complex (composed of a p85 and a p110 subunit) is recruited to the receptor by the SH2 domain of p85. Prior to its activation, p85 exerts an inhibitory effect on p110. The RTK-p85 interaction relieves this inhibition, and also positions p110 in close proximity to its lipid substrates at the cell membrane. Levels of intracellular PIP_3 increase as a result of the increased catalytic activity of p110.

Newly generated PIP_3 acts as a second messenger that activates downstream signaling proteins in the AKT family. The three closely related AKT proteins are encoded by the cellular homologs of the viral oncogene *V-AKT*, originally isolated from a mouse thymus tumor. AKT proteins binds PIP_3 via a protein domain originally defined in the cytoskeletal protein *pleckstrin*. As a result of the pleckstrin homology domain-PIP3 interaction, AKT is recruited to the inner surface of the cell membrane, where it is phosphorylated and activated by the phosphoinositide-

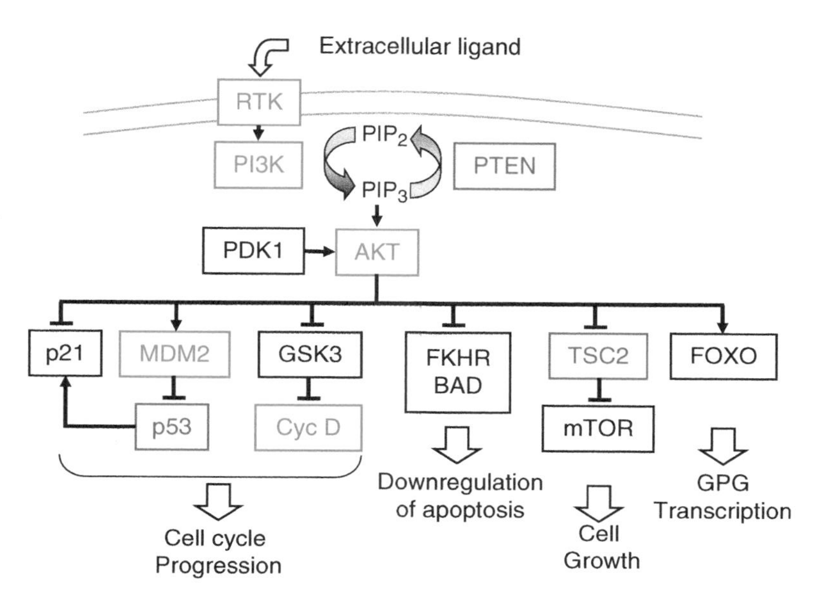

Fig. 6.15 The PI3K/AKT pathway. Ligand-dependent activation of RTK signaling causes the activation of PI3K, and the generation of PIP_3. Via its pleckstrin homology domain, AKT binds PIP_3 and is thus recruited to the inner surface of the cell membrane. AKT is activated by a dual regulatory mechanism that requires translocation and subsequent phosphorylation by PDK1. Active AKT phosphorylates numerous downstream substrates; several representative regulators are shown. Cell cycle progression is stimulated by the AKT-dependent phosphorylation of the cyclin-dependent kinase inhibitor p21. Expression of p21 is also inhibited by the MDM2-dependent inhibition of p53. The activity of cyclin D is increased by the AKT dependent inhibition of glycogen synthetase kinase 3B (GSK3). Apoptosis is downregulated by inhibitory signaling to several proapoptotic proteins, including BAD. AKT inhibits the mTOR pathway via inhibition of TSC2, and thereby promotes protein biosynthesis. The expression of growth-promoting genes (GPG) is increased by the activation of the FOXO family of transcription factors

dependent protein kinases (PDKs). While the activation of PI3K activity appears to be the major mode of AKT phosphorylation and activation, several PI3K-independent pathways to AKT tyrosine phosphorylation have been identified.

AKT proteins are serine/threonine protein kinases that are involved in multiple downstream pathways that control cell survival (Fig. 6.15):

Promotion of cell cycle progression. AKT inhibits negative regulators of cell cycle progression. Among these is p21, the product of the *CDKN1A* gene. High levels of p21 inhibit the cyclin-dependent kinases that promote the progression of the cell cycle. Phosphorylation of p21 by AKT causes the sequestration of p21 in the cytoplasm, thereby preventing it from exerting its regulatory effect in the nucleus. The inhibition by AKT of glycogen synthetase 3 (GSK3) is another mechanism by which AKT regulates cyclin-dependent kinase activity. Cyclin D is directly inhibited by GSK3; this inhibition is relieved by AKT-dependent inhibition of GSK3. Direct activation of a family of transcription factors known as FOXO causes the increase in the expression of growth promoting genes, while activation of MDM2 antagonizes p53 and thus prevents the expression of growth inhibitory genes.

Downregulation of apoptosis. AKT inhibits some transcription factors (eg. FKHR) that promote cell death, and positively regulates other factors that induce the expression of pro-survival genes. AKT also directly phosphorylates several substrates that are more directly involved in apoptosis. Among these are BAD, a proapoptotic member of the BCL2 family, which is inhibited by AKT-dependent phosphorylation.

Control of Cell Growth and Energetics: The mTOR Pathway

An important downstream target of PI3K/AKT signals is the pathway controlled by the mammalian target of rapamycin (mTOR). Rapamycin is an antifungal drug synthesized by a bacterium originally isolated from Easter Island, known locally as Rapa Nui. Studies in yeast showed that rapamycin could cause cycling cells to arrest prior to S-phase, the phase of the cell cycle during which DNA is replicated. This mode of cell cycle arrest was mediated by the specific interaction between rapamycin and several proteins that were subsequently shown to be centrally involved in cell growth, mobility and proliferation, and which ultimately contribute to cell survival. The mammalian ortholog of these yeast regulators, mTOR, was discovered independently by two research teams: David Sabatini and Solomon Snyder and Robert Abraham and Stuart Schreiber.

mTOR is a serine/threonine kinase that regulates the increase the synthesis of macromolecules on the basis of the availability of nutrients and optimal growth conditions. Evolutionarily, mTOR signaling is a mechanism by which an organism can efficiently negotiate the transition between anabolic and catabolic states, thus allowing it to survive under conditions of variable nutrient availability. Accordingly, the mTOR pathway is highly responsive to growth factors, nutrients such as amino acids and the levels of ATP and oxygen.

The activity of mTOR is regulated by the assembly and function of two large, distinct mTOR-containing protein complexes, known as mTORC1 and mTORC2. The first complex, mTORC1, integrates a diverse array of environmental cues and signaling pathways and is the master regulator of cell growth and macromolecular biosynthesis. In contrast, the mTORC2 complex is activated by growth factors and RTKs but is relatively insensitive to other environmental cues. mTORC2 is less well understood, but this complex can apparently upregulate AKT and interact with the actin cytoskeleton in a manner that promotes cellular motility (Fig. 6.16).

A key negative regulator of the mTORC1 complex is a heterodimer that contains two proteins: tuberous sclerosis 1 (TSC1) and tuberin (TSC2). The TSC1/2 complex is a substrate of the effector kinases induced by the growth factors and RTKs that stimulate the PI3K and RAS pathways, and is inhibited by these phosphorylation events. These effectors include AKT, ERK1 and ERK2, and ribosomal S6 kinase (RSK1). The TSC1/2 complex is activated in response to low energy states by adenosine monophosphate-activated protein kinase (AMPK), a metabolic master switch that promotes ATP generation. AMPK is activated in the context of low energy and nutrient levels by the serine/threonine kinase STK11, in a process that also appears to involve a protein called foliculin. TSC1/2 is also receptive to inhibitory signals from pro-inflammatory cytokines and developmental pathways that are recurrently dysregulated in cancer, including the WNT and Hedgehog pathways (see sections below). TSG1/2 inhibition by any of these mechanisms results in the activation of mTOR signaling via the mTORC1 complex.

A prominent effect of mTORC1 activation is increased protein translation. The relevant substrates of mTORC1 include the eukaryotic translation initiation factor 4E binding protein (4E-BP1) and S6 kinase 1 (S6K1). Activated mTORC1 also increases the levels of lipid biosynthesis, cellular metabolism and ATP production. These activities fulfill many of the key requirements for optimal cell growth and survival.

Genetic Alterations in the PI3K/AKT and mTOR Pathways Define Roles in Cell Survival

The unified pathway that links upstream PI3K/AKT signaling to downstream effectors in the mTOR pathway is populated by proto-oncogenes and tumor suppressor genes (Fig. 6.16). The frequent mutational activation of these pathways in diverse cancers attests to their critical roles in the regulation of cell survival.

PIK3CA encodes a p110 subunit of the PI3K heterodimer. As described in Chap. 2, *PIK3CA* is a proto-oncogene that is mutated at high frequency in many common types of cancer, including colorectal, breast, brain, bladder and ovarian cancers. *PIK3CA* is activated primarily by point mutations in one of two regions that determine overall enzyme structure and lipid kinase activity (Fig. 6.17). In addition, amplification of *PIK3CA* is a frequent occurrence in several solid tumors, including lung, ovarian and esophageal cancer. Oncogenic mutations and genetic amplification increase PIK3CA kinase activity and trigger constitutive activation of AKT. Inactivating mutations occur in *PIK3R1*, which encodes the p85 adapter protein that mediates the association of the p110 catalytic subunit to the plasma membrane. These mutations are found in a high proportion of uterine cancers.

The phosphorylation of PIP_2 by PI3K is antagonized by the lipid phosphatase encoded by *PTEN* (Fig. 6.14). As described in Chap. 3, *PTEN* is a tumor suppressor gene that is frequently inactivated in many sporadic cancers. Additionally, germline mutations of *PTEN* cause a heritable predisposition to cancer. Although PTEN can function as a protein kinase, it appears that its tumor suppressor function is primarily linked to its role in the dephosphorylation of PIP_3.

Mutation or amplification of the AKT family member *AKT1* is observed in a small proportion of bladder and breast cancers. Amplification of the related gene

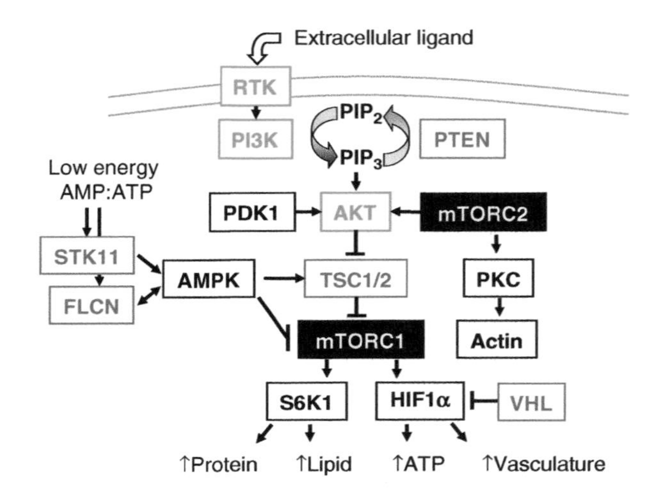

Fig. 6.16 The control of biosynthetic and energetic pathways by mTOR complexes. mTOR activity is controlled by multiple regulatory proteins. AKT promotes activation of the mTORC1 complex via the inactivation of the TSC1/2 heterodimer. A second complex, mTORC2, promotes the activity of AKT. mTORC2 also interacts with the cytoskeleton by a promoting an interaction between protein kinase C (PKC) and actin. The TSC1/2 complex is activated in response to the 5′-adenosine monophosphate-activated protein kinase (AMPK), an evolutionarily conserved metabolic master switch that senses fluctuations in the AMP:ATP ratio via signals from the STK11 kinase. A complex of proteins containing foliculin (FLCN) also appears to be involved in energy and nutrient sensing by AMPK. Downstream targets of mTORC1 include S6K1, which promotes the biosynthesis of proteins and lipids, and HIF1α, which promotes ATP generation by glucose metabolism. HIF1α is negatively regulated by the tumor suppressor VHL. Proteins encoded by proto-oncogenes are shown in *red*; tumor suppressor gene products are shown in *blue*

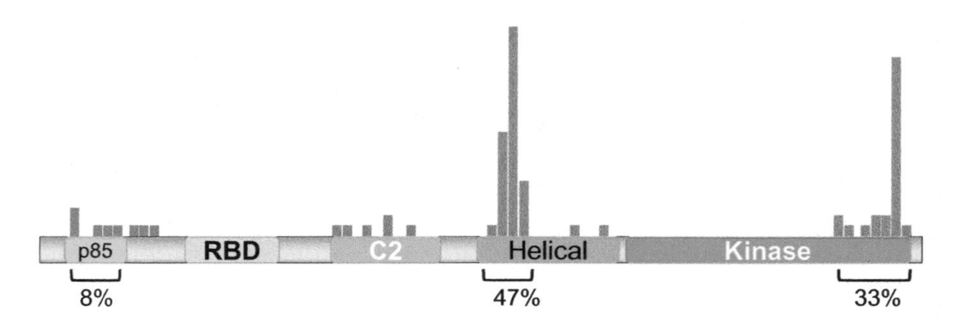

Fig. 6.17 Mutations of *PIK3CA* in colorectal cancers. The *PIK3CA*-encoded protein contains multiple functional domains, including a binding site for the PI3K regulatory subunit (p85), a RAS-binding domain (RBD), a membrane anchoring domain (C2), a helical domain, and a lipid kinase domain that comprises the catalytic activity of the protein. The *bars* indicate the relative numbers of missense mutations and their respective positions within the coding region. The driver mutations in *PIK3CA* are recurrent, and predominately occur at within one of the three hotspots indicated (Data from Samuels *et al. Science* 2005, 304:554.)

AKT2 has been observed in diverse cancers, including tumors in the pancreas, ovary, uterine cervix, and lung.

In the downstream pathways (Fig. 6.16), the mTOR regulators TSC1 and TSC2 are encoded by tumor suppressor genes. Germline inactivation of *TSC1* or *TSC2* results in a rare autosomal dominant genetic disorder called *tuberous sclerosis* (TSC). TSC is characterized by the proliferation of benign tumors, including hamartomas, in the brain, kidneys, heart, eyes, lungs and skin. These tumors develop into cancers very rarely, but the benign tumors in the central nervous can cause severe neurological symptoms that include seizures, cognitive disability, developmental delay and behavioral disturbances. The majority of TSC cases are sporadic rather than inherited, and accordingly caused by *de novo* germline mutations. The mutational loss of TSC1/2 activity causes the constitutive activation of mTORC1.

Originally purified from liver tissue as liver kinase B1 (LKB1), the primary activator of AMPK is the serine/threonine kinase STK11. STK11 is encoded by a tumor suppressor gene that is mutated in a significant proportion of adenocarcinomas of the lung. Germline mutations in *STK11* cause *Peutz-Jeghers syndrome* (alternatively known as hereditary intestinal polyposis syndrome), a rare autosomal dominant disorder that is characterized by the development of benign hamartomas (see Chap. 3) throughout the gastrointestinal tract and pigmented macules on the lips and oral mucosae. While these lesions are invariably benign, patients affected by Peutz-Jeghers syndrome have a significantly increased risk of developing intestinal cancers. Germline mutations in the gene that encodes foliculin, *FLCN*, are the cause of *Birt-Hogg-Dubé* syndrome, a heritable form of cancer in the kidney.

As described in Chap. 3, *von Hippel-Lindau* (VHL) disease is an inherited kidney cancer syndrome caused by mutations in the eponymous tumor suppressor gene *VHL*. The VHL protein is a component of an enzyme complex that possesses ubiquitin ligase activity. An important substrate of the VHL-associated ubiquitin ligase is the hypoxia-inducible factor HIF1α, a regulator of gene expression that is highly responsive to the levels of oxygenation (Fig. 6.18). HIF1α promotes cell survival in growing tumors by inducing the expression of genes that control a process known as *angiogenesis*, the formation of new blood vessels. The prototypical HIF1α target gene is *VEGFA*, which encodes the vascular endothelial growth factor A. In cancers, new vasculature promotes the exchange of nutrients, and increases cell survival. The role of VHL as a suppressor of HIF1α-mediated angiogenesis explains why hemangiomas, neoplastic growths composed of new blood vessels, feature prominently in the clinical presentation of VHL disease.

The STAT Pathway Transmits Cytokine Signals to the Cell Nucleus

The Signal Transducer and Activator of Transcription (STAT) pathway is an important component of innate and adaptive immune regulation. This evolutionarily-conserved signaling system is highly responsive to cytokines, small secreted proteins that transmit signals to and from cells of the immune system. The STAT

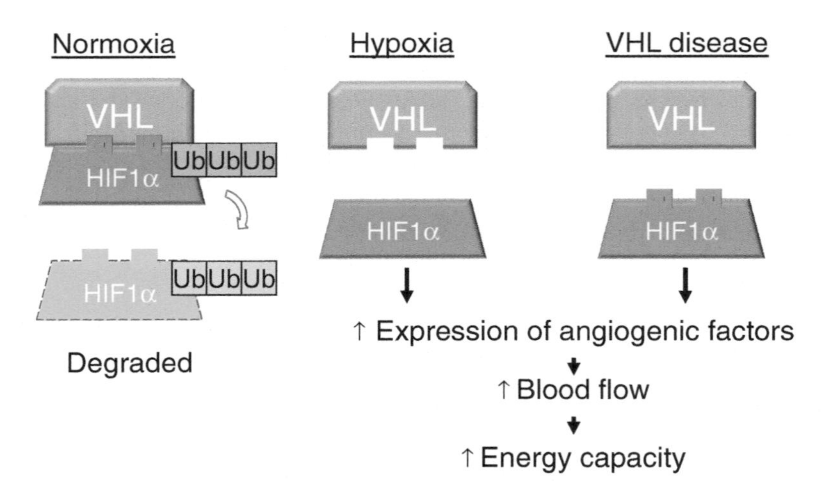

Fig. 6.18 The regulation of HIF1α by VHL. HIF1α is a transcription factor that is highly responsive to the microenvironmental oxygen concentration. At normal oxygen levels (normoxia), two proline residues on HIF1α are covalently modified and facilitate its interaction with a specific site on VHL. This interaction results in the poly-ubiquitination of HIF1α, and its subsequent degradation by the proteasome. Under conditions of hypoxia, which are frequently encountered in growing tumors, the specific proline residues on HIF1α are unmodified and VHL is therefore not bound. The mutations that cause VHL disease commonly alter the HIF1α binding site. In the stable VHL-unbound state, HIF1α induces the expression of genes, including VEGFA, that promote angiogenesis and increase local blood flow

pathway is composed of a cytokine receptor on the cell surface, an intracellular protein tyrosine kinase called JAK, and a STAT effector protein. The biochemical function of the JAK family of related enzymes was unknown at the time of their discovery, and these proteins were accordingly designated 'Just Another Kinase'. The JAKs are now called Janus kinases, from the two-faced Roman god of beginnings and endings. This new name reflects the two interactive kinase domains that are characteristic of these proteins.

The STAT pathway is triggered by the binding of a cytokine to a receptor on the cell surface. Antiviral proteins known as interferons are important intercellular activators of this pathway. The intracellular domains of the bound receptor undergo conformation changes that stimulate the catalytic activity of JAK. JAK, in turn, phosphorylates the receptor and thereby creates a docking site for the STAT family of proteins, which are encoded by seven distinct genes. Bound at these phosphotyrosine docking sites, STAT proteins are also phosphorylated by JAK. These modifications create new docking sites on the STAT proteins that allow them to partner with one another, forming active homo- and hetero-dimers. These active STAT dimers translocate to the cell nucleus and activate target genes that potentiate immune responses. In addition to cytokine-responsive receptors, STAT proteins can also be activated by RTKs such as EGFR, and by the non-receptor tyrosine kinase SRC. The STAT pathway is negatively regulated by protein tyrosine phosphatases and proteins that competitively inhibit the binding of STAT for phospho-tyrosine binding.

Mutations that affect upstream RTKs can cause constitutive STAT signaling. *KIT*, an RTK gene originally discovered by Axel Ulrich and colleagues as a cellular homolog of the feline sarcoma viral oncogene *v-kit*, encodes a receptor that recognizes growth promoting ligands involved in hematopoiesis. Amplification of *KIT* causes ligand-independent STAT pathway activation, and is a frequent driver of acute myeloid leukemias. Similarly, gain-of-function mutations in the cytokine receptor protein encoded by *CRLF2* contribute to acute lymphoblastic leukemia.

Downstream of the receptors, a recurrent V617F mutation in *JAK2* that causes cytokine-independent activation of its kinase activity is frequently found in myeloproliferative neoplasms, including acute myeloid leukemia. Similar hotspot mutations in *JAK1* and *JAK3* contribute to acute forms of leukemia such as T-cell acute lymphoblastic leukemia, and are found rarely in solid tumors. Inactivating mutations in a tumor suppressor gene that functions as a Suppressor of cytokine signaling (*SOCS1*) are found in Hodgkin's lymphoma. This loss of function enhances JAK-STAT activity, and causes cells to become hypersensitive to growth factors.

Morphogenesis and Cancer: The WNT/APC Pathway

Communication between neighboring cells is vital for the normal development of multicellular organisms. In adult humans, mutations that affect cell to cell communication can cause a loss of tissue homeostasis that leads to cancer. A signaling pathway that is important in embryonic development and is also inactivated in some types of cancer is triggered by ligands known as *WNTs*. WNTs are secreted proteins that become soluble and active upon the covalent attachment of a lipid moiety. In their lipid-modified form, WNTs function as ligands that trigger evolutionarily-conserved morphogenic pathways. The WNTs comprise a large family of proteins that control cell fates during mammalian development.

The first insights into the role of WNT signaling and the structure of the downstream WNT-dependent pathways were gained from studies of development in *Drosophila*. A ligand required for wing development, designated Wg, activates a pathway that mediates fundamental developmental processes that include embryonic induction, generation of cell polarity and the specification of cell fate.

The mammalian homologs of Wg were originally identified as genes that were called INTs because they were found near the sites of murine retrovirus insertion. Tumors were found to form in mice in which retrovirus integration caused INT genes to become overexpressed. Significant sequence homology between Wg and INT led to the re-designation of the mammalian genes as WNTs. These evolutionarily-conserved ligands revealed a link between altered developmental processes and cancer.

There are several distinct pathways that are triggered by the large family of WNT ligands. The WNT-dependent pathway that is populated by cancer genes is alterna-

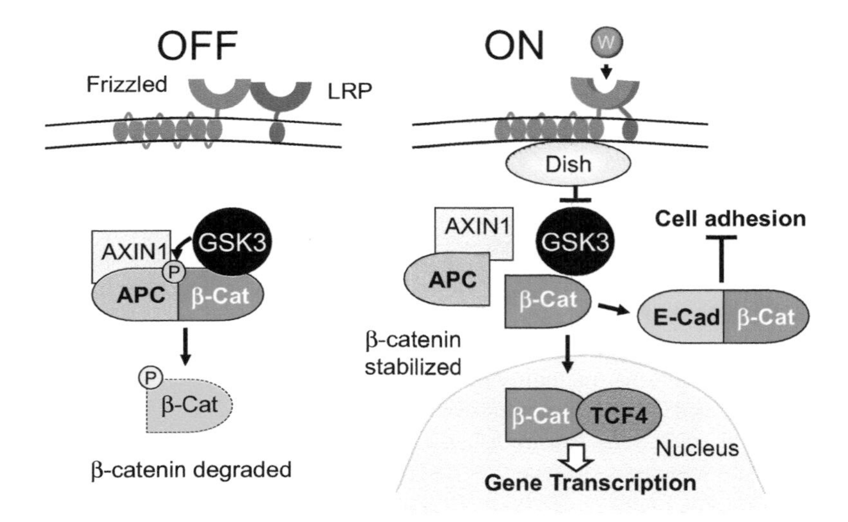

Fig. 6.19 The canonical WNT signaling pathway. In the absence of WNT ligand (OFF; *left panel*), phosphorylation of β-catenin by the GSK3 kinase favors the formation of a complex composed of APC and AXIN. β-catenin is targeted for degradation when the WNT pathway is OFF. When the pathway is turned on by ligand, Frizzed and LRP cooperatively activate Disheveled at the cell membrane, which functions to inactivate GSK3. In the absence of GSK3-mediated phosphorylation, the degradation complex is dissociated and β-catenin is stabilized, translocates to the nucleus and, in cooperation with the TCF family of transcription factors, activates the expression of growth promoting genes. Cytoplasmic β-catenin can also associate with E-cadherin, which mediates cell adhesion

tively referred to as the *canonical* WNT pathway or the WNT/APC pathway (Fig. 6.19). The upstream receptor of the WNT/APC pathway is a transmembrane protein known as Frizzled, which like other proteins in the pathway is named after its *Drosophila* homolog. Frizzled proteins are a class of G protein-coupled receptors with extracellular WNT binding domains and seven transmembrane domains. Upon ligand binding, Frizzled associates with a second type of transmembrane lipid-modified protein called the liporeceptor-related protein (LRP). It is believed that LRP functions as a co-receptor complex with Frizzled. Together, the two proteins activate an intracellular protein called Dishevelled.

An important consequence of WNT/APC pathway activation is the stabilization of a protein known as β-catenin. In the absence of upstream signals, β-catenin is phosphorylated by the protein kinase GSK3 (Fig. 6.19). Phosphorylation of β-catenin promotes the formation of a physical complex containing the tumor suppressor protein APC and a protein called AXIN1. This complex functions in the ubiquitin-dependent degradation of β-catenin by the proteasome. When WNT signaling is triggered by ligand binding, the activation of Dishevelled by the membrane-associated signaling complex leads to the inhibition of GSK3 kinase activity. As a result, β-catenin dissociates from the degradation complex and, thus stabilized, translocates to the cell nucleus. Nuclear β-catenin associates with and activates the

T-cell factor (TCF) known as TCF4, a transcription factor. Studies in genetically engineered mice have demonstrated that TCF4 is required for normal stem cell proliferation in the adult intestine. The growth promoting targets of β-catenin-activated TCF transcription include the transcription factor MYC and the cell cycle regulator Cyclin D.

β-catenin is a multifunctional protein that is involved in multiple cellular processes. In addition to the TCF transcription factors in the nucleus, β-catenin also associates with a transmembrane protein called epithelial-cadherin, or E-cadherin. *Cadherins* are a class of transmembrane proteins that mediate adhesion between cells and their surrounding matrix of structural proteins. The interaction between β-catenin and E-cadherin demonstrates a distinct role for WNT/APC signaling in the regulation of cellular organization and homeostasis.

Dysregulation of the WNT/APC Pathway in Cancers

Inactivating mutations in *APC* occur frequently in colorectal cancers. As detailed in Chap. 3, APC is the gatekeeper that prevents neoplastic growth in the colorectal epithelia. Germline mutations in *APC* cause polyposis and confer a markedly increased lifetime risk of cancer, while somatic mutations of *APC* initiate the growth of the majority of sporadic colorectal tumors. The role of the canonical WNT pathway in colorectal tumorigenesis is strongly supported by the central regulatory role of APC in this pathway, and by the observation that colorectal cancer cells typically exhibit upregulated TCF4 activity.

APC is biallelically inactivated in most, but not all, colorectal cancers. Some colorectal cancers retain wild type *APC* alleles, but harbor mutations in other genes that disrupt canonical WNT signaling at other points in the pathway (Fig. 6.20). The elucidation of the canonical WNT pathway demonstrated the regulatory role played by several proteins, including β-catenin and AXIN1. Mutations in the genes that encode these proteins contribute to a small fraction (5–10 %) of colorectal cancers.

β-catenin, encoded by the *CTNNB1* gene, is phosphorylated by GSK3 kinase on several n-terminal serine and threonine residues. Phosphorylation of these residues enhances the binding of β-catenin to APC. *CTNNB1* is a proto-oncogene that is activated by mutations that affect the association between β-catenin and APC. Point mutations or small deletions that alter *CTNNB1* codons 30, 33, 37 and 45, which encode the GSK3 phosphorylation sites, have been found in cancers with wild type *APC*. The form of β-catenin encoded by cancer-associated mutant *CTNNB1* alleles exhibits reduced APC-binding. Cells that harbor oncogenic *CTNNB1* therefore exhibit WNT ligand-independent stabilization of β-catenin and increased activation of TCF-mediated transcription. The mutant form of β-catenin thereby causes constitutive activation of the canonical WNT pathway.

Mutations in *CTNNB1* and *APC* are mutually exclusive. Loss of APC or mutation of the GSK3 phosphorylation sites on β-catenin each prevent the binding of

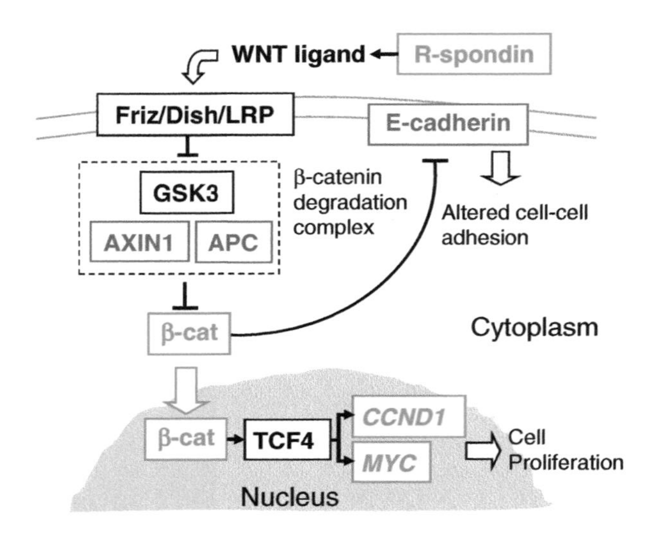

Fig. 6.20 Constitutive WNT signaling in cancer. Several types of mutations can mimic or enhance the effects of activated WNT signaling. The secreted R-spondin proteins appear to interact with WNT ligands on the cell surface and promote upstream pathway activation. Mutations in *APC* in colorectal cancers very frequently disrupt the β-catenin degradation complex, leading to WNT ligand-independent stabilization of β-catenin. Oncogenic mutations that affect the APC binding site of β-catenin have the same effect. Inactivating mutations in AXIN-encoding genes can also disrupt the β-catenin degradation complex. Stabilized β-catenin alters cell adhesion via interactions with cytoplasmic E-cadherin, and also promotes transcriptional transactivation by TCFs. Among the targets of β-catenin/TCF transcription are the proto-oncogenes *CCND1*, which encodes the cell cycle regulator cyclin D, and *MYC*. Proteins and genes affected by oncogenic mutations are shown in *red*, tumor suppressors are shown in *blue*

APC to β-catenin. Accordingly, disruption of this binding event can be achieved either by truncating mutations in *APC* or activating point mutations in *CTNNB1*. A second type of gene that is mutated in colorectal cancers with normal *APC* alleles is a proto-oncogene that encodes secreted proteins called R-spondins. These proteins are secreted, and appear to function together with WNT ligands to promote downstream signaling. Recurrent gene fusions involving the R-spondin family members *RSPO2* and *RSPO3* result in the potentiation of signaling initiation by WNT ligands.

In addition to APC, the AXIN proteins function to negatively regulate the canonical WNT signaling pathway. One of two genes that encode AXIN proteins, *AXIN1* is a tumor suppressor that is inactivated by truncating mutations. Loss of AXIN1 inhibits the binding of the GSK3 kinase and causes the destabilization of the β-catenin degradation complex. The epithelial cadherin (E-cadherin) is encoded by *CDH1*, a tumor suppressor gene. Loss of E-cadherin during tumorigenesis appears to increase cellular motility, a frequently observed trait of cancer cells.

The genetic alterations that initiate colorectal tumorigenesis are also found at lower frequency in other types of cancer. Mutations in *APC* occur in relatively small numbers of cancers of many types. But most of these mutations do not truncate the open reading frame and are therefore passenger mutations. As discussed in Chap. 5, genes such as *APC* tend to accumulate increased numbers of mutations just because they are large. The germline truncating mutations in APC that cause colorectal cancer also predispose carriers to several other types of cancer (see Chap. 3). Conversely, somatic mutations in the β-catenin gene *CTNNB1* are more common in cancers outside the gastrointestinal tract. *CTNNB1* mutations occur in about one quarter of liver cancers, and are also found in a significant fraction of melanomas, uterine cancers, adrenocortical carcinomas and tumors in the brain called medulloblastomas. Inactivating mutations affecting *AXIN1* have been found in liver cancers. Inactivating somatic *CDH1* mutations are found in a significant fraction of breast cancers, and in sporadic stomach cancers. Germline inactivation of *CDH1* is the cause of a rare, familial form of stomach cancer called *hereditary diffuse gastric cancer*. These findings demonstrate that the WNT pathway is disrupted in different ways in different types of cancer.

Notch Signaling Mediates Cell-to-Cell Communication

The Notch signaling pathway transmits signals between neighboring cells, a mode of communication known as *juxtacrine signaling*. This pathway is normally regulated in many tissues during embryonic development and accordingly deregulated in many types of cancer.

Signals at the cell surface are generated by one of four different NOTCH proteins, which are single-pass transmembrane receptors. These receptors are activated upon direct cell-to-cell contact, by ligands on the surface of neighboring cells. The binding of ligand to the extracellular domain of the NOTCH receptor induces the proteolytic cleavage and release of an intracellular domain. This cleaved protein product then enters the nucleus, where it affects gene expression by interactions with transcription factors such as GATA proteins, which are involved in blood formation. The GATA proteins also function as downstream elements of the TGF-β signaling pathway.

As described in Chap. 3, *NOTCH1* can be activated by mutations in some types of cancer, but inactivated in others. This dual role as a context-dependent proto-oncogene/tumor suppressor gene is highly unusual, and also highly illustrative of the unique selective forces that must shape the process of tumorigenesis in different tissues. *NOTCH2* is required for B-cell development, and is a tumor suppressor gene mutated in splenic lymphomas.

FBXW7 encodes a ubiquitin ligase that controls the stability of several NOTCH receptor proteins. Inactivating mutations in *FBXW7*, found in about 20 % of colorectal cancers and also in uterine, stomach and cervical cancers, lead to increased levels of receptor and enhanced Notch pathway activity. Downstream, inactivating mutations in *GATA1* and activating mutations in *GATA2* can alter pathway activity in several malignancies, including non-small cell lung cancer and acute myeloid leukemia.

Morphogenesis and Cancer: The Hedgehog Pathway

The tumor suppressor gene *PTCH1* was discovered on the basis of its evolutionarily conserved role as a receptor for the hedgehog ligand. The interaction between Patched proteins and extracellular hedgehog ligands is a fundamental element of embryonic pattern formation. Detailed analysis of the underlying mechanism of PTCH1 function in mammalian cells by Matthew Scott, Phillip Beachy and others has led to the elucidation of a pathway that is activated in many malignancies (Fig. 6.21).

In the absence of hedgehog ligands, Patched receptors primarily function as repressors of a type of G protein-coupled receptor (GPCR) that is evolutionarily related to a *Drosophila* protein called Smoothened. Like other GPCRs, Smoothened and its mammalian ortholog SMO are signaling proteins that possess seven transmembrane domains and are therefore integral components of cellular membranes. The signaling activity of SMO is repressed by PTCH1, a 12-pass transmembrane

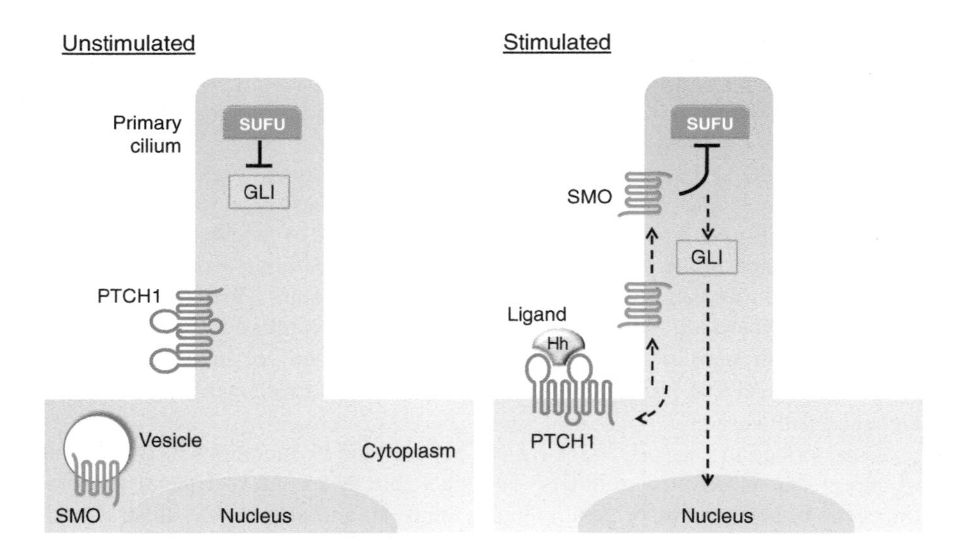

Fig. 6.21 Activation of canonical hedgehog signaling within the primary cilium. In mammals, hedgehog signaling occurs within a non-motile projection from the cell surface known as the primary cilium. In the absence of ligand (*left panel*), the transmembrane protein PTCH1 is located near the base of the cilium, where it prevents the entry of SMO, which is also a transmembrane protein. The GLI transcription factors are held in check by SUFU, while SMO remains inactive and associated with intracellular vesicular membranes. The pathway can be stimulated by the presence of hedgehog ligands (*right panel*). The interaction between PTCH1 and Hh ligand causes a repositioning of PTCH1 and facilitates the ciliary entry of SMO. Within the cilium, SMO suppresses SUFU and thereby causes GLI proteins to be de-repressed. The GLI transcription factors are then actively transported down the cilium and can subsequently enter the nucleus. The effects of the canonical hedgehog pathway are caused by the GLI-mediated transcription of genes that promote cell growth and inhibit differentiation

protein. This repression is relieved when PTCH1 is bound by a hedgehog ligand. The negative regulation of SMO by PTCH1 does not involve a direct protein-protein interaction between these two proteins, but rather is based on changes in their subcellular localization.

In mammalian cells, hedgehog signals are primarily generated in a compartment called the primary cilium. Primary cilia are non-motile tubulin-based structures that function as hubs for signal transduction. Physically and conceptually, primary cilia resemble antennae that pick up external signals and channel them to a receiver, the cell nucleus. Several other signaling pathways, most notably the WNT/APC pathway, also signal through the primary cilium, but the hedgehog pathway is uniquely reliant on this structure.

When no ligand is available for binding, PTCH1 resides on the cell surface near the base of the primary cilium and prevents SMO from entering (Fig. 6.21). PTCH1 is believed to function as a sterol pump that prevents small regulatory molecules from activating SMO, but the precise biochemical activity of PTCH1, the identity of these regulatory molecules, and the nature of SMO inhibition remain incompletely understood. In the absence of local SMO, the GLI transcription factors are maintained within the primary cilium in a sequestered, inactive state by a regulator called SUFU (a name derived from the *Drosophila* ortholog Suppressor of fused). SUFU protein also competes with an E3 ubiquitin ligase called SPOP for binding to GLI2 and GLI3, and thereby prevents their degradation.

Signaling is activated when PTCH1 is bound by a hedgehog ligand. When this receptor-ligand interaction occurs, the repression of SMO by PTCH1 is relieved, and SMO is thus permitted to move to the ciliary membrane. At this new location, SMO blocks the function of SUFU and thereby causes GLI proteins to be actively transported out of the primary cilium. The ultimate destination of these transcription factors is the cell nucleus, where they affect a transcriptional program that mediates cell proliferation and differentiation.

Both PTCH1 and SMO have been reported to mediate a variety of cellular functions in addition to the regulation of GLI proteins. The pathway that is involved in GLI regulation is sometimes referred to as the *canonical hedgehog signaling pathway* to distinguish it from these other, more obscure activities. The canonical hedgehog signaling pathway is populated by cancer genes. The relevance of the other activities of PTCH1 and SMO to tumorigenesis remains uncertain.

Hedgehog ligands are not present in most normal differentiated tissues, but they are expressed in a wide range of human cancers. These ligands can activate hedgehog signaling in tumor cells, and also in the normal cells of the surrounding stroma. In most cases, the molecular basis of SHH expression is unknown, and the overall effect of the resulting signals on tumor evolution is difficult to quantify.

Hedgehog signaling can be constitutively activated by cancer-associated mutations in *PTCH1*. Mutant PTCH1 proteins fail to repress SMO; in cancers that harbor these mutations, the activity of SMO is ligand-independent. As detailed in Chap. 3, germline mutations in *PTCH1* are the cause of Basal Cell Nevus Syndrome (also known as Gorlin syndrome), a disease that predisposes affected individuals to basal cell carcinomas of the skin, cerebellar brain tumors known as medulloblastomas, and rhabdomyosarcomas, a form of pediatric sarcoma that arises in skeletal muscle. Somatic mutations in *PTCH1* are found in the sporadic forms of these cancers, and in malignant peripheral nerve sheath tumors, melanomas, and cancers of the uterus and lung.

While inactivation of *PTCH1* is the primary mode of genetic activation of hedgehog signaling in evolving tumors, small numbers of cancers harbor mutations in other pathway components. Activating mutations in *SMO* or amplifications of the *SMO* locus have been observed in small proportions of lung and ovarian cancers, and in melanomas. *SUFU* is inactivated in some prostate tumors while the SUFU antagonist encoded by *SPOP* is activated in others. Germline mutations in *SUFU* reportedly contribute to medulloblastoma predisposition.

Interestingly, a role for the GLI family of transcription factors in cancer was suggested in 1987, long before the mammalian hedgehog pathway was elucidated. Kenneth Kinzler and Bert Vogelstein discovered a novel gene that was amplified and highly expressed in a single glioma, a highly malignant form of brain cancer. The proto-oncogene within the amplicon was accordingly named *gli*. This gene, since designed *GLI1*, is amplified in about 10 % of gliomas.

TGF-β/ SMAD Signaling Maintains Adult Tissue Homeostasis

Cell proliferation and apoptosis are two of the most critical determinants of cell survival. These processes are accordingly highly regulated. A cytokine called transforming growth factor β1 (TGF-β1) is one of three related secreted protein ligands that function to preserve tissue homeostasis in developed tissues, and which are involved in many basic disease processes, including cancer. Genes that populate the signal transduction pathways downstream of TGF-β are frequently altered in several common forms of cancer.

The receptors that interact with TGF-β ligands are single-pass transmembrane serine/threonine protein kinases, enzymatically distinct from the RTKs. There are three general types of TGF-β receptors, known as types I II, and III. The receptors are variably comprised of several distinct proteins and isoforms, but each has high binding affinity for TGF-β1.

Signaling by TGF-β family members is initiated by binding of ligand to one of their specific receptors on the surface of the cell. TGF-β proteins in the form of homodimers induce the assembly of a receptor complex that can include multiple receptor proteins and various accessory receptor proteins (Fig. 6.22). Upon receptor complex assembly, the constitutively active type II receptor is brought into proximity of the type I receptor, which is then phosphorylated. Thus activated, the type I receptor phosphorylates the signaling proteins SMAD2 and SMAD3. These proteins form several different multimeric complexes with SMAD4. SMAD4 is accordingly referred to as a *co-SMAD* to reflect this cooperative feature. SMAD2/3-SMAD4

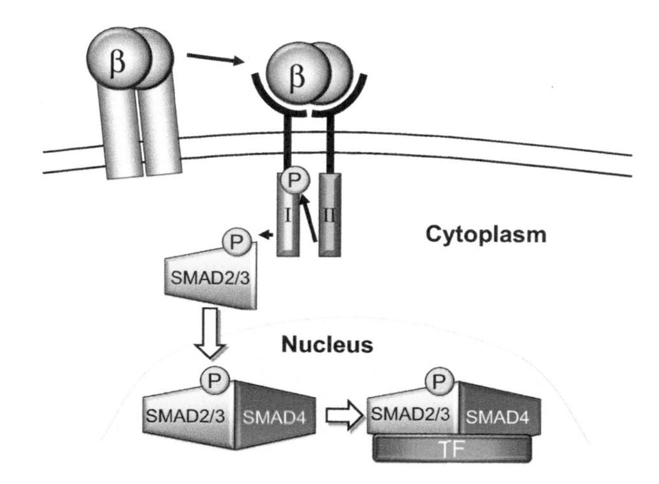

Fig. 6.22 Activation of canonical TGF-β signaling. Accessory receptors (shown in *gray*) bind homodimeric TGF-β ligand molecules and present them to TGF-β receptors. Upon ligand binding, the type I and type II TGF-β receptors form a complex, causing the phosphorylation of the type I receptor on specific serines and threonines by the type II receptor. The activated type I receptor phosphorylates SMAD2 and SMAD3 proteins in the cytoplasm. SMAD2 and SMAD3 then form multimeric complexes with SMAD4 in the nucleus. These complexes associate with transcription factors and function to both transactivate and repress downstream genes

complexes shuttle into the nucleus via the nuclear pore complex. In the nucleus, SMAD2/3-SMAD4 complexes cooperate with nuclear transcription factors to regulate the expression of a wide variety of genes involved in cell proliferation and death.

Despite the apparent simplicity of the TGF-β/SMAD pathway, the canonical TGF-β signaling pathway can respond to numerous ligands and generate diverse cellular responses. In contrast with the best-characterized RTK pathways, the TGF-β pathways appear to be differentially sensitive to varying concentrations of extracellular ligand. In addition, many intracellular proteins not directly required for signaling can promote or inhibit SMAD-complex formation. SMAD4 is the substrate of several regulatory proteins associated with other pathways, including GSK3 and ERK1/2. Many of the TGF-β responses are cell type-specific. For example, the same ligand might cause one type of cell to proliferate, but trigger a second type of cell to undergo apoptosis. The molecular mechanisms that underlie the wide range of TGF-β responses are accordingly complex.

Canonical TGF-β signaling suppresses the growth of most normal cells. Several downstream genes that are regulated at the transcriptional level by TGF-β/SMAD pathway activation actively suppress growth (Fig. 6.23). The genes *CDKN1A* and *CDKN2B* encode the cyclin-dependent kinase inhibitors, p21 and

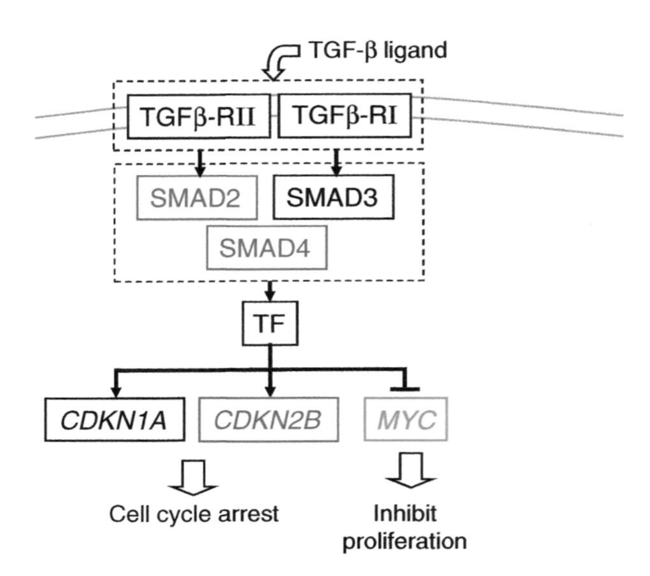

Fig. 6.23 Disruption of the TGF-β/SMAD signaling pathway by tumor suppressor gene mutations. The SMAD signaling complexes can be disrupted by mutations in either *SMAD2* or *SMAD4*. Due to their close proximity on chromosome 18q, these genes are frequently inactivated by deletions in the same cancers. Normal signaling promotes growth inhibition via cell cycle arrest. Inactivation of TGF-β/SMAD signaling in cancers results in a loss of cell cycle arrest mediated by *CDKN1A* and *CDKN2B*, and the promotion of proliferation caused by the disinhibition of *MYC*. Proteins and genes affected by oncogenic mutations are shown in *red*, tumor suppressors are shown in *blue*

p15 respectively, that function to arrest cell cycle progression. In addition, activated SMAD complexes also appear to repress the transcription of pro-growth target genes, including *MYC*.

Many types of cancer cells are resistant to canonical TGF-β signaling, and proliferate and remain undifferentiated despite the presence of TGF-β ligand. Several genes that compose the TGF-β/SMAD pathway are targets of inactivating mutations in cancers. *SMAD4* is a tumor suppressor gene that is inactivated in a significant fraction of colorectal and pancreatic cancers and also in about one half of all the rare cancers of the bile ducts, called cholangiocarcinomas. *SMAD2* is located in close proximity to *SMAD4* on chromosome 18q, and is therefore lost in many of the large deletions that affect *SMAD4*. In some cancers, *SMAD2* is affected by mutations that do not appear to affect *SMAD4*, indicating that *SMAD2* also functions as a tumor suppressor. Heritable germline mutations in *SMAD4* cause Juvenile Polyposis Syndrome, a disease that confers cancer predisposition (Chap. 3).

MYC Is a Downstream Effector of Multiple Cancer Gene Pathways

The *MYC* proto-oncogene encodes a transcription factor that regulates the expression of a very large number of downstream genes in response to both extracellular and intracellular signals. In general, MYC enhances cell survival by inducing genes that are required for progression of the cell cycle, and represses genes that are involved in the maintenance of tissue homeostasis. It has been estimated that 15 % of all human protein-coding genes are either induced or repressed by MYC. MYC target genes are involved in diverse cellular processes including metabolism, cell cycle regulation, apoptosis, protein synthesis, angiogenesis and cell-cell adhesion. These broad cellular effects probably explain why *MYC* is amplified or activated by translocations in many cancers of all types. MYC is widely expressed across human tissue types. The other MYC family members are expressed in a more tissue specific manner, and are accordingly involved in fewer types of cancer.

MYC-encoded proteins are transcriptional trans-activators that bind specific promoter sequences upstream of pro-growth target genes. Each member of the MYC protein family contains two domains that are highly characteristic of transcription factors. At the n-terminus of the MYC proteins is a transactivation domain that is involved in the recruitment of other essential transcription factors. A c-terminal domain known as a *basic helix-loop-helix leucine zip*per facilitates both protein-protein interactions as well as sequence specific DNA binding.

MYC proteins function in complex with one of several factors known as *MYC-associated protein X* (MAX) proteins. MAX proteins also contain a basic helix-loop-helix leucine zipper motif that facilitates MYC/MAX heterodimer formation. In partnership with a MAX protein, MYC binds to a defined DNA sequence motif known as an E box (Fig. 6.24). The E box sequence 5′CACGTG-3′ is a very common protein-binding motif, and is located in my places throughout the human genome.

MYC proteins are constantly degraded and thus have a half-life of only 15–20 min. The levels of MYC therefore decrease quickly when the gene is no longer active. In contrast, MAX proteins are constitutively expressed at high levels and are highly stable. The transcriptional activity of the MYC/MAX heterodimer is primarily limited by the intracellular concentration of MYC protein.

The MYC/MAX heterodimer increases the expression of many of its target genes, but in some cases target gene expression is repressed. The mechanism by which MYC proteins repress the transcription of specific genes involves a third category of proteins known as MADs. Like MYC proteins, MAD proteins form heterodimers with MAX and these appear to compete with MYC/MAX complexes for DNA binding.

In normal (non-cancer) cells, *MYC* expression is tightly regulated and highly sensitive to upstream signals. *MYC* transcripts and MYC proteins are highly labile, and so decreased levels of *MYC* transcription can lead to a rapid decrease in MYC protein activity. The half-life of MYC protein can be affected by upstream signals

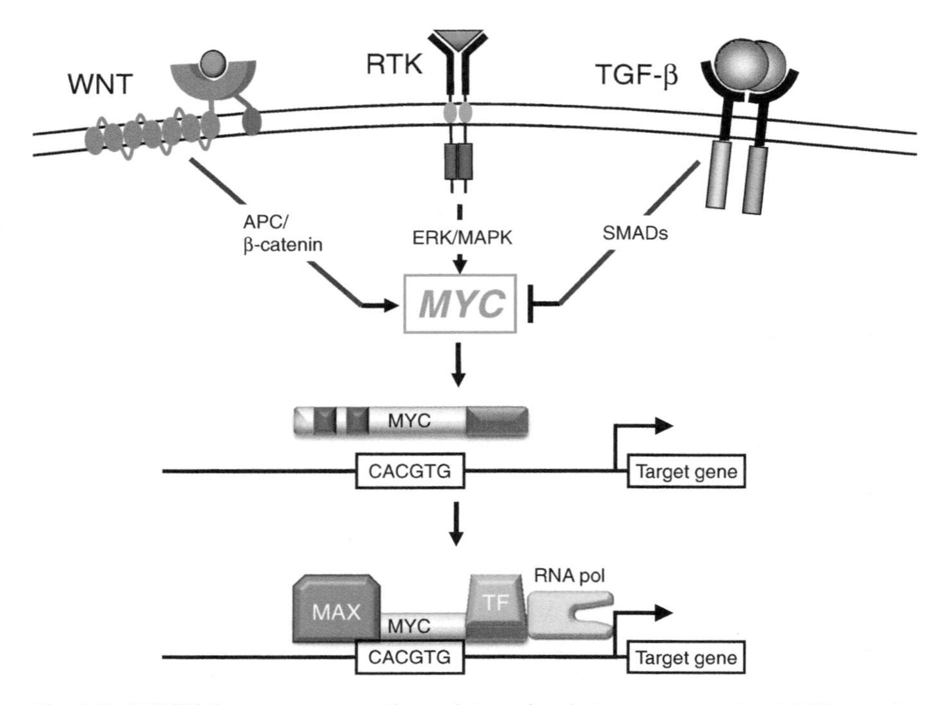

Fig. 6.24 MYC links upstream growth regulatory signals to gene expression. MYC normally functions downstream of several cell surface receptor signaling pathways that are recurrently functionally altered in cancers. The canonical WNT and RTK pathways and their respective downstream mediators promote expression of the *MYC* gene; the TGF-β pathway transmits an inhibitory signal that inhibits *MYC* expression. MYC protein dimerizes with its MAX binding partner via two specific c-terminal binding sites (shown in *blue*) and associates with DNA sequences that conform to the consensus 5′-CACGTG-3′, a binding site known as the E box. The n-terminal bHLHLZ domain (shown in *gray*) of MYC interacts with transcription factors that recruit RNA polymerase. MYC can also promote gene repression by displacing specific transcription cofactors (not shown)

from the receptor tyrosine kinase pathways. Like many highly regulated proteins, MYC is post-translationally modified. Phosphorylation of a specific residue in the n-terminus, serine 62, has been found to increase MYC stability. Serine 62 phosphorylation occurs upon RAS/RAF activation, via ERK. A second phosphorylation event, on threonine 58 can trigger MYC degradation by the proteasome. Phosphorylation at this site is inhibited by PI3K signaling, probably via inhibition of GSK3 kinase. In normal cells, these pathways likely serve to ensure that any activation in MYC activity is transient in nature.

MYC is highly regulated at the level of its transcription (Fig. 6.24). As described in the previous sections, the engagement of the WNT receptor with ligand ultimately promotes *MYC* gene expression, whereas the pathway triggered by TGF-β and its downstream pathways inhibit *MYC* transcription (Fig. 6.25). The downstream pathways triggered by receptor tyrosine kinases also converge on the MYC

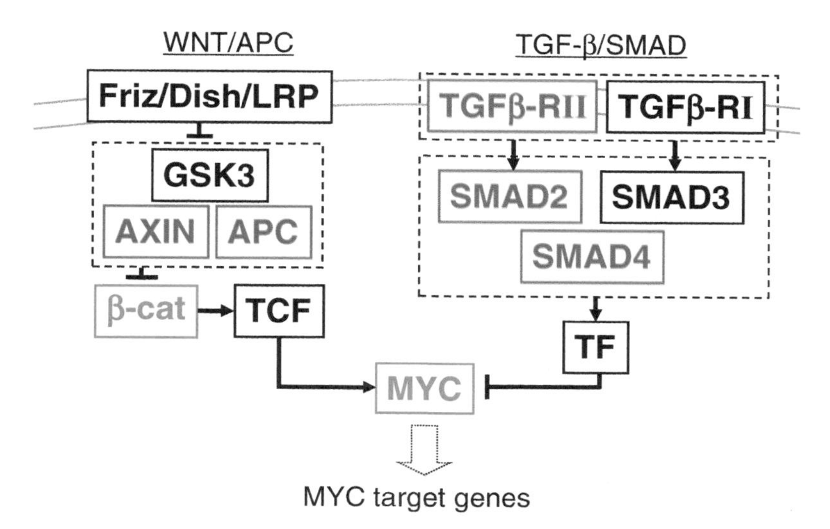

Fig. 6.25 Transcription of *MYC* is differentially regulated by the canonical WNT and TGF-β pathways. WNT/APC signaling promotes *MYC* transcription via the downstream activation of β-catenin. In contrast, TGF-β/SMAD signaling activates transcription complexes that repress the transcription of *MYC*

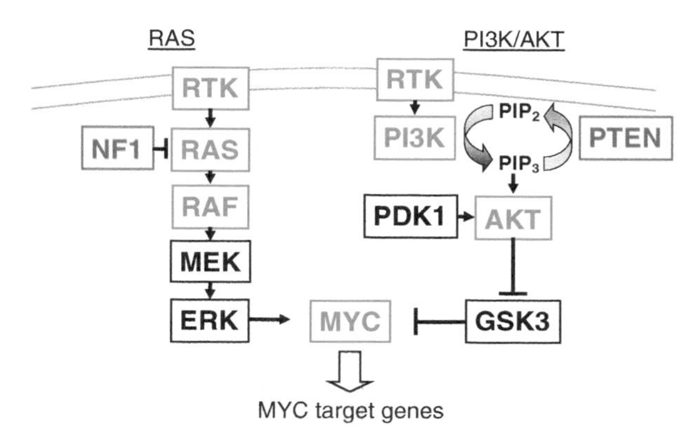

Fig. 6.26 Transcription of *MYC* is induced by RTK-mediated pathways. The RTK-RAS-RAF-MEK-ERK and RTK-PI3K-AKT pathways each lead to increased *MYC* expression

gene, increasing its expression and thereby promoting a pro-growth transcriptional program (Fig. 6.26).

MYC is most commonly activated in cancers by amplification or by translocations that place the MYC open reading frame in a more actively transcribed context. Less commonly, the *MYC* proto-oncogene can be activated by point mutations in functionally important hot spots. Mutations in the *MYC*-encoded threonine 58 and serine 62 sites that are involved in protein stabilization are frequently found in

Burkitt lymphoma, a cancer of the lymphatic system associated with the Epstein-Barr virus.

Whether activated by amplification, translocation or point mutation, *MYC* promotes the transcriptional transactivation of E box-containing target genes. The transcriptional targets of MYC are highly diverse. Among the most consistently upregulated are genes involved in biosynthetic processes that include nucleotide metabolism, ribosome biogenesis, RNA processing and DNA replication. Numerous studies suggest that a primordial function of MYC is to increase cellular biomass and promote cell cycle transitions.

p53 Activation Is Triggered by Damaged or Incompletely Replicated Chromosomes

Mutations that inactivate *TP53* are highly prevalent in cancers. In accordance with this central role in tumor suppression, p53 participates in numerous functions related to cell survival and genome maintenance. Unlike the signal transduction pathways that originate at the cell surface, the p53 pathways appear to primarily respond to intracellular stimuli.

The most proximal trigger of p53 activation is the presence in the cell of a DNA strand break or a collapsed DNA replication fork. Such changes can be the result of either DNA damage or interrupted DNA replication or repair.

Many perturbations in the cellular microenvironment can lead directly or indirectly to the damage or structural deformation of chromosomal DNA. Exogenous factors, such as ionizing radiation as well as endogenous processes such as aerobic respiration, generate highly reactive species that can directly create single and double strand DNA breaks, the latter of which represent a potentially lethal form of DNA damage.

A particularly vulnerable period in the division cycle of a cell is S-phase, the interval in which chromatin is replicated. Many metabolic states can cause inhibition of DNA replication and result in the accumulation of DNA replication intermediates. Various agents that damage the DNA directly, particularly double helix-altering lesions such as crosslinks, or limit the building blocks of chromatin can cause the stalling of the molecular machines that replicate chromosomes. Agents such as ultraviolet light and many types of toxins can create DNA adducts. Such adducts represent physical obstacles that can effectively block replication fork progression. Nutrient deprivation and the accumulation of metabolic byproducts can affect the pathways of biosynthesis that produce chromatin precursors, thereby impeding the efficient replication of the genome. Low levels of oxygen, a state called *hypoxia*, can also inhibit DNA replication and cause increases in p53 levels. In summary, diverse conditions that cause suboptimal conditions for DNA replication can be manifest as DNA breaks or stalled replication forks. These DNA structures can activate the enzyme-mediated pathways that regulate p53.

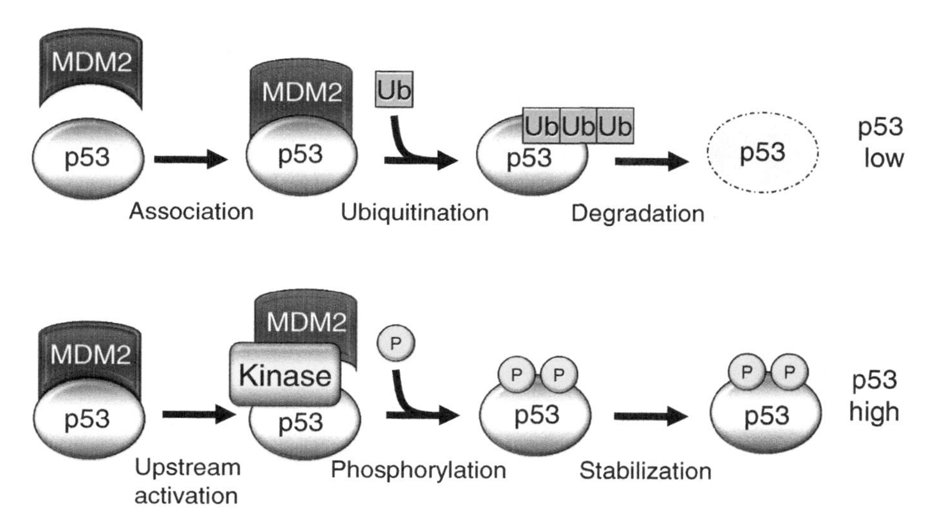

Fig. 6.27 p53 is stabilized upon phosphorylation. Under unperturbed growth conditions, p53 protein is associated with the MDM2 protein. MDM2 is a component of an enzyme complex that covalently attaches ubiquitin moieties to p53, and thus marks it for degradation by the proteasome. By this mechanism, proliferating cells maintain low levels of p53. After sensing DNA strand breaks or stalled DNA replication forks, upstream kinases catalyze the phosphorylation of p53 at multiple sites. These modifications are associated with the physical separation of p53 and MDM2, and the resulting stabilization of p53 protein, a potent inhibitor of cell growth

The p53 pathway is highly responsive to many changes in chromatin structure and integrity. In acknowledgment of the central role of p53 as a suppressor of tumorigenesis and responder to DNA damage, Arnold Levine aptly described p53 as the '*guardian of the genome*'.

The p53 protein is extensively modified after its translation. By a mechanism that is the best understood, the activity of p53 is controlled by coupled phosphorylation and ubiquitination reactions. Under conditions that favor cell growth, the majority of p53 molecules in the cell are physically bound to the protein product of the *MDM2* proto-oncogene (Fig. 6.27). The MDM2 protein is a ubiquitin ligase, and is part of a multi-enzyme process that covalently adds ubiquitin moieties to protein substrates, including p53. Modified with ubiquitin, MDM2 substrates are tagged for degradation by the proteasome. As a consequence of this constitutive degradation process, the half-life of p53 in the cell is short – approximately 5–20 min. The interaction with MDM2 therefore is a mechanism for keeping p53 levels low under conditions in which cell growth and survival are favored.

Changes in the intracellular or extracellular environment that cause chromosomal breaks or stalling of DNA replication forks lead to the phosphorylation of p53 by upstream serine/threonine protein kinases. Phosphorylation of p53 at several critical serine residues accompanies a conformational change that disrupts the p53-MDM2 interaction. The disruption of p53-MDM2 complexes prevents ubiquitin-mediated degradation, causes a several-fold increase in protein half-life and thereby leads to an increase in the intracellular concentration of p53. The multi-site phosphorylation of p53 regulates its activity by controlling its abundance.

The control of p53 concentration by MDM2 is an important mechanism of regulation, but there are clearly additional ways in which covalent modifications affect p53 function. In response to various types of growth inhibitory stress, p53 can be phosphorylated and dephosphorylated on as many as 10 different serine and threonine residues. In addition, p53 is acetylated and conjugated to SUMO. Many of these modifications appear to affect p53 conformation and activity in ways that are MDM2-independent. The multitude of posttranslational modifications that affect p53 function are concentrated in the N- and C-termini.

p53 Is Controlled by Protein Kinases Encoded by Tumor Suppressor Genes

Protein kinases clearly play a key role in the responses of p53 to DNA damage and related stimuli. But which kinases perform this critical function? From an experimental standpoint, identifying the kinase or kinases that are responsible for the phosphorylation of any given substrate is challenging. Cell-free biochemical systems that employ purified proteins can be used to establish kinase-substrate interactions. However, relationships observed *in vitro* may not accurately represent what actually occurs *in vivo*. Another complicating factor is the fact that protein kinases often modify many substrates. This characteristic, sometimes referred to as *enzymatic promiscuity*, makes it difficult to determine which substrates are physiologically relevant to the function under investigation. In the case of p53, *in vitro* studies have identified a large number of kinases that can effectively modify p53 on the residues known to be affected by DNA damage *in vivo*.

A major breakthrough in understanding the mechanisms of p53 regulation came in 1992, when Michael Kastan and colleagues reported that cells from patients affected by an autosomal recessive cancer predisposition syndrome called *Ataxia telangiectasia* (AT) exhibited defective stabilization of p53 after treatment with ionizing radiation. It was subsequently demonstrated that the gene mutated in AT, designated *ATM*, encodes a kinase that directly phosphorylates p53 on a regulatory serine residue *in vivo* and *in vitro*. This phosphorylation site (serine 15) is within the p53 domain that physically interacts with MDM2. This seminal series of experiments thus proved that ATM could phosphorylate p53 and that this single modification has a strong effect on p53 activation. *ATM*, like *TP53*, is a tumor suppressor gene. The demonstration of a direct functional interaction between their encoded proteins indicates that *ATM* and *TP53* suppress tumorigenesis by participating in a common pathway in the DNA damage response.

ATM kinase activity increases very rapidly after cells are exposed to DNA damaging agents, such as ionizing radiation, that cause double strand DNA breaks. Detailed biochemical studies have revealed that ATM is activated at the site of DNA

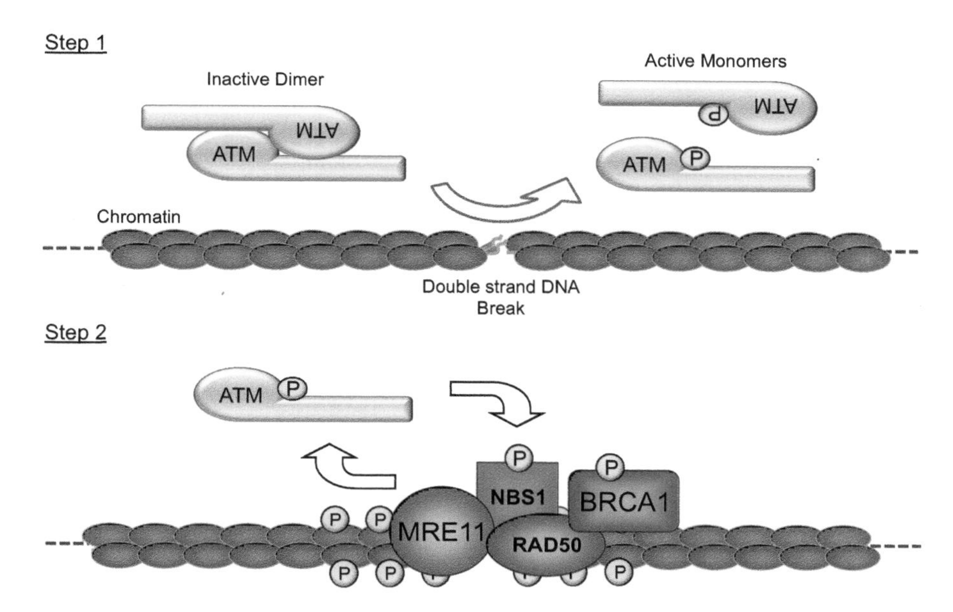

Fig. 6.28 Activation of ATM at the site of a double-strand DNA break. Endogenous cellular processes, such as stalled replication forks, and exogenous environmental agents, such as ionizing radiation, can cause double strand DNA breaks. The changes in chromosome structure caused by such lesions rapidly activate ATM in a two-step process. Initially present in inactive, dimeric form, ATM is concurrently phosphorylated (shown in *yellow*) and dissociated into monomers. Thus activated, ATM phosphorylates a chromatin component known as histone H2AX in the vicinity of the double strand break, as well as proteins in the MRN (MRE11, RAD50, NBS1) complex and BRCA1. These protein/DNA complexes actively recruit and retain ATM at the double strand break site, facilitating the activation of downstream effectors, including the Fanconi anemia proteins and p53

breaks in two defined steps (Fig. 6.28). In the absence of a break, inactive ATM molecules exist in bound pairs, known as homo-dimers. Within minutes after a DNA break occurs, the ATM dimers dissociate into monomers with catalytic kinase activity. The ATM kinase activity level does not reach its full potential until the ATM monomers interact with a multiprotein complex encoded by *MRE11*, *NBS1* and *RAD50* (accordingly known as the MRN complex), and with the protein encoded by the tumor suppressor *BRCA1*. The MRN complex binds DNA and has multiple biochemical properties that include the cutting, unwinding and bridging the ends of the damaged double helix. BRCA1 protein is involved in a repair process known as non-homologous DNA end joining. The MRN complex and the BRCA1 protein are required for the efficient recruitment and retention of ATM monomers at the sites of double strand DNA breaks.

Activated ATM is a serine/threonine protein kinase that can phosphorylate numerous downstream substrates. Cumulatively, ATM and the other proteins activated in response to DNA damage and DNA replication intermediates compose the *DNA damage signaling network*. This signaling network resembles a web of interconnected molecular circuits that integrate many upstream stimuli and numerous

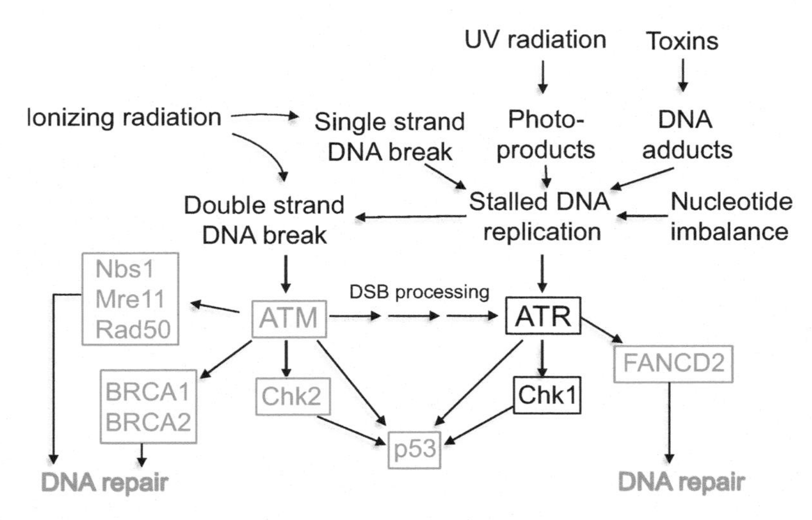

Fig. 6.29 Activation of the DNA damage response network by ATM and ATR. Diverse types of environmental agents and cell states can cause DNA damage and stalling of DNA replication complexes. These diverse stimuli activate ATM and ATR, the apical kinases of the DNA damage response network. A major function of this signaling network is to inhibit growth and promote DNA repair. Signals generated by ATM and ATR are amplified by the checkpoint kinases, Chk1 and Chk2. Each of these kinases has been shown to phosphorylate p53 on activating sites, under some conditions. Proteins encoded by tumor suppressor genes are highlighted in red. ATM and ATR can together phosphorylate over 700 cellular proteins; only a small illustrative subset of highly studied substrates is shown

several downstream targets, including p53. Via this complex network, perturbations to chromosomes can trigger many diverse cellular responses, including the critical processes of DNA repair (Fig. 6.29). Comprehensive protein profiling studies have revealed that over 700 proteins are phosphorylated by ATM and the related kinase ATR at more than 900 distinct phosphorylation sites.

Many protein kinases associated with cancer gene pathways can modify p53 on sites known to be important to its regulation. In addition to ATM and ATR, the ERKs, GSK3β, the JNKs can all phosphorylate p53 in response to genotoxic stimuli such as ultraviolet light. Mutations in *ATM* do not recapitulate all of the cancer-related phenotypes seen upon mutation of *TP53*, nor do mutations in any other of the diverse p53 kinase genes. These observations imply that many kinases and pathways, including those in the DNA damage signaling network function together to upregulate p53, in response to diverse stimuli. It is also possible that different kinases may be of primary importance in different tissues, and in response to different types of chromosome-damaging stimuli.

Several of the most highly studied components of the DNA damage signaling network are:

Checkpoint kinase 2 (CHEK2). CHEK2 encodes a serine/threonine kinase known as Chk2 that is phosphorylated and thus activated by ATM. Chk2 amplifies the ATM signal and transduces it to cellular compartments that may be distant from the DNA strand break. Chk2 can directly phosphorylate p53 and many other substrates. Cells that lack Chk2 are nonetheless able to stabilize p53 in response to DNA damage, demonstrating that Chk2 is not required for p53 activation. Germline *CHEK2* mutations contribute to familial breast cancers, and have been associated with modest increases in breast cancer risk. *CHEK2* is therefore cancer predisposition gene in the breast epithelium. The penetrance of *CHEK2* mutations is lower than that of *BRCA1* and *BRCA2*.

Ataxia telangiectasia- and Rad3-related (*ATR*). *ATR* is a gene in the same family of kinase genes as *ATM,* and encodes a protein kinase that triggers a parallel signaling pathway. *ATR* is not involved in AT, nor is it mutationally inactivated in sporadic tumors. In contrast to ATM, which is biochemically activated by double strand DNA breaks, ATR is primarily activated by DNA structures that accumulate when DNA replication forks stall. ATR is therefore triggered by ultraviolet light and other types of agents that cause DNA adducts, as well as by agents that deplete the nucleotide pools required for DNA replication. The activity of ATM at double strand DNA breaks can also create DNA structures that are recognized by ATR.

Checkpoint kinase 1 (CHEK1). CHEK1 was originally discovered as a homolog of a checkpoint kinase gene that is conserved in yeast that acts as a central regulator of growth control. Structurally unrelated to Chk2, the *CHEK1*-encoded protein Chk1 is a serine/threonine protein kinase that is an extensively studied component of the pathway that includes ATR. ATR directly phosphorylates Chk1 on several c-terminal serine residues. Thus activated, Chk1 can phosphorylate p53 on sites that are important for its activation. *CHEK1* itself is not a tumor suppressor gene.

p53 Induces the Transcription of Genes That Suppress Cancer Phenotypes

TP53 encodes a protein that primarily functions as a transcription factor. Upon its stabilization by upstream DNA damage signals, p53 regulates genes that inhibit growth and facilitate cellular repair processes.

When stabilized and activated by posttranslational modifications, p53 becomes more abundant and assembles into tetramers. In this configuration, p53 binds tightly to DNA that contains a consensus binding sequence (Fig. 6.30). This sequence motif is commonly found in the promoter regions of functionally diverse genes involved in growth suppression. When bound to a promoter element, p53 is a strong inducer of gene expression.

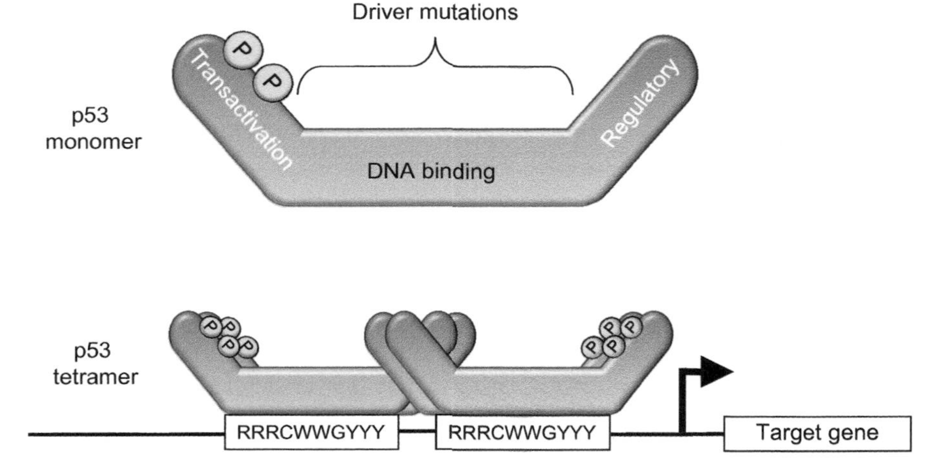

Fig. 6.30 p53 transactivates transcription. The p53 protein has a central core domain that is required for sequence-specific DNA binding, an n-terminal transactivation domain that mediates interactions with other transcription factors, and a c-terminal domain that is required for protein oligomerization and other modes of regulation. The driver mutations that inactivate *TP53* most commonly occur in the exons that encode the central DNA binding domain. The terminal regions are predominantly affected by post-translational modifications catalyzed by numerous enzymes, including protein kinases. Shown are representative phosphate groups that are associated with reduced binding to the p53 regulator MDM2. Activated p53 assembles into tetramers that bind a bipartite promoter element that contains two half sites with the consensus RRRCWWGYYY DNA sequence motif separated by 0–13 nonspecific bases. R=purines A or G; W=A or T; Y=pyrimidines C or T; only one DNA strand is shown. The binding of tetrameric p53 increases promoter activity (*arrow*) and target gene expression

Most of the single base substitutions that inactivate *TP53* are located in the exons that encode a large central DNA binding domain. Proteins encoded by cancer-associated mutant *TP53* genes therefore fail to bind normally to promoter sequences. While other biochemical functions have been attributed to the p53 protein, it is the transcriptional transactivation function that is most universally inactivated in cancers that harbor *TP53* mutations. The preponderance of mutations in the DNA binding region suggests that the tumor suppressor function of p53 is closely related to its role as a transcription factor.

Many genes can be switched on by activated p53. There are an estimated 1600 copies of the p53 DNA binding consensus sequence scattered throughout the genome. This number includes many sites that would not be expected to affect the transcription of protein coding genes. The diverse gene transcripts are induced by activated p53 can be collectively referred to as the *p53-dependent transcriptome*.

The p53-dependent transcriptome encodes proteins that function in downstream pathways that regulate cell survival, and function to maintain a stable genome (Fig. 6.31). The mutations that frequently inactivate *TP53* in cancers disrupt these pathways and thereby cause significant changes in the ways that mutant cells respond to environmental stressors and DNA damaging agents. The normal cellular response

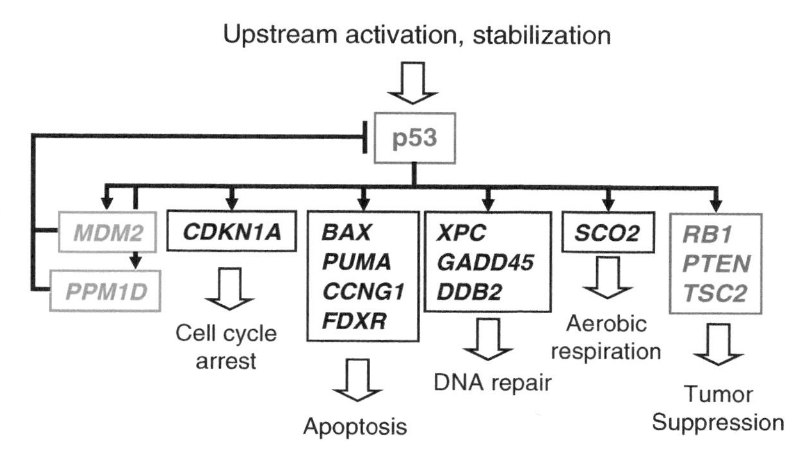

Fig. 6.31 Representative genes and pathways activated by p53. Following its stabilization and activation, p53 transactivates the transcription of numerous target genes. These genes, in turn, control many aspects of cell proliferation. By regulating the expression of the proto-oncogenes *MDM2* and *PPM1D*, p53 induces feedback loops that attenuate its activity. The genes shown are a representative subset of the >100 genes that are regulated by p53 in various cell types

to stressful changes in the microenvironment is to stop growing and to attempt to repair genomic DNA. Cell clones that have lost p53 are less reliant on aerobic metabolism, fail to properly undergo cell cycle arrest, and therefore continue to proliferate. These surviving clones often fail to appropriately initiate DNA repair, and therefore can exhibit genomic instability.

Several target genes and pathways provide a representative view of the functions that are lost when p53 is inactivated during tumorigenesis:

Cell cycle arrest. Several p53 target genes function to control the progression of the cell division cycle. The p21 protein, encoded by *CDKN1A*, binds and thereby inactivates several of the cyclin-dependent kinases that drive the cell cycle forward.

Programmed cell death (apoptosis). p53 controls multiple regulators of programmed cell death, also known as apoptosis. The genes in this category that are most robustly induced by p53 include *BAX*, *PUMA*, *FDXR*, and *CCNG1*. The proteins encoded by these genes collectively destabilize mitochondria and thereby decrease the apoptotic threshold. The loss of p53 function decreases the ability of cells to trigger apoptosis.

DNA repair. TP53 participates in several DNA repair processes that are triggered in response to DNA damage. Genes such as *XPC*, *GADD45* and *DDB2* are commonly induced by p53, along with the genes that control cell cycle arrest. P53 can thus facilitate the tight coordination of cell cycle arrest and DNA repair.

Glucose metabolism. Normal cells employ the highly efficient process of *aerobic respiration* to convert the energy of glucose into adenosine triphosphate (ATP). In contrast, cancer cells preferentially rely on the anaerobic pathway known as *glycolysis* to provide ATP. This metabolic change is termed the Warburg effect (Chap. 1). The enhancement of glycolysis provides a distinct selective advantage to cells growing in regions of low oxygen concentration, such as those that occur around growing tumors. The p53 target gene *SCO2* encodes the synthesis of cytochrome C oxidase 2 protein, a regulator of the cytochrome oxidase C complex, the major site of oxygen utilization in eukaryotic cells. *SCO2* expression is upregulated by p53. The loss of p53 function reduces *SCO2* expression, resulting in a metabolic switch from respiration to glycolysis. Cells with mutated *TP53*, therefore have a survival advantage in regions of low oxygenation. The increased local production of lactic acid and other metabolites that arise via the glycolytic pathway may also contribute to cloncal selection.

Tumor suppression by other pathways. In addition to directly controlling cell growth and survival, p53 can also activate genes that populate other tumor suppressor pathways. p53 has been shown to regulate the expression of the tumor suppressor genes *RB1*, *PTEN* and *TSC2*, and to thereby exert control over their respective tumor suppressive functions.

Feedback Loops Dynamically Control p53 Abundance

The p53 protein is activated in response to DNA damage and subsequently deactivated when DNA is eventually repaired. Two transcriptional targets of p53 cooperatively mediate a dynamic process that functions to tightly regulate the temporal abundance of p53 protein.

When a cell experiences DNA damage, upstream kinases in the DNA damage signaling network are activated and immediately catalyze the phosphorylation of p53 protein, thereby leading to its stabilization. The *MDM2* gene contains the p53 DNA binding consensus sequence in its promoter, and is transcriptionally activated by bound p53 tetramers. MDM2 RNA and protein are therefore increased in abundance after p53 levels increase.

Ultimately, the activation of p53 is transient and dependent on persistent upstream signals. The levels of p53 in the cell are predominantly controlled by the association between p53 and MDM2. As increased levels of p53 cause the elevated expression of MDM2, this ubiquitin ligase increasingly targets p53 for degradation. If DNA strand breaks persist, newly synthesized p53 will be continually phosphorylated and activated. However, if the DNA strand breaks are successfully repaired, the upstream kinase signals subside, and the high levels of MDM2 protein cause a reduction in p53 levels and a concomitant downregulation of p53 activity (Fig. 6.32).

A second transcriptional target of p53 that is relevant to the dynamic regulation of p53 regulation is *PPM1D*, which encodes a protein phosphatase called WIP1 (originally designated as the wild-type p53-induced protein phosphatase 1D). WIP1 catalyzes the dephosphorylation of p53, and therefore functions in direct opposition to the upstream protein kinases of the DNA damage response network. By dephosphorylating p53, WIP1 promotes the association of p53 with MDM2 and thereby

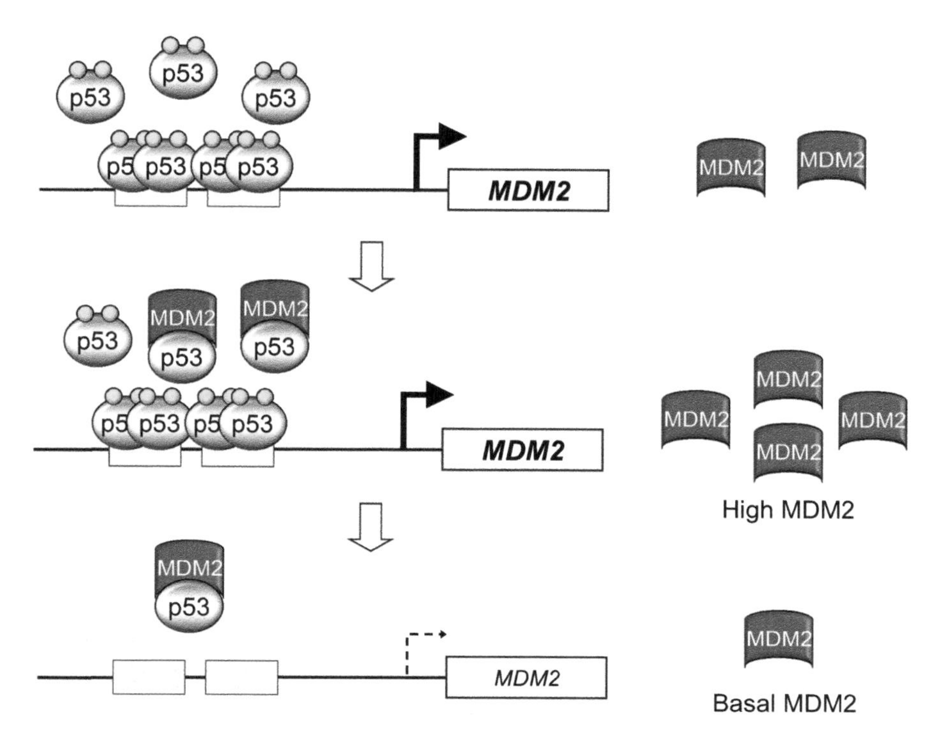

Fig. 6.32 Attenuation of p53 activity by MDM2. Phosphorylated p53 is stabilized and assembles into tetramers that bind the p53 consensus binding sites in the *MDM2* promoter. High levels of MDM2 protein thus accumulate after p53 is stabilized. As upstream signals subside, MDM2 associates with unphosphorylated p53 molecules, targeting them for degradation. Lower levels of p53 eventually cause *MDM2* expression to return to basal levels

promotes the subsequent degradation of p53. Together, the p53-dependent activation of *MDM2* and *PPM1D* expression constitutes a negative feedback loop that functions to attenuate p53 activity (Fig. 6.33). Consistent with the role of WIP1 as a negative regulator of p53, *PPM1D* is a proto-oncogene. So is *MDM2*.

The interconnected feedback loops that control p53 abundance provide critical insight into how *MDM2* and *PPM1D* can promote tumorigenesis. In some types of cancer, most commonly sarcomas, *MDM2* is converted from a proto-oncogene to an oncogene by gene amplification. As a result of this amplification in cancers, *MDM2* is expressed at significantly higher levels, independent of the levels of p53. The high abundance of MDM2 protein in cancer cells with *MDM2* amplification causes the inhibition of p53 function. An alternative pathway to increasing p53 function that is activated in some cases is the amplification of an *MDM2*-related gene called *MDM4*, which also encodes a ubiquitin ligase.

Other cancers, including papillary thryroid carcinomas and gliomas, target the p53 pathway by unusual, gain-of-function truncating mutations in *PPM1D*. Germline truncating mutations in *PPM1D* are associated with a rare predisposition

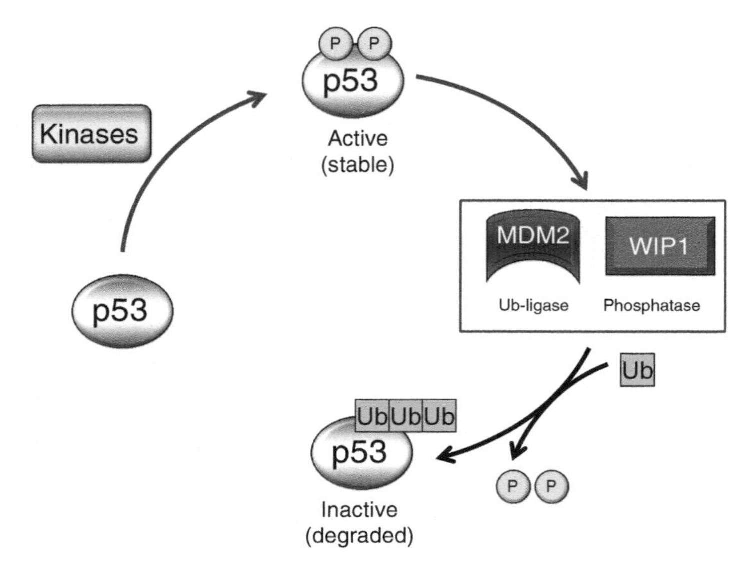

Fig. 6.33 p53 is controlled by multiple feedback loops. Newly translated p53 can be phosphorylated and thereby activated by the kinases that mediate the DNA damage responses. Active p53 induces the expression of the WIP1 protein phosphatase, encoded by *PPM1,* and the ubiquitin ligase encoded by *MDM2*. These enzymes catalyze the respective ubiquitination and dephosphorylation of p53, which cooperatively trigger its degradation. Thus, the duration of the p53 responses to DNA damage are limited by its turnover

to breast and ovarian cancer. As would be predicted, the cancer-associated alterations to *MDM2* and *PPM1D* are mutually exclusive to one another and to *TP53* mutations.

The DNA Damage Signaling Network Activates Interconnected Repair Pathways

The genes that cause the rare, autosomal recessive diseases that link genetic instability with cancer (discussed in Chap. 4) are generally involved in the repair of damaged DNA. Different types of DNA damage are repaired by distinct multi-protein complexes. The activity of these repair complexes is stimulated by the same DNA damage signaling network that causes the upregulation of p53 (Fig. 6.34).

The cellular hallmark of Fanconi anemia (FA) is a marked sensitivity to the effects of DNA crosslinking agents. Accordingly, the FA gene-encoded proteins have been found to function in repair complexes that process DNA crosslinks. Of the 17 FA genes that have been identified, eight are components of a multi-protein FA core complex. The FA core complex, formed by FANCA, FANCB, FANCC, FANCE, FANCF, FANCG, FANCL and FANCM, functions in the nucleus to add a

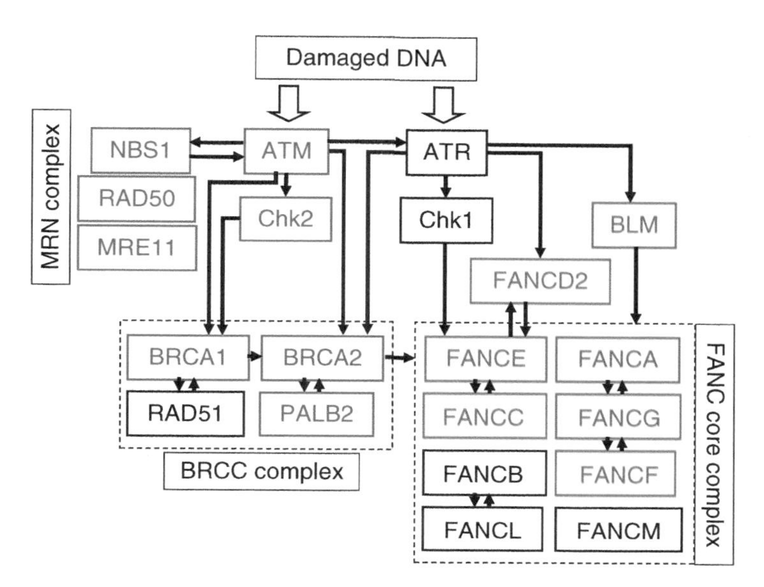

Fig. 6.34 The DNA damage signaling network activates DNA repair complexes. The DNA damage responses triggered by activation of the ATM and ATR kinases involve multiple DNA repair pathways. These pathways involve genes that are mutated in the germlines of many cancer-prone individuals and families. Components of the Fanconi anemia (FA) core complex, the Mre11/Rad50/NBS1 (MRN) core complex, and the BRCA1/BRCA2 containing (BRCC) complex are directly activated by upstream signaling kinases. Insight into the physical relationships between the components of these complexes has been gained by biochemical studies that have revealed multiple pairwise associations; only the most highly illustrative of these are shown. Proteins highlighted in *blue* are encoded by genes that are associated with cancer predisposition

single ubiquitin moiety to the FANCD2 protein. The mono-ubiquitination of FANCD2 allows it to associate with chromatin at sites of DNA crosslinks. At these damaged sites, FANCD2 co-localizes with the ATR protein kinase, the DNA helicase encoded by *BLM*, and the BRCA1/2-complex, which all contribute to a complex repair process.

The BRCA1 and BRCA2 genes function in a distinct multi-protein complex that has been termed the BRCA1- and BRCA2-containing (BRCC) complex. At the FA repair foci, BRCA2 is partnered with PALB2, a protein required for homologous recombination-mediated DNA repair. PALB2 appears to be required for BRCA2 localization. BRCA1 associates with a binding partner called BARD1, which contributes to the mono-ubitquitation of FANCD2.

NBS1, the gene mutated in Nijmegan breakage syndrome, encodes a protein called NBS1 or nibrin, a component of the MRN complex that also includes MRE11 and RAD50. The MRN protein complex is important for the recruitment and retention of ATM to the sites of DNA double strand breaks.

The proteins required for DNA repair are encoded by genes mutated in recessive cancer predisposition syndromes, but mutations in these genes can also confer cancer predisposition in a dominant manner. Germline mutations in *BRCA1*, *BRCA2* and *PALB2* cause familial breast cancers; *PALB2* has also been identified as a susceptibility gene for familial pancreatic cancer. These genetic findings underscore the central importance of DNA repair to the maintenance of genetic stability and the suppression of tumorigenesis.

Inactivation of the Pathways to Apoptosis in Cancer

The maintenance of tissue homeostasis depends not only on the rate of cell proliferation, but also on the rate of cell death. The anatomical stability of adult tissues is largely dependent on highly conserved signaling pathways that cause a form of cell death known as *apoptosis*. Apoptosis is genetically programmed, associated with specific morphological changes, and unlike other forms of cell death, occurs in the absence of any apparent physical trauma or injury.

The selective elimination of cells by apoptosis is critical to processes as diverse as the development of the extremities and the modulation of immune responses. Apoptotic pathways appear to be functional in all normal cells of the human body, and tens of billions of cells are programmed to die each day. In many cancers, the pathways that lead to apoptosis are disrupted by either proto-oncogene activation or by tumor suppressor gene inactivation. As a result, cancer cells often fail to respond normally to death signals. They may also be relatively resistant to the forms of anticancer therapy that rely on apoptotic induction.

Two distinct categories of stimuli can cause apoptosis. Extracellular signaling molecules, including highly specific cytokines, hormones and growth factors, can activate what is known as the *extrinsic pathway*. Via this pathway, cell surface receptors generate signals upon binding death-inducing ligands (Fig. 6.35). The receptors that can trigger apoptosis include the tumor necrosis factor (TNF) receptor superfamily, the TNF-related apoptosis inducing ligand (TRAIL) and the First apoptosis signal (Fas). The use of recombinant ligands to activate these receptors and induce apoptosis in cancer cells will be described in Chap. 8.

Alternatively, death receptor-independent apoptosis can be caused by various forms of intracellular stress, including chromosomal DNA damage and failure to complete mitosis. Such events activate what is known as the *intrinsic pathway* to apoptosis (see Fig. 6.36). A key component of the intrinsic pathway is the mitochondrion, and the intrinsic pathway is sometimes referred to as the mitochondrial pathway.

The main site of cellular ATP generation, the mitochondrion is also the target of both anti- and pro-apoptotic mediators which respectively function to stabilize and destabilize a crucial barrier called the mitochondrial outer membrane. Activation of the intrinsic pathway causes permeabilization of the mitochondrial outer membrane and the attendant release of molecules from the intermembrane space into the cytoplasm. Among the molecules normally sequestered in the mitochondrion are reactive oxygen species and the electron transport protein cytochrome C. When released

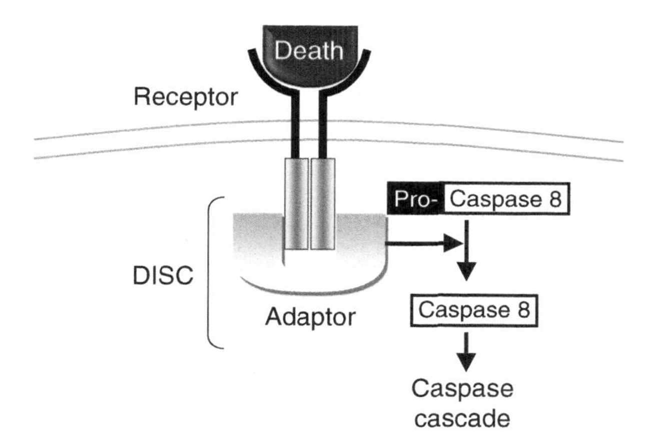

Fig. 6.35 The extrinsic pathway to apoptosis. Also known as the death receptor pathway, the extrinsic pathway is triggered by extracellular ligands. Receptor molecules – including the TNF-receptor superfamily, Fas, and the TNF-related apoptosis inducing ligand (TRAIL) – form multimers in response to death ligand binding. Adaptor proteins associate with the intracellular domains of multimerized death receptors and recruit the pro-enzyme (inactive) form of the caspase 8. Together, these components form the death-inducing signaling complex (DISC) that triggers the cleavage of pro-caspase-8 and thereby initiates a downstream cascade of caspase activation

into the cytoplasm, cytochrome C binds to a protein called Apaf-1, forming a complex known as the *apoptosome*.

The outcome of activation of either the external or internal apoptosis pathways is the onset of marked cellular changes that include disruption of cellular and nuclear membranes and the breakdown of chromatin. Cellular proteins are digested by a class of cysteine proteases that cleave polypeptides at aspartic acid residues, or *caspases*. Many of the characteristic features of apoptosis can be blocked by chemical inhibitors of the caspases, demonstrating their central role as the major effectors of apoptotic pathways.

Caspases are translated as inactive pro-enzymes called *pro-caspases*. Cleavage of pro-caspases results in their activation. A ligand-activated death-inducing signaling complex (DISC) facilitates the proteolytic activation of caspase 9 by the extrinsic pathway, while the apoptosome causes the proteolytic activation of caspase 8 by the intrinsic pathway. These upstream caspases, also known as *initiator caspases*, then cleave and activate downstream caspases, also known as *effector caspases*. The rapid and irreversible activation of the effector caspases by the initiator caspases, a process known as the *caspase cascade*, ultimately results in the proteolytic degradation and destruction of the cell.

The pathways to apoptosis are frequently inhibited by mutations that drive tumorigenesis. Pro-caspase 8 is encoded by a tumor suppressor gene, *CASP8*, mutationally inactivated in 5–10 percent of head and neck squamous cell cancers. More commonly, cancer genes affect the intrinsic pathway (Fig. 6.37) and thus disable the apoptotic responses that are normally triggered when cells are damaged or fail to

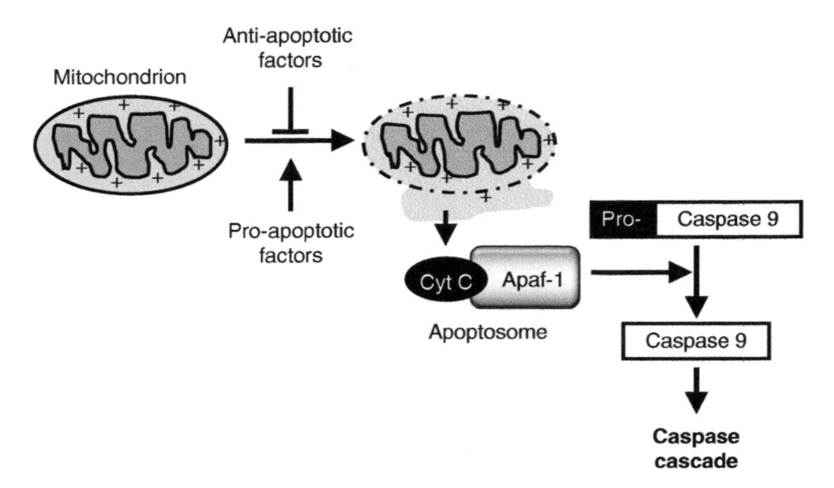

Fig. 6.36 The intrinsic pathway to apoptosis. Apoptotic stimuli cause the permeabilization of the mitochondrial outer membrane. This disruption causes the contents of the mitochondrial intermembrane space results to be released into the cytoplasm. These contents include toxic, charged radicals (+) and cytochrome C. Cytochrome C forms a complex with Apaf-1, a component of the apoptosome. This multiprotein complex facilitates the cleavage and activation of pro-caspase 9. Mitochondrial outer membrane permeability (MOMP) is ultimately determined by the net balance of anti- and pro-apoptotic factors

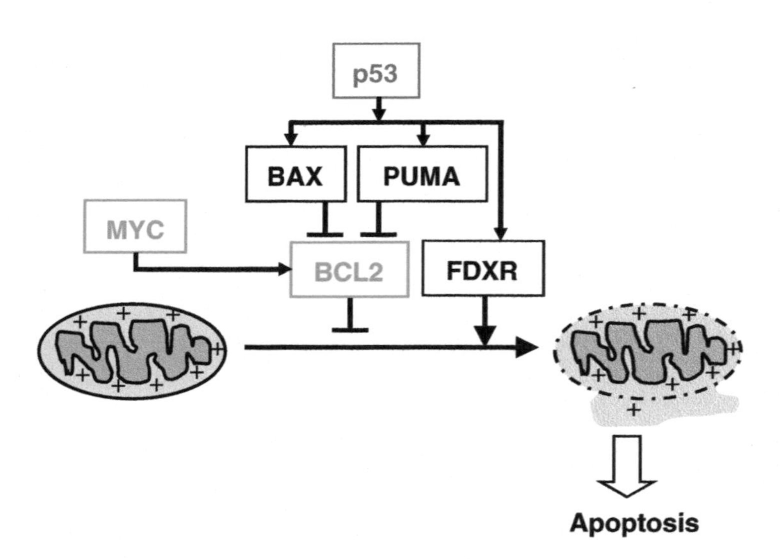

Fig. 6.37 Cancer genes affect mitochondrial outer membrane permeability. Upstream signaling pathways that induce transcription by MYC increase the levels of the apoptosis inhibitor BCL2. BCL2 is antagonized by the proapoptotic BCL2-family members BAX and PUMA, which are induced by p53. p53 also increases the expression of ferredoxin reductase (FDXR), which directly destabilizes the mitochondrial outer membrane

divide properly. The intrinsic pathway is also activated by many of the anticancer therapeutics that cause DNA damage, inhibit DNA synthesis or otherwise impair cell proliferation.

The threshold for the initiation of apoptosis via the intrinsic pathway is governed by the extent to which the mitochondrial outer membrane is permeable, a state-dependent characteristic known as *MOMP*. Cells with high MOMP are more prone to initiate apoptosis. The first identified regulator of MOMP is the protein encoded by the *BCL2* gene. *BCL2* was originally cloned in 1984, by Carlo Croce and coworkers, as an oncogene activated by a common translocation in B-cell lymphomas. While all oncogenes known at that time could be demonstrated to cause increased cell proliferation when experimentally introduced into cultured cells, *BCL2* did not have this expected effect. Upon further study, overexpression of *BCL2* was shown to confer resistance to stimuli that would otherwise cause apoptosis. Thus, *BCL2* defined a new type of oncogene, one that functioned not by increasing proliferation, but by inhibiting cell death.

BCL2 is a member of an eponymous family of highly interactive proteins that affect the apoptosis threshold by controlling MOMP. The BCL2 family contains both pro-apoptotic that increase MOMP and anti-apoptotic members that prevent this increase; all of the proteins in this family share characteristic protein motifs. It is the net balance between the two types of BCL2 proteins that determines the MOMP, and therefore the threshold for initiation of apoptosis. BCL2 proteins have been detected in close physical proximity to the mitochondrial outer membrane. Structural homologies between pro-apoptotic BCL2-family proteins and bacterial proteins that function in membrane pore formation suggest a potential mechanism of action.

In addition to its many other functions, p53 plays a central role in apoptosis (Fig. 6.37). Apoptotic signals cause the stabilization and activation of p53, which then functions as a potent mediator of mitochondrial permeabilization. Among the apoptotic targets of activated p53 are the BCL2 family members BAX and PUMA. These pro-apoptotic proteins antagonize the anti-apoptotic effects of BCL2, and increase MOMP. Wild type p53 also activates transcription of the *FDXR* gene. *FDXR* encodes ferredoxin reductase, which targets mitochondrial membrane stability independently of the BCL2 family. Cancer cells with inactivating mutations in *TP53* have decreased MOMP and are therefore resistant to apoptotic signals.

RB1 and the Regulation of the Cell Cycle

The counterbalance to cell death, in terms of tissue homeostasis, is cell proliferation. Proliferating cells undergo repeated iterations of synthetic growth and division, a process known as the *cell cycle*. The cell cycle is composed of four discrete phases (Fig. 6.38). The replication of the genome occurs during S-phase, a period of DNA synthesis. Chromosomes are segregated and cells physically divide into daughter cells during mitosis. Cells increase in mass during two gap phases called

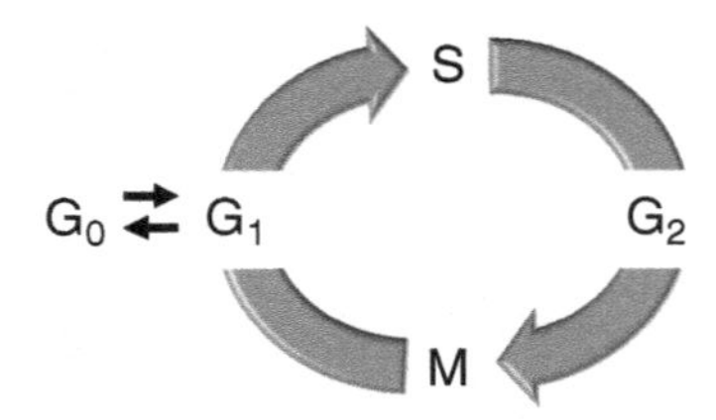

Fig. 6.38 The phases of the cell cycle. DNA replication occurs during S-phase (S). Mitosis (M) results in chromosome segregation and cell division. These two phases are separated by two gap periods (G_1 and G_2), during which increases in cell mass occur. Cells can exit the cell cycle from G_1 and reversibly enter a non-proliferative state known as G_0

G_1 and G_2 that occur prior to S-phase and prior to mitosis, respectively. It is during G_1 and G_2 phases that cells are highly responsive to proliferative and anti-proliferative stimuli. An additional phase known as G_0 is characterized by proliferative quiescence, and represents a state of potentially reversible exit from the cell cycle.

The basic mechanisms by which cells progress from one phase of the cell cycle to subsequent phases have been elucidated in model organisms, including yeasts, amphibians and sea urchins. Pioneering studies conducted during the 1970s and 1980s revealed that transitions through the phases of the cell cycle are promoted by increases in protein kinase activity. Phase-specific kinase activation is initiated by a class of proteins called *cyclins*, so named because the prototypes in model organisms were found to increase and decrease in abundance with the distinct phases of the cell cycle. During each phase, a characteristic cyclin binds and activates a distinct serine/threonine protein kinase called a *cyclin-dependent kinase* (CDK). Thus activated, the cyclin-CDK complex phosphorylates phase-specific substrates that promote cell cycle progression (Fig. 6.39). Specific cyclin-CDKs prepare the cell to undergo DNA replication during late G_1; S-phase specific cyclin-CDKs promote progression of replication forks and coordinate the firing of replication origins; mitotic cyclin-CDKs promote the creation of the bipolar mitotic spindle and the concomitant dissolution of the nuclear membrane. These mechanisms of cell cycle progression are highly conserved in all eukaryotic cells.

The first molecular connection between cancer genes and the regulation of the cell cycle was appreciated with the cloning and characterization of *RB1*, the gene mutated in sporadic and heritable forms of retinoblastoma (see Chap. 3). The RB1 protein plays a critical role in the regulation of the $G_1 \rightarrow S$ transition (Fig. 6.40). RB1 directly controls the activity of a transcription factor called E2F, which promotes the expression of several genes required for S-phase. Among these is a gene that encodes a type E cyclin, that defines S-phase. Prior to S-phase, E2F is bound to unphosphorylated RB1 protein. In this bound state, E2F is inactive and does not associate with gene promoters. This inactive form of E2F is thus maintained by RB1.

Transcription of the cyclin D gene *CCND1* is highest in early G_1. By late G_1, accumulating cyclin D stimulates the activation of CDK 4 and CDK 6, which can each phosphorylate RB1. Phosphorylation of RB1 disrupts the RB1-E2F complex. Thus liberated, E2F can transactivate target genes including *CCNE1*, a gene that

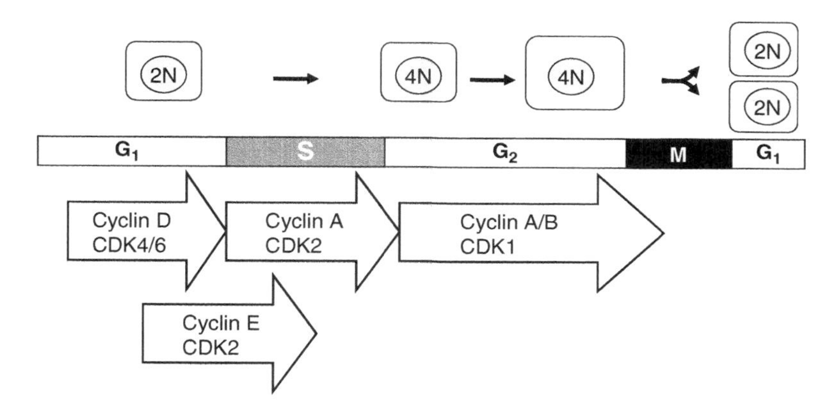

Fig. 6.39 Cell cycle progression is driven by sequentially activated cyclin-dependent kinase complexes. A single cell cycle is illustrated in linear form. Cells in G_1 have a diploid DNA content (2 N) which becomes 4 N up completion of S-phase. The transition between phases of the cell cycle is driven by the sequential assembly and activation of cyclin-CDK complexes. Each activated cyclin-CDK complex phosphorylates phase-specific substrates. Note that several cyclins and CDKs can associate with different partners as the cell cycle progresses

encodes cyclin E. Cyclin E/CDK2 complexes also phosphorylate RB1, accelerating the production of cyclin E and the resultant transition into S phase. By this mechanism, the accumulation of cyclin D during G_1 stimulates a subsequent wave of cyclin E expression that commits a cell to enter into S-phase and replicate its chromosomes.

Cyclin D proteins are important targets of several upstream mitogenic signaling pathways. In cancers, loss of RB1 function renders the $G_1 \rightarrow S$ transition cyclin D independent and growth is therefore mitogen-independent. *CCND1* is a proto-oncogene that is amplified at low frequency in several types of cancer, including cancers of the esophagus and of the head and neck.

Cancer cells frequently contain increased levels of cyclin D. This observation can be attributed to the regulation of cyclin D levels by several upstream cancer gene pathways (Fig. 6.41). The RAS pathway promotes *CCND1* expression, while the WNT/APC pathway has been shown to inhibit *CCND1* expression via the inhibition of β-catenin. *CCND1* is also a direct target of MYC. The PI3K/AKT pathway prevents the inhibition of targeted cyclin D protein inactivation by the GSK3 kinase. In summary, cyclin D levels can increase via multiple cancer gene pathways, as a result of either the inactivation of tumor suppressor genes or the activation of oncogenes.

Uncontrolled proliferation is one of the universal hallmarks of cancer. The seminal discovery and characterization of RB1 provided unparalleled insight into how human cells proliferate, and how this process can be dysregulated at the most fundamental level in cancer cells.

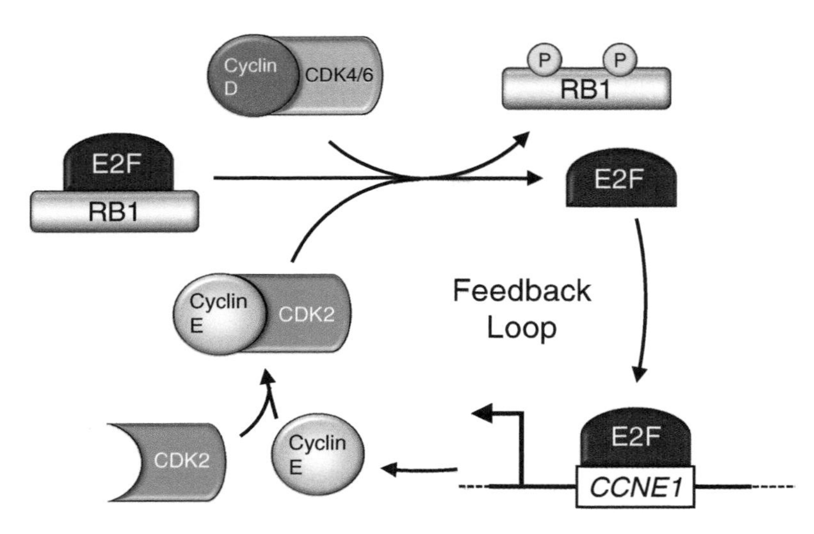

Fig. 6.40 RB1 mediates the sequestration of E2F and suppresses S-phase entry. During G_1, RB1 is bound to the transcription factor E2F. Phosphorylation of RB1 by cyclin D/CDK4/6 complexes disrupts this association and thus frees E2F to stimulate the transcription of *CCNE1*, which encodes cyclin E. The accumulating cyclin E-CDK2 complexes also phosphorylate RB1, and thereby create a positive feedback loop that results in the progression of the cell into S-phase

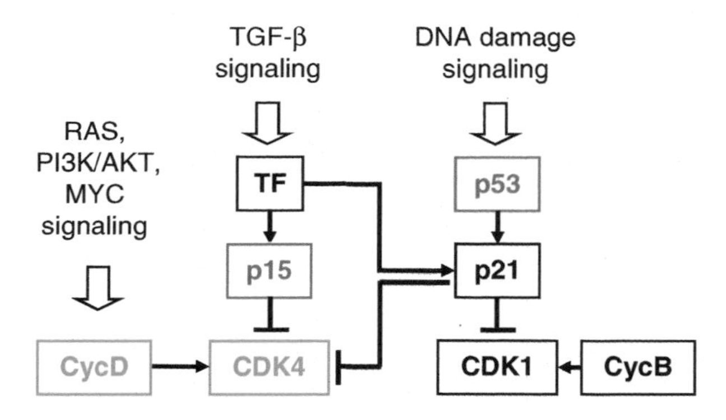

Fig. 6.41 Upregulation of CDKIs by cancer gene pathways. Several cancer gene pathways, including the TGF-β/SMAD and the p53 pathways, induce the expression of CDKI genes. TGF-β ligand results in the upregulation of *CDKN2B* transcription and p15 expression. p15 is an INK4 protein that inhibits the activity of CDK4 and CDK6 complexes, thus blocking transit between G_1 and S phase. The activation of p53 results in the transcriptional upregulation of *CDKN1A* and increased expression of its encoded protein, p21. The p21 protein is a universal inhibitor of CDKs, including CDK1 which controls entry into mitosis. In contrast, oncogenic pathways such as RAS and PI3K/AKT induce the expression of the proto-oncogene *CCND1* and its encoded protein cyclin D, and thereby promote progression of the cell cycle

Several Cancer Gene Pathways Converge on Cell Cycle Regulators

The cell division cycle is tightly controlled. Accordingly, the cyclin-CDK complexes that mediate cell cycle transitions are subject to multiple layers of regulation (Fig. 6.42). The most basic mechanism of regulation is the limiting abundance of cyclin. Indeed, CDKs are defined as such by their requirement for cyclin binding.

A second mode of CDK regulation involves post-translation modification. Active CDK complexes can be inhibited by the phosphorylation of the CDK catalytic subunit by highly conserved tyrosine kinases, including Wee1 and Mik1. These kinases normally function to regulate cell size. Phosphorylation on specific tyrosine residues renders CDKs catalytically inactive. In the reverse reaction, these inhibitory phosphates can be removed by a class of protein phosphatases belonging to the

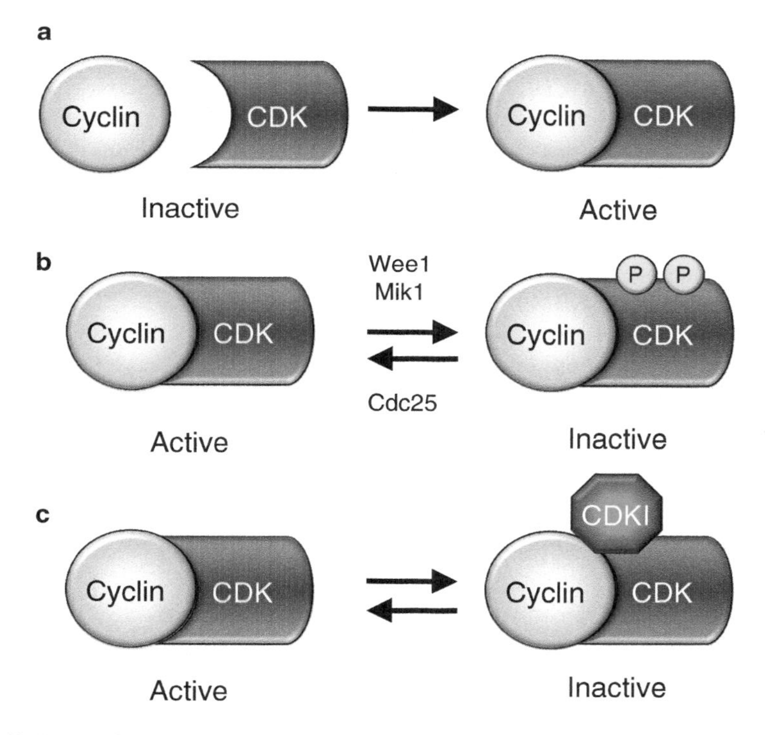

Fig. 6.42 Mechanisms of CDK regulation. (**a**) Monomeric cyclin-dependent kinases (CDKs) are essentially devoid of enzymatic activity. The association of cyclins with partner CDKs triggers the transition between cell cycle phases during unperturbed growth. (**b**) Cyclin-CDK complexes can be inactivated by tyrosine phosphorylation (shown in *yellow*). Protein kinases that limit cell growth, such as Wee1 and Mik1, directly phosphorylate CDKs, rendering them catalytically inactive. Removal of the inhibitory phosphates is catalyzed by the protein tyrosine phosphatases in the Cdc25 family. (**c**) Cyclin-CDK complexes can be reversibly inactivated by physical association with cyclin-dependent kinase inhibitor proteins (CDKIs), including p15, p16, p16ARF, p18 and p21

CDC25 family. The balance between tyrosine kinase and phosphatase activities sets the threshold for CDK activation and cell cycle progression. None of these genes are mutationally inactivated in a significant number of tumors, and so his mode of regulation is functionally intact in cancer cells.

A third means of regulating cyclin/CDK complexes is the binding of inhibitory subunits known as *cyclin-dependent kinase inhibitors* (CDKIs). Human cells express two distinct classes of CDKIs. *Universal* CDKIs associate with all cyclin-CDK complexes and therefore function to inhibit all cell cycle transitions. The three members of this class are designated by molecular weight: p21, p27 and p57. Proteins belonging to the second class of CDKIs bind exclusively to the CDK4 and CDK6 complexes that specifically mediate the transition from G_1 to S phase. These include the two protein products of the *CDKN2A* locus, p16 and p14 (ARF), and the neighboring gene *CDKN2B*, which encodes p15 (see Chap. 3). *CDKN2C*, at a physically separate locus on chromosome 1, encodes a CDKI designated p18. These four functionally-related CDKIs are sometimes referred to as *INK4 proteins*, reflecting their ability to specifically inhibit CDK4.

Many types of cancers develop defects in CDK regulation or CDKI induction. Germline mutations in *CDK4* are involved in a subset of kindreds with Familial Multiple Mole and Melanoma (FAMMM, see Chap. 3). This syndrome can also be caused by germline mutants in *CDKN2A*. The *CDKN2A* and neighboring *CDKN2B* genes are frequently inactivated by somatic deletions in several types of cancer, including a highly lethal form of brain tumor known as glioblastoma multiforme (GBM). Malignant peripheral nerve sheath tumors and melanomas also harbor a significant number of deletions that involve *CDKN2A/CDKN2B. CDKN2C* is frequently inactivated in GBM by deletion; point mutations in *CDKN2C* that interfere with the binding of p18 to CDK6 have also been reported. Interestingly, GBM samples often exhibit deletions involving both *CDKN2A/CDKN2B* as well as *CDKN2C*, suggesting that co-deletion of both regions provides an additive selective advantage. Cancer cells that lose *CDKN2ACDKN2B* and/or *CDKN2C* will exhibit a loss of control over the $G_1 \rightarrow S$ transition.

Alternatively, the upstream pathways that lead to induction CDKI can be disrupted by upstream mutations in one of several cancer gene pathways that induce the transcription of CDKI genes. The TGF-β and p53 pathways are two examples of cancer gene pathways that directly control CDKI gene expression. Among the target genes of the TGF-β pathway is *CDKN2B*. In most normal cells, TGF-β ligand induces the expression of *CDKN2B* and a concomitant increase in p15 protein, which then associates with and inhibits CDK4 and CDK6 complexes. Inhibition of CDK4/6 blocks cell cycle progression by preventing the $G_1 \rightarrow S$ transition. Cancer cells that have developed mutations that disrupt the TGF-β signaling pathway fail to upregulate p15 and thus have reduced control over entry into S-phase. This is a common functional defect in cancer cells.

A direct connection between p53 and the regulation of the cell cycle became apparent with the discovery in 1993 that *CDKN1A* is a transcriptional target of p53. *CDKN1A* encodes p21, a universal CDKI that regulates multiple cell cycle transitions. In most proliferating cells, p21 protein is present at very low levels. Upon activation by DNA strand breaks or DNA replication intermediates, p53 engages its binding sites in the *CDKN1A* promoter and dramatically increases *CDKN1A* transcription. Cancer cells that have acquired *TP53* mutations have impaired induction of *CDKN1A* transcription, and therefore fail to restrict the progression of the cell cycle in response to damaged and incompletely replicated chromosomes.

Many Cancer Cells Are Cell Cycle Checkpoint-Deficient

Genetically programmed growth arrest occurs at defined points in the cell cycle, known as *checkpoints*. First described in yeasts, checkpoints function to ensure that the events of the cell cycle begin and end in their proper sequence. For example, a checkpoint in late G_1 prevents damaged chromosomes from being replicated. A distinct checkpoint in late G_2 prevents incompletely replicated chromosomes from being segregated during mitosis. After DNA damage, the G_1/S and G_2/M checkpoints provide a means for cells to halt their growth in a coordinated fashion and initiate DNA repair. In organisms as diverse as humans and yeast, checkpoints function to protect cells from the deleterious effects of failed DNA replication and incomplete chromosomal segregation.

Cell cycle checkpoints are pathways that functionally inhibit CDKs. CDKs can be inhibited by tyrosine phosphorylation or by interactions with CDKI proteins (Fig. 6.42). Both of these events are controlled by checkpoint pathways. The DNA damage signaling network directly implements checkpoints by the inactivation of Cdc25 family members. The most prominent of these is Cdc25A. Phosphorylation of Cdc25A by upstream kinases results in its rapid degradation by ubiquitin-dependent proteolysis. The loss of a CDK phosphatase tips the balance in favor of CDK inhibitory phosphorylation.

The G_2/M checkpoint is subject to several modes of regulation (Fig. 6.43). The degradation of CDC25A is the first phase of checkpoint activation. The second phase of checkpoint activation is mediated by p21, which accumulates as a result of p53 activation. In the presence of DNA damage, p21 binds CDK proteins and ensures that they remain inactive, thus stabilizing checkpoint-mediated growth arrest. An additional p53-induced gene, *SFN*, encodes a protein,14-3-3σ, a binding protein that functionally sequesters phosphorylated CDK complexes and prevents them from entering the nucleus. The fact that this major checkpoint in the cell cycle is implemented by functionally overlapping mechanisms is an indicator of its central importance in maintaining cell genetic stability and viability.

During the evolution of cancers, mutations that cause checkpoint deficiencies allow clonal populations of cells to escape growth arrest normally triggered by signaling molecules or adverse environmental conditions. Thus, checkpoint defects can provide a selective proliferative advantage. However, this advantage comes at a price. While checkpoint-deficient cancer cells can escape growth controlling stimuli, they are apparently diminished in their ability to survive more severe forms of DNA damage. Effective DNA repair requires a coordinated halt of cell cycle processes, a function lost in many cancer cells. Indeed, cancer cells have been observed to continue replicating their genomes and to undergo failed mitoses following treat-

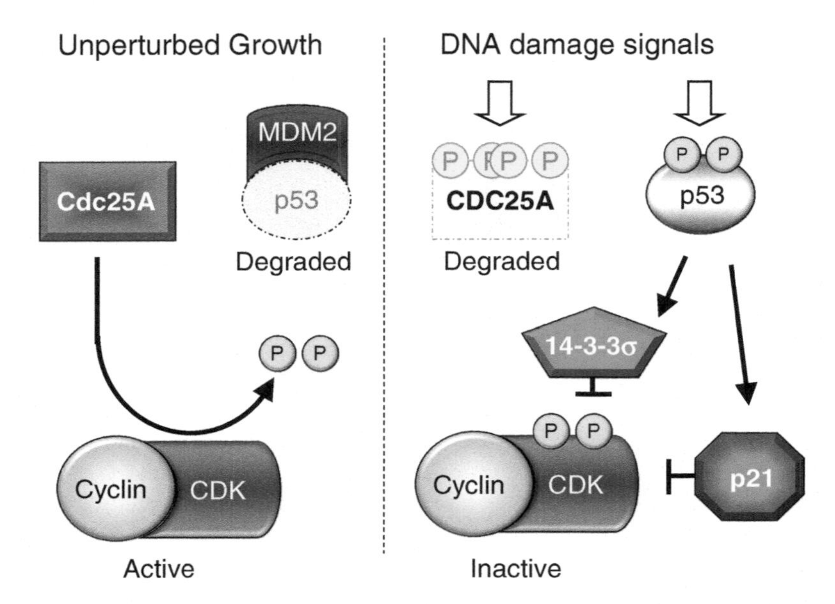

Fig. 6.43 Activation of cell cycle checkpoints in response to DNA damage. During unperturbed cell growth (*left*), the Cdc25A phosphatase removes inhibitory phosphates from conserved tyrosine residues on CDKs. Under these conditions, p53 is present at very low levels due to MDM2-dependent protein degradation. Upon sensing damaged chromosomal DNA, the DNA damage signaling network causes the phosphorylation of Cdc25A on at least four serine/threonine residues (*right*). These modifications effectively target Cdc25A for degradation by the proteasome. In the absence of Cdc25A, the phosphorylated (inactive) form of a CDK quickly becomes predominant. At the same time, stabilized, activated p53 induces expression of the CDKI p21 and a protein called $14-3-3\sigma$, which sequesters CDKs and prevents them from functioning in the nucleus

ment with DNA damaging agents such as ionizing radiation. A loss of checkpoint control is thought to underlie the inherent sensitivity of many kinds of cancer cells to the effects of DNA-damaging forms of therapy. The roles of cancer genes in therapeutic responses will be discussed in detail in Chap. 8.

Chromatin Modification Is Recurrently Altered in Many Types of Cancer

Human chromosomes are highly dynamic stores of genetic and epigenetic information. Chromosomal loci are accordingly regulated by many diverse enzymes and biochemical processes. As the control of gene expression and genetic stability are both altered in some way in virtually all cancers, it was not surprising that the deep analysis of cancer genomes revealed many mutations that affect the interactions between chromosomal proteins, including histones, and chromosomal DNA.

A prominent and highly studied aspect of chromatin modification is the extensive remodeling of histones that occurs in concert with the activation of gene transcription. Histones can be directly altered by driver mutations. For example, the variant histone H3 encoded by the *H3F3A* gene is altered by mutations in one-third of the pediatric cases of glioblastoma. This variant, known as H3.3, is normally deposited on chromatin at transcriptionally active loci and telomeric regions by proteins called ATRX (which is unrelated to the ATR protein kinase) and DAXX. The pattern of H3.3 deposition and its pattern of post-translational modifications (known in this context as 'marks') influence global DNA methylation and global gene expression. The cancer-associated mutations in *H3F3A* cause amino acid substitutions near the K27 and K36 residues at which H3.3 is normally post-translationally modified. Mutations at these sites define two epigenetically distinct subgroups of the disease. In pediatric tumors, the deregulation of H3.3 deposition is often the result of mutations in *ATRX* or *DAXX*. Interestingly, the G34 mutation in *H3F3A* and the mutations in ATRX and DAXX are associated with the Alternative Lengthening of Telomeres (ALT) phenotype, which is present in the small proportion of cancers that do not express the telomere maintenance enzyme telomerase (Chap. 4).

Adult brain tumors, particularly glioblastomas that evolve from lower-grade tumors (a subtype categorized as secondary glioblastomas), frequently harbor recurrent point mutations in the genes *IDH1* and *IDH2*. These proto-oncogenes encode isoforms of the metabolic enzyme *isocitrate dehydrogenase*. Isocitrate dehydrogenase enzymes catalyze a critical step of the citric acid (TCA) cycle, in which isocitrate is oxidatively decarboxylated to concomitantly produce 2-oxoglutarate (2-OG, alternatively called α-ketoglutarate) and the reduced form of nicotinamide adenine dinucleotide phosphate (NADPH). 2-OG is a co-factor for numerous cellular processes, including the removal of methyl groups from histones; NADPH is a cofactor in lipid and glucose metabolism, and also provides a defense against oxidative damage. The three NADP-dependent isocitrate dehydrogenase isoforms have the same catalytic activity, but IDH1 functions in the cytoplasm whereas IDH2 and IDH3 are located in the mitochondrion.

Most of the mutations that affect the citric acid cycle occur in *IDH1*, at the codon for the amino acid R132. About 10 % of mutations in this pathway hit the functionally corresponding amino acid in *IDH2*, R172. These conserved arginine residues occur at a site involved in isocitrate binding. Mutations decrease isocitrate binding and increase the binding of NADPH; this change causes reduced isocitrate decarboxylation. Importantly, these mutated enzymes gain a new catalytic activity: the production of 2-hydroxyglutarate (2-HG) from 2-OG, accompanied by the consumption of NADPH. This reverse reaction is incomplete in nature, in that 2-OG is reduced but not carboxylated to generate isocitrate. Cells with a mutant IDH gene therefore have extremely elevated levels of 2-HG.

2-HG triggers epigenetic chromatin modifications that interfere with normal cellular methylation processes, and thereby promote altered gene expression. These epigenetic changes contribute to the selective growth of cells that harbor *IDH1* or *IDH2* mutations. 2-HG has therefore been referred to as an *oncometabolite*. The high intracellular concentrations of 2-HG in IDH-mutant cancer cells causes a global increase in CpG-island DNA methylation.

Mutations in *H3F3A* and *IDH1* occur in a mutually exclusive pattern in glioblastomas, suggesting that these genes mediate a common process or pathway. Indeed, the oncometabolite 2-HG has been observed to promote the methylation of histone H3.3 on residue K27. In addition to the mutations in adult glioblastomas, mutations in *IDH1* and *IDH2* are found in myeloid disorders, including acute myeloid leukemia (AML) and in a rare type of sarcoma that affects cartilage, called chondrosarcoma.

Diverse types of genetic mutations can impact the epigenetic states of chromatin and thereby influence gene expression and chromosomal stability. Examples of these alterations include:

Chromatin packaging. An evolutionarily conserved multi-protein chromatin remodeling complex called SWI/SNF, a designation derived from yeast phenotypes mating type switching and sucrose non-fermenting, alters nucleosome positioning. These multiprotein complexes have ATPase and DNA helicase activities, and appear to alter the chromatin structure around genes that are actively transcribed. Central components of the SWI/SNF complex are a family of proteins that avidly bind AT-rich regions of DNA via a shared domain called the AT-rich interaction domain (ARID), and thereby serve to localize and organize these complexes. Genes that encode the ARID proteins include the tumor suppressors *ARID1A*, which is mutated in many stomach, pancreatic and ovarian cancers, *ARD1B* and *ARID2*. Additional components of the SWI/SNF complexes that are mutated in cancers are encoded by tumor suppressor genes that include *SMARCA4*, *SMARCB1*, and *PBRM1*.

Histone modification. Enzymes that leave regulatory, post-translational modifications on histones called 'marks', are the targets of driver mutations. The histone methyltransferases encoded by *MLL2, MLL3, SETD2* are mutated in leukemias.

DNA methylation. Patterns of global DNA methylation at cytosine residues are abnormal in most cancers (Chap. 1). Epigenetic states are highly interconnected; patterns of DNA methylation can be affected by changes in histones or metabolites. More directly, global DNA methylation can be impacted by cancer-associated mutations in *DNMT1* and *DNMT3A*, which encode DNA methyltransferases.

Summary: Putting Together the Puzzle

Cancer genes populate cellular pathways that collectively maintain a stable genome, determine cell fates and modulate cell survival. The elucidation of these pathways has provided insight into how normal cells are transformed by mutations into cancers. Cancer genes encode proteins that are functionally or structurally related and in many cases biochemically interconnected. These interconnections provide an explanation as to why cancers with distinct sets of cancer genes can often appear clinically similar. But the diversity of cancer genes and pathways also underscores the many unique ways that cancers can develop and respond to therapy.

In several illustrative cases, cancer gene pathways have provided a roadmap for the discovery of novel cancer genes. For example, the RAS family of proto-oncogenes was discovered with the use of *in vitro* transformation assays. Subsequent biochemical studies revealed the interaction between RAS and RAF proteins and prompted the close genetic analysis of *BRAF*, which is mutated in several cancers at a high frequency. Likewise, *PTEN* pointed the way to *PIK3CA* and *APC* revealed the role of *CTNNB1*.

The international effort to understand the genetic basis of cancer has at times seemed like the assembly of a large jigsaw puzzle. The first pieces are difficult to link together because there are so many pieces, and it is therefore difficult to imagine how they might fit together to create a comprehensive picture. But as pieces are brought together into small assemblies, patterns begin to emerge. With progress, smaller assemblies can be linked to one another, and there remain fewer unlinked pieces left to choose from. Analogously, the pace of discovery in basic cancer research dramatically increased as more cancer-related genes and pathways came to light. Early discoveries by pioneering cancer scientists created a basic framework for understanding how cancer genes fit together into complex and interactive protein networks. Subsequent high-throughput approaches rapidly provided the missing pieces to the cancer genetics puzzle.

Mutated tumor suppressor genes and oncogenes serve to highlight the cellular functions that are most relevant to the clonal evolution of cancers (Table 6.3). The twelve pathways or biochemical processes altered in cancer: Notch, hedgehog, APC, chromatin modification, transcriptional regulation, cell cycle control/apoptosis, RAS, PI3K, STAT, MAPK, TGF-β and DNA damage control together account

Table 6.3 Cell signaling pathways altered in cancers and in the germline of individuals predisposed to cancer

Process	Signaling pathway	Cancer genes
Cell fate	Notch	*EP300, FBXW7, GATA1, GATA2, NOTCH1, NOTCH2*
	Hedgehog	*EXT1, EXT2, PTCH1, SMO, SPOP, SUFU*
	APC	*APC, AXIN1, CDH1, CTNNB1, EP300, FAM123B, GNAS, HNF1A, NF2, PRKAR1A, RNF43, SOX9*
	Chromatin modification	*ARID1A, ARID1B, ARID2, ASXL1, ATRX, CREBBP, DNMT1, DNMT3A, EP300, EZH2, H3F3A, HIST1H3B, IDH1, IDH2, KDM5C, KDM6A, MEN1,MLL2, MLL3, NCOA3, NCOR1, PAX5, PBRM1, SETD2, SETBP1, SKP2, SMARCA4, SMARCB1, SPOP, TET2, WT1*
	Transcriptional regulation	*AR, BCOR, CREBBP, DAXX, DICER1, GATA3, IKZF1, KLF4, LMO1, PHOX2B, PHF6, PRDM1, RUNX1, SBDS, SF3B1, SRSF2, U2AF1*

(continued)

Table 6.3 (continued)

Process	Signaling pathway	Cancer genes
Cell survival	Cell cycle regulation/ apoptosis	*ABL1, BCL2, CARD11, CASP8, CCND1, CDC73, CDK4, CDKN2A, CDKN2C, CYLD, DAXX, FUBP1, MDM2, MDM4, MED12, MYC, MYCL1, MYCN, MYD88, NFE2L2, NPM1, PPM1D, PPP2R1A, RB1, TNFAIP3, TRAF7, TP53*
	RAS	*ALK, B2M, BRAF, CBL, CEBPA, CSF1R, CIC, EGFR, ERBB2, FGFR2, FGFR3, FH, FLT3, GNA11, GNAQ, GNAS, HRAS, KIT, KRAS, MAP2K1, MAP3K1, MET, NRAS, NF1, PDGFRA, PTPN11, RET, SDH5, SDH8, SDHC, SDHD, VHL*
	PI3K	*AKT1, ALK, B2M,CBL, CEBPA, CSF1R, EGFR, ERBB2, FGFR2, FGFR3, FH, FLCN, FLT3, GNA11, GNAQ, GNAS, GPC3, KIT, MET, NKX21, PRKAR1A, PIK3CA, PIK3R1, PDGFRA, PTEN, RET, SDH5, SDH8, SDHC, SDHD, STK11, TSC1, TSC2, TSHR, VHL, WAS*
	STAT	*CRLF2, FGFR2, FGFR3, FLT3, JAK1,JAK2, JAK3,KIT, MPL, SOCS1, VHL*
	MAPK	*B2M, CEBPA, ERK1, GNA11, GNAQ, MAP2K4, MAP3K1, NKX21, TNFAIP3, TSHR, WAS*
	TGF-β	*ACVR1B, BMPR1A, FOXL2, GATA1, GATA2, GNAS, EP300, MED12, SMAD2, SMAD4*
Genome maintenance	DNA damage control	*ATM, BAP1, BLM, BRCA1, BRCA2, BRIP1, BUB1B, CHEK2, ERCC2, ERCC3, ERCC4, ERCC5, FANCA, FANCC, FANCD2, FANCE, FANCF, FANCG, MLH1, MSH2, MSH6, MUTYH, NBS1, PALB2, PMS1, PMS2, RECQL4, STAG2, TP53, WRN, XPA, XPC*

The source of this list is Vogelstein et al. *Science* (2013), and the Cancer Gene Census (www.sanger.ac.uk/genetics/cgp/Census/)

for virtually all of the observed phenotypic abnormalities of cancer cells. While currently undiscovered genetic drivers of cancer may eventually prove the involvement of additional pathways or processes, such pathways would be relevant only to highly unusual or very rare cancers.

Further Reading

Bakkenist CJ, Kastan MB (2004) Initiating cellular stress responses. Cell 118:9–17

Bensaad K, Vousden KH (2007) P53: new roles in metabolism. Trends Cell Biol 17:286–291

Berger S (2010) Keeping p53 in check: a high-stakes balancing act. Cell 142:17–19

Blume-Jensen P, Hunter T (2001) Oncogenic kinase signalling. Nature 411:355–365
Cohen P (2002) The origins of protein phosphorylation. Nat Cell Biol 4:E127–E130
Dang CV (2012) MYC on the path to cancer. Cell 149:22–35
Fish EN, Platanias LC (2014) Interferon receptor signaling in malignancy: a network of cellular pathways defining biological outcomes. Mol Cancer Res 12:1691–1703
Giaccia AJ, Kastan MB (1998) The complexity of p53 modulation: emerging patterns from divergent signals. Genes Dev 12:2973–2983
Giacinti C, Giordano A (2006) RB and cell cycle progression. Oncogene 25:5220–5227
Hajra KM, Fearon ER (2002) Cadherin and catenin alterations in human cancer. Genes Chromosom Cancer 34:255–268
Hanahan D, Weinberg RA (2000) The hallmarks of cancer. Cell 100:57–70
Hanahan D, Weinberg RA (2011) Hallmarks of cancer: the next generation. Cell 144:646–674
Horn HF, Vousden KH (2007) Coping with stress: multiple ways to activate p53. Oncogene 26:1306–1316
Kastan MB, Bartek J (2004) Cell-cycle checkpoints and cancer. Nature 432:316–323
Kastan MB, Lim DS (2000) The many substrates and functions of ATM. Nat Rev Mol Cell Biol 1:179–186
Laplante M, Sabatini DM (2012) mTOR signaling in growth control and disease. Cell 149:274–293
Linding R et al (2007) Systematic discovery of in vivo phosphorylation networks. Cell 129:1415–1426
Losman J-A, Kaelin WG Jr (2013) What a difference a hydroxyl makes: mutant IDH, (R)-2-hydroxyglutarate, and cancer. Genes Dev 27:836–852
Massague J, Gomis RR (2006) The logic of TGFbeta signaling. FEBS Lett 580:2811–2820
Nelson WJ, Nusse R (2004) Convergence of Wnt, beta-catenin, and cadherin pathways. Science 303:1483–1487
Polakis P (2007) The many ways of Wnt in cancer. Curr Opin Genet Dev 17:45–51
Raabe EH, Eberhart CG (2012) Methylome alterations "mark" new therapeutic opportunities in glioblastoma. Cancer Cell 22:417–418
Samuels Y, Ericson K (2006) Oncogenic PI3K and its role in cancer. Curr Opin Oncol 18:77–82
Sansal I, Sellers WR (2004) The biology and clinical relevance of the PTEN tumor suppressor pathway. J Clin Oncol 22:2954–2963
Scott JD, Pawson T (2000) Cell communication: the inside story. Sci Am 282:72–79
Sears RC (2004) The life cycle of C-myc: from synthesis to degradation. Cell Cycle 3:1133–1137
Shields JM, Pruitt K, McFall A, Shaub A, Der CJ (2000) Understanding Ras: 'it ain't over til it's over'. Trends Cell Biol 10:147–154
Simpson L, Parsons R (2001) PTEN: life as a tumor suppressor. Exp Cell Res 264:29–41
Solomon DA, Kim JS, Jean W, Waldman T (2008) Conspirators in a capital crime: co-deletion of p18INK4c and p16INK4a/p14ARF/p15INK4b in glioblastoma multiforme. Cancer Res 68:8657–8660
Toledo F, Wahl GM (2006) Regulating the p53 pathway: in vitro hypotheses, in vivo veritas. Nat Rev Cancer 6:909–923
Venkitaraman AR (2005) Medicine: aborting the birth of cancer. Nature 434:829–830
Vivanco I, Sawyers CL (2002) The phosphatidylinositol 3-Kinase AKT pathway in human cancer. Nat Rev Cancer 2:489–501
Vogelstein B, Kinzler KW (2004) Cancer genes and the pathways they control. Nat Med 10:789–799
Vogelstein B, Lane D, Levine AJ (2000) Surfing the p53 network. Nature 408:307–310
Vogelstein B, Papadopoulos N, Velculescu VE, Zhou S, Diaz LA Jr, Kinzler KW (2013) Cancer genome landscapes. Science 339:1546–1558
Vousden KH, Lane DP (2007) P53 in health and disease. Nat Rev Mol Cell Biol 8:275–283

Wiley HS (2014) Open questions: the disrupted circuitry of the cancer cell. BMC Biol 12:88
Zhao JJ, Roberts TM (2006) PI3 kinases in cancer: from oncogene artifact to leading cancer target. Sci STKE 2006:pe52
Zhou BB, Elledge SJ (2000) The DNA damage response: putting checkpoints in perspective. Nature 408:433–439

Chapter 7
Genetic Alternations in Common Cancers

Cancer Genes Cause Diverse Diseases

Each of the roughly 100 types of human cancer is caused by the activation of proto-oncogenes and the loss of tumor suppressor genes. Although cancer genomes are complex, some clear mutational patterns are apparent. Several cancer genes are observed very frequently in some types of cancer, but rarely found in other types. Other cancer genes are much more widespread across many types of cancer. Analysis of many cancer genomes has shown that nearly 150 genes are recurrently altered by mutations to provide tumor cells a selective growth advantage. These studies have shown that there are many potential combinations of cancer genes that can cooperatively allow the growth of different types of neoplasia.

One measure of the relative importance of a cancer gene and its corresponding pathway in a given cancer type is the frequency at which it is mutated. *APC* is mutated at a very high frequency in colorectal cancers and must therefore participate in a critical pathway that maintains homeostasis in the epithelial tissue of the colon and rectum. This pathway is apparently less essential in other tissues. In contrast, recurrent mutations affecting *TP53* and *KRAS* have been observed at significant frequency in many types of cancer. From these observations, one can infer that loss of p53 and KRAS mediate pathways that are fundamental to cell survival in many diverse epithelial tissues.

Studies of diseases such as retinoblastoma and colorectal cancer have provided fundamental insights into the nature of cancer genes. Each of these cancers has a unique attribute that facilitated cancer gene discovery. Retinoblastoma is a relatively homogenous disease that has readily distinguishable hereditary and sporadic forms. The two-hit hypothesis developed by Knudson provided the first model for understanding cancer predisposition and the role of tumor suppressor genes. In comparison with retinoblastomas, colorectal tumors are plentiful and can be found in individuals at different ages. Because tumor samples can be obtained during routine colonoscopy, all stages of growth – including the critical premalignant stages typified by adenomas – have been subject to detailed genetic

F. Bunz, *Principles of Cancer Genetics*, DOI 10.1007/978-94-017-7484-0_7

analysis. The multi-stage model of tumorigenesis that emerged from studies of colorectal cancers provided a highly useful paradigm for understanding how cancer clones evolve and expand.

Most cancers are not understood at quite the same evolutionary level of detail as retinoblastoma and colorectal cancer. Complicating factors for some cancer types include clinical heterogeneity, access by geneticists to insufficient numbers of clinical samples representing different stages of disease, and a lack of a clearly diagnosable hereditary form of the disease that allows the mapping of a predominant gatekeeper gene and pathway. Despite these early obstacles to progress, we now have a nearly complete understanding the cancer genes and pathway abnormalities that underlie most common types of cancer.

Cancer Incidence and Prevalence

According to statistics compiled by the National Cancer Institute, it is projected that more than 1.6 million people will be diagnosed with cancer in the US each year, and 590,000 people will die of cancer. A moderate but significant downward trend in the rates of cancer incidence and mortality over the past 10 years provides some encouragement (Fig. 7.1).

The *incidence* of a specific cancer is defined as the number of newly diagnosed cases that will occur during a given time period, typically one year. This number may include multiple primary cancers that occur in a single patient, but does not typically include recurrences after treatment. The *mortality* is the rate of deaths that are directly attributed to a given cancer during that same time period. Cancer incidence and mortality are most often expressed as rates per 100,000 people at risk for one year. The most lethal forms of cancer are those in which the mortality rate approaches the incidence rate (Table 7.1). Another term frequently used to describe

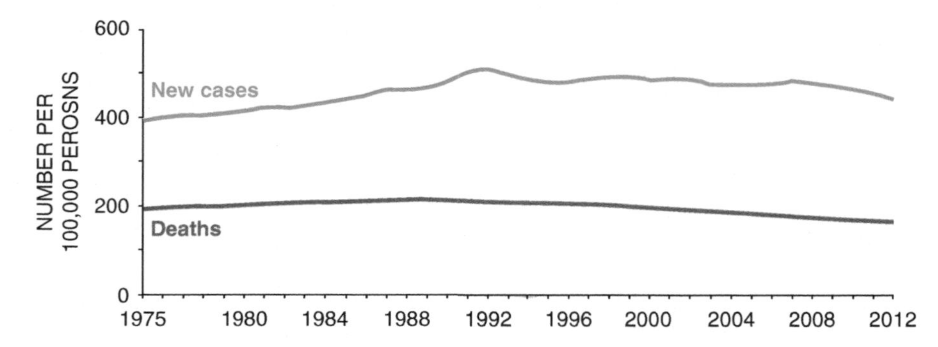

Fig. 7.1 Changes in cancer incidence and mortality, over time. Rates for new cancers at all sites have been declining by an average of 0.9 % per year for the past 10 years. Data from the Surveillance, Epidemiology, and End Results Program (SEER), conducted by the National Cancer Institute

Table 7.1 The most commonly diagnosed cancers in the US population, by incidence. Excluded are non-melanoma skin cancers, which are very common but rarely lethal

Cancer site	Incidence rate (per 100,000)	Survival at 5 years[b] (%)	Mortality rate (per 100,000)	Lifetime risk[c] (%)	Trend[d] (%)
Prostate	137.9[a]	99	21.4	14	−4.3
Breast	124.8[a]	89.4	21.9	12.3	0
Lung	58.7	17.4	47.2	6.6	−1.7
Colon and rectum	42.4	64.9	15.5	4.5	−3.1
Uterine endometrium	25.1[a]	81.7	4.4	2.8	0
Melanoma of the skin	21.6	91.5	2.7	2.1	+1.4
Bladder	20.3	77.4	4.4	2.4	−0.6
Lymphoma (non-Hodgkin)	19.7	70	6.2	2.1	0
Kidney	15.6	73.2	3.9	1.6	+1.4
Thyroid	13.5	97.9	0.5	1.1	+5.0
Leukemia (all types)	13.3	58.5	7.0	1.5	+0.2
Pancreas	12.4	7.2	10.9	1.5	+0.8
Ovary	12.1[a]	45.6	7.7	1.3	−1.1
Oral cavity and pharynx	11.0	63.2	2.5	1.1	0
Liver	8.2	17.2	6.0	0.9	+4.0
Uterine cervix	7.7[a]	67.8	2.3	0.6	−1.0
Stomach	7.4	29.3	3.4	0.9	−1.5
Brain and nervous system	6.4	33.3	4.3	0.6	−0.2

Data collected and curated by the Surveillance, Epidemiology, and End Results program of the National Cancer Institute, from 2008 to 2012

[a]For cancers that occur in only one sex (e.g. prostate cancer in men) only the at-risk population is considered

[b]At any stage, from the time of diagnosis

[c]Based on rates from 2002 to 2012, the percentage of people born today who will be diagnosed with cancer during their lifetime

[d]Change in incidence rate per year, over the 10 years from 2002 to 2012

the impact of cancer upon a population is the *prevalence*. Cancer prevalence is defined as total number of new and pre-existing cases of cancer, and reflects the number of people living with disease. *Survival* is a measure of the proportion of patients who are alive subsequent to the diagnosis of their cancer. The prevalence of a cancer is a function of both incidence and survival.

There are striking differences in cancer incidence and mortality among different subpopulations. These disparities negatively impact people with low income and those who live in geographically isolated areas. Access to healthcare and screening services and exposure to carcinogens related to diet and lifestyle are but a few of the many non-genetic factors that are known to strongly influence both incidence and mortality.

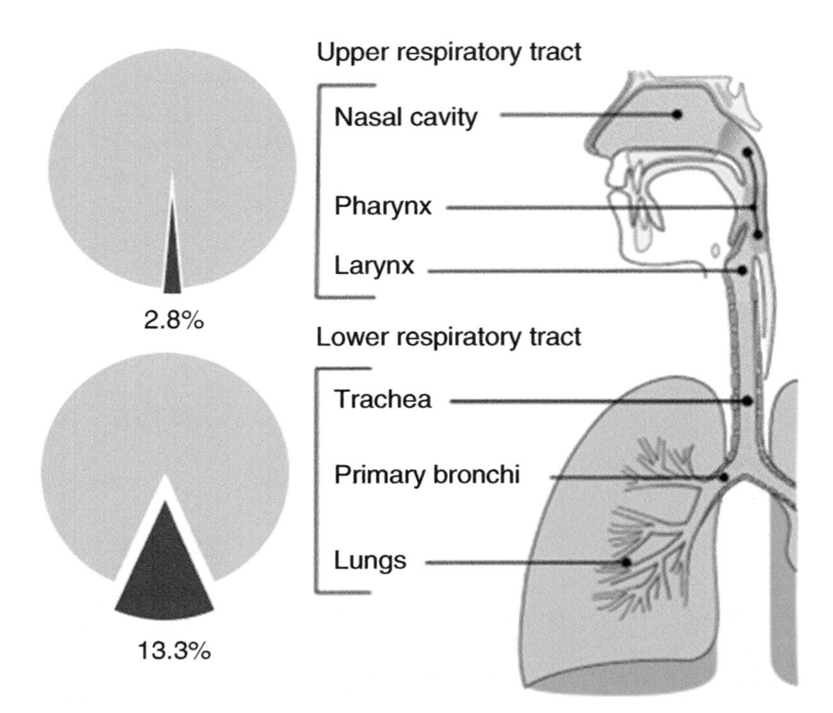

Fig. 7.2 Cancers in the upper and lower respiratory tract. Large airways become smaller as they progressively branch, ultimately terminating in the alveoli. Upper airway cancers occur primarily in the oropharynx. Cancers in the lung are among the most common human malignancies, and account for over 13 % of the total cancer burden. Illustration from the National Cancer Institute

Lung Cancer

Lung cancer is the leading cause of cancer death in both men and women in the US and worldwide. More than 90 % of lung cancers develop as a direct result of exposure to tobacco smoke, whether directly from smoking or from exposure to second hand smoke. Trends in lung cancer incidence and mortality closely track patterns of smoking in the population. These patterns also contribute to cancer health disparities between different ethnic and socioeconomic groups. Approximately 10 % of smokers eventually develop lung cancer.

Tumors in the lung arise from epithelial cells that line the alveoli, bronchioles and bronchi (Fig. 7.2). There are four histologic types of lung cancer that fall into two broad treatment groups. Squamous cell carcinoma, adenocarcinoma of the lung, and large cell carcinoma are collectively referred to as non-small cell lung carcinomas (NSCLC), which together compose 75 % of lung tumors. Because this group of cancers tends to metastasize at a later point in the disease, early detection and surgical resection result in many cures. The remaining one quarter of lung cancers are small cell lung carcinomas (SCLC), the most aggressively metastatic tumors and therefore the most difficult to effectively treat. Cigarette smoking has been conclusively shown to be causally related to both groups of lung cancers. As described in Chap. 5, chronic exposure to the carcinogens in tobacco smoke cause high numbers of mutations; the tumors found in non-smokers have far fewer mutations.

Unlike some of the other common cancers, lung cancer does not occur in a classical familial form. Therefore, there is no obvious gatekeeper gene that is known to strongly affect predisposition. Nonetheless, there is ample evidence that genetic factors do influence the incidence of lung cancer in at-risk smokers. For example, patients diagnosed with retinoblastoma have been found to have an increased incidence of lung cancer later in life compared with the normal population. While the penetrance of *RB1* mutations with respect to the development of retinoblastoma is nearly 100 %, the penetrance of *RB1* mutations with respect to lung cancer is much lower but still significant. A very rare germline mutation in *EGFR*, at position T790M, has been associated with an inherited susceptibility to lung adenocarcinomas.

Several cancer genes have been found at high frequency in sporadic lung cancers. The gene mutated most frequently in lung cancers is *TP53*. *TP53* mutations are found in about 50 % of NSCLC and in 90 % of SCLC. As described in Chap. 1, many smoking-associated mutations are G→T transversions that occur in known hotspots of the *TP53* open reading frame. These characteristic mutations can be directly attributed to bulky adducts caused by exposure to BPDE, a carcinogen in cigarette smoke. Amplification of *MDM2* occurs in 5–10 % of NSCLC, highlighting the importance of the p53 pathway in this tissue.

Somatic *RB1* mutations are found in a significant proportion of sporadic lung cancers. *RB1* is inactivated in 30–40 % of NSCLC and in two thirds all SCLC tumors. Among NSCLC, *RB1* mutations are associated with more advanced tumors, implying that *RB1* loss occurs during later stages of tumorigenesis. Deletions affecting *CDKN2A* and *CDKN2B* are found in about 20 % of NSCLC. Similarly, the gene that encodes cyclin D, *CCND1*, is amplified in a proportion of NSCLC. The receptor tyrosine kinase encoded by *EGFR* is activated by mutations in about 10 % of patients. For reasons that are unclear, *EGFR* mutations are more common in female patients; these mutations present a target for newly developed drugs (see Chap. 8).

A clinically distinct subset of patients with NSCLC harbor a chromosomal translocation that causes a gene fusion called *EML4-ALK*. *ALK* is a proto-oncogene that encodes a receptor tyrosine kinase. ALK, first discovered in an anaplastic lymphoma, can activate several intracellular signal transduction pathways, including the RAS pathway. Accordingly, the *EML4-AML* fusion gene is mutually exclusive to mutations in *KRAS* and *EGFR*. Lung tumors that contain *EML4-ALK* (which are referred to as ALK-positive) are associated with never or light smoking history, younger age and a unique histology. Only 3–4 % of NSCLC are ALK-positive, but these tumors are highly responsive to a drug called crizotinib, a drug that targets ALK activity (see Chap. 8).

Tumor suppressor mutations in *TP53*, *STK11*, *CDKN2A* and *SMARCA4* occur frequently in lung adenocarcinomas. Mutations in *KRAS* are found in about one third of these tumors. Other oncogenes are found less frequently, including *ERBB2* and *MET*. Gene expression data obtained from lung adenocarcinomas indicate that the MAPK and PI3K pathways are commonly activated in this tumor type, but in many cases a genetic mechanism of activation remains obscure.

Prostate Cancer

Prostate cancer is the most commonly diagnosed cancer in men, after non-melanoma skin cancer. Over 35 % of all cancers affecting men are prostate cancers and approximately one in seven men will eventually be diagnosed with this disease. The high incidence of prostate cancer has contributed to a prevalence that is nearly three million in the US. To a great extent, prostate cancer is associated with aging and thus rare in men below the age of 45. Prostate cancer tends to develop very slowly, and many men with the disease eventually die from other causes.

The prostate is a walnut-sized gland located near the base of the urinary bladder (Fig. 7.3). Most of the lesions that develop into prostate malignancies arise in the periphery of the gland, while approximately 20 % of premalignant lesions occur in the region that surrounds the urethra, known as the *transition zone*. The transition zone frequently undergoes hypertrophy, causing a common condition known as

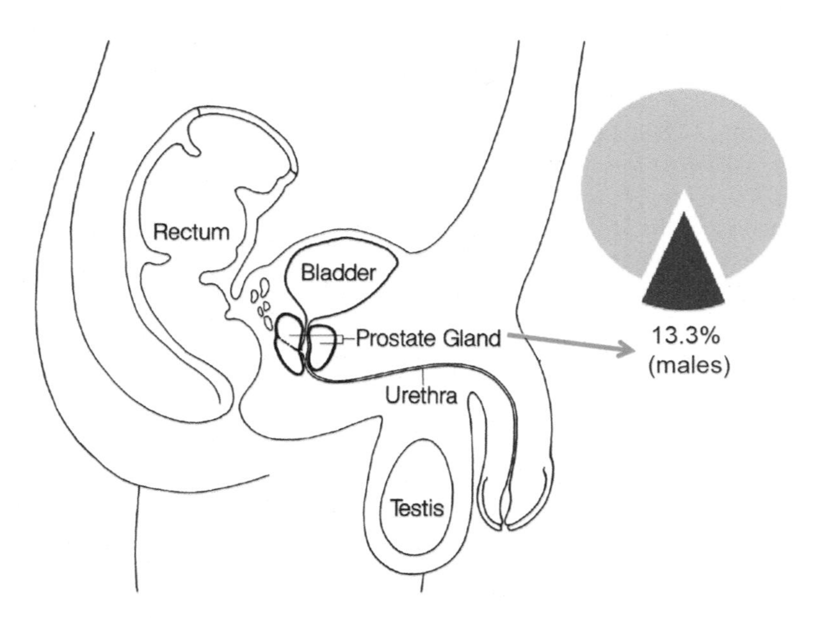

Fig. 7.3 Cancer in the prostate gland. Positioned near the base of the urinary bladder, the prostate surrounds the urethra. Tumors or benign hypertrophy can cause urinary obstruction. Illustration from the National Cancer Institute

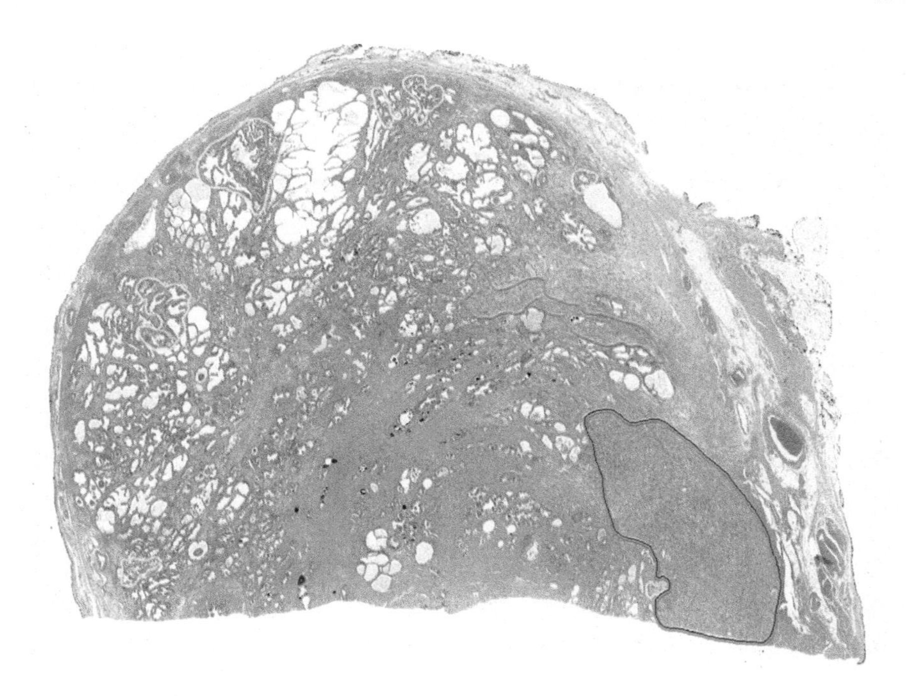

Fig. 7.4 Multifocal neoplasia in the prostate. Prostate intraepithelial neoplasia (PIN; circled in *yellow*) and prostate cancer (circled in *red*) can be seen in a single section of prostate tissue viewed under low magnification. Image by Angelo De Marzo, MD, PhD, The Johns Hopkins University

benign prostatic hyperplasia (BPH). BPH can coexist with prostate cancer, but is not a premalignant condition.

The initiation of tumors in the prostate gland is a very frequent event. Nearly one-third of all men over the age of 45 have histologically identifiable prostate cancer precursor lesions known as *prostatic intraepithelial neoplasia* (PIN). Many PIN lesions are multifocal (Fig. 7.4), suggesting that they represent multiple lesions that arose independently. PIN lesions are thought to be the precursors of prostate cancer, but the majority of PIN lesions do not progress to clinically detectable prostate tumors.

The evolution of prostate tumors clearly has a highly variable course. While the rate of PIN development is similar throughout the world, the rates of prostate cancers in different populations are highly dependent on race and geographic location. This variability is probably due to a combination of genetic and environmental factors, most of which remain unidentified.

Also variable is the genetic etiology of prostate cancer, which varies significantly from case to case. No single gene has been found to be mutated in the majority of prostate cancers, but mutations in *TP53* occur in about one half of cases of metastatic disease. The *TMPRSS-ERG* gene fusion is also very common, occurring in over 40 % of cases.

The cells of the prostate are highly responsive to male hormones called *androgens*. Accordingly, androgens such as testosterone are physiologic drivers of prostate tumor growth. The *TMPRSS-ERG* gene fusion causes alterations to the androgen signaling pathway that causes cells to become androgen-independent. The androgen receptor itself is frequently overexpressed via amplification of its corresponding gene, *AR*.

About 15 % of metastatic cases of prostate cancer feature inactivation of *PTEN*. Somatic mutations in *BRCA2* and *APC* are also found in a significant proportion of cases.

Cases of prostate cancer have been found to cluster in high-risk families. Studies of familial aggregation suggest that 5–10 % of prostate cancers are attributable to the inheritance of autosomal dominant cancer genes. Men that have a family history of the disease reportedly have an approximately threefold increased relative risk for prostate cancer, as do men that carry germline mutations in *BRCA1* or *BRCA2*, which are commonly associated with breast cancer in women. While such epidemiological evidence suggests that prostate cancer has a strong hereditary component, alleles that strongly predispose carriers to prostate cancer have not been identified. About 100 genetic variants known as single-nucleotide polymorphisms (SNPs) have been associated with familial risk of prostate cancer in populations of European ancestry; these variants cumulatively account for one third of the familial risk. African American men have a significantly higher incidence of prostate cancer and nearly double the mortality, compared with men from other ethnic groups. However, non-genetic factors are thought to predominantly contribute to this disparity.

Breast Cancer

Breast cancer is the most commonly diagnosed cancer in women and the leading cause of cancer mortality. Nearly three million women in the US have a history of breast cancer; approximately 30 % will ultimately die of the disease. Men also develop breast cancer, albeit rarely. After increasing over a period of several decades, the rates of breast cancer incidence and mortality have been stable for the past 10 years.

The majority of breast cancers arise from the epithelia that line the milk-producing lobules and ducts of the mammary gland (Fig. 7.5). All women have a similar number of these cells, regardless of overall breast size. For this reason, breast size is not a significant risk factor for breast cancer. Approximately 80 % of breast cancers are ductal in origin, between 5 and 10 % are infiltrating lobular carcinomas and the remainder arise from diverse cell types.

Like several common types of cancer, breast cancer begins with histologically defined precursor lesions. Small, noninvasive lesions, typified by *ductal carcinomas in situ* (DCIS), are believed to progress to first invasive and then metastatic lesions. In contrast, small lesions found in the lobular epithelia, known as *lobular carcino-*

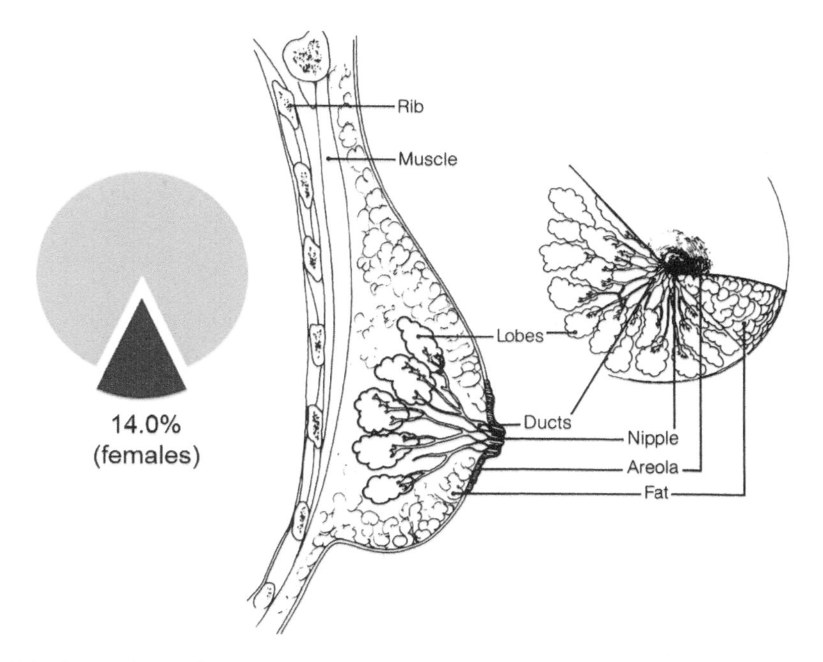

Fig. 7.5 Cancer in the female breast. Milk produced in the lobules is transported to the nipple by the breast ducts. The bulk of breast mass is composed of stromal and fatty tissue. Illustration from the National Cancer Institute

mas in situ (LCIS), are not believed to be precursor lesions that progress, although their appearance is associated with subsequent disease.

There are many risk factors for the development of breast cancer, the single most significant of which is a positive family history. About 5–10 % of breast cancers are hereditary in nature, arising as a consequence of germline alleles that confer cancer predisposition. Two high-penetrance tumor suppressor genes have been described, *BRCA1* and *BRCA2* (Chap. 3). Together, these two genes account for about one quarter of familial breast cancers. Mutations in *BRCA1* have been identified in 15–20 % of women with a family history of breast cancers. The median age of breast cancer onset in *BRCA1* mutation carriers is 42 years, which is 20 years younger than what is observed in sporadic cases.

BRCA1 and BRCA2 proteins function in pathways involved in DNA repair and cell cycle regulation (see Chap. 5). Defects in these pathways lead to elevated rates of mutagenesis and accordingly decreased genetic stability. Other DNA repair proteins that functionally interact with BRCA1 and BRCA2, such as Chk2 and the FANC proteins, are encoded by breast cancer susceptibility genes. Breast cancer is a major component of the clinical spectrum of Li-Fraumeni syndrome, Cowden disease and ataxia telangiectasia, demonstrating that germline mutations in *TP53*, *PTEN* and *ATM*, respectively, confer a significant risk (Chap. 4).

Several genes that are widely found to be mutated in other common cancers are also mutated in sporadic breast cancers. Over 20 % of breast cancers harbor *TP53* mutations. A similar proportion harbors somatically acquired mutations in *PIK3CA*. Mutations in *ATM, GATA3* and *CDH1* are also recurrently observed. Gene amplification appears to be a major molecular component of breast cancer. Significant proportions of tumors harbor amplified regions involving *MYC, CCND1* and *ERBB2* (formerly known as *HER2/neu*).

Colorectal Cancer

Cancer that starts in the colon and rectum (Fig. 7.6), also called the large intestine or large bowel, is the third most common cancer type in the US, behind only lung and prostate cancers in men and lung and breast cancers in women. Colorectal cancer is the second leading cause of cancer mortality, and accounts for 8 % of cancer deaths. The lifetime risk of cancer in the general population is about 5 %.

As described in the earlier chapters of this text, benign colorectal lesions typically progress to invasive and metastatic cancers in distinct histopathological stages that correlate with highly characteristic genetic mutations. The unraveling of the stepwise genetic basis of colorectal cancer has greatly influenced our broader understanding of cancer in all of its forms.

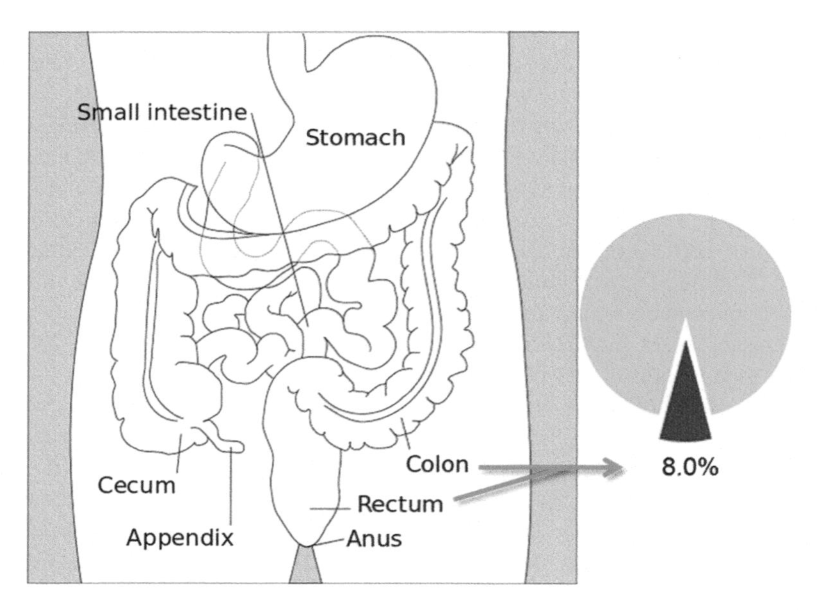

Fig. 7.6 Cancer in the colon and rectum. Colorectal cancers arise from precursor lesions throughout the large bowel, and contribute to approximately 8 % of cancer deaths. Illustration from the National Cancer Institute

Colorectal cancers arise from precursor lesions called *polyps*. These macroscopic growths in the epithelial lining of the colon and/or rectum can be associated with heritable cancer syndromes, but most commonly arise in the absence of predisposing mutations. There are several types of polyps that confer varying levels of risk. Hyperplastic polyps are benign, with low potential for becoming malignant. In contrast, adenomas are pre-malignant neoplasia. Adenomas can be further categorized according to their histologic patterns of cell growth. Tubular adenomas are rounded, villous adenomas have fingerlike projections and serrated polyps have a saw-like appearance under the microscope. Large adenomas (>1 cm) are more advanced than smaller ones and according carry a higher risk of eventually becoming a cancer. In many cases, larger polyps can be removed during endoscopy, substantially reducing the risk of a future malignancy. It has been estimated that full implementation of screening by colonoscopy could reduce the incidence of colorectal cancer by up to 80 %.

In contrast to polyps that arise in the epithelia, hamartomas are a distinct type of polyp, composed of several tissue types including connective tissue and mucus-filled glands. As described in Chap. 3, hamartomas arise in large numbers the heritable disorder juvenile polyposis syndrome. These lesions have low malignant potential but are indicative of a constitutional landscaper defect that can increase cancer risk.

Most colorectal cancers are sporadic in nature and therefore not attributable to a hereditary predisposition. But about 5 % of cases occur in the context of an underlying tumor suppressor mutation. Familial adenomatous polyposis (FAP) is caused by dominant germline mutations in *APC* or, more rarely, recessive mutations in *MUTYH*. Affected individuals develop large numbers of pre-malignant adenomas; their greatly increased risk of cancer is a product of the individual risk conferred by each polyp. In contrast, people affected by hereditary non-polyposis colorectal cancer (HNPCC) have small numbers of polyps, but the underlying genetic instability caused by mismatch repair deficiency greatly accelerates their growth and therefore their malignant potential.

Most colorectal cancers (90 %) harbor truncating mutations in *APC*. Activating mutations in *CTNNB1* are found in some of the tumors that retain wild type *APC*. Other *APC*-wild type tumors recurrently harbor unique gene fusions that affect the function of a family of secreted proteins called R-spondins. These genes, *RSPO2* and *RSPO3*, have been shown to interact with WNT ligands to promote canonical WNT/APC signaling. The mutually exclusive pattern of mutations of *APC*, *CTNNB1* and genes that encode the R-spondin proteins, which cumulatively occur in essentially all colorectal cancers, underscores the primary importance of suppressing WNT signaling in this tissue. Mutations in *TP53* and *KRAS* are found in more than one half of all tumors. *PIK3CA* and *FBXW7* are the remaining mountain peaks in the colorectal cancer landscape (Chap. 5). Among the many hills in this terrain are mutations in *SMAD4*, *BRAF*, *PTCH1* and *ATRX*.

Endometrial Cancer

Endometrial cancer is the most common malignancy of the female genital tract. The endometrium that lines the interior of the uterus (Fig. 7.7) is composed of both epithelial and stromal cells. While cancers can arise from both of these cell types, more than 95 % of endometrial cancers are carcinomas that arise from epithelial cells. Endometrial carcinomas, can be further categorized by histological criteria into endometroid carcinoma and uterine serous carcinoma. Endometrioid carcinoma arises in a stepwise manner from a noninvasive precursor lesion called *complex atypical hyperplasia*. The less common uterine serous carcinoma develops in the setting of epithelial atrophy, from a precursor lesion called *endometrial intraepithelial carcinoma* (CAH). These lesions are distinguishable both clinically and at the molecular level.

Although most cases are sporadic, about 5 % have a known, heritable etiology. Endometrial cancer is the most common extra-colonic cancer associated with hereditary nonpolyposis colorectal cancer (HNPCC). Women who carry HNPCC alleles have a relative risk of endometrial cancer that is 10-fold higher than the general population and an absolute risk of 40–60 %. Of sporadic cancers, many exhibit microsatellite instability that is indicative of defective DNA mismatch repair

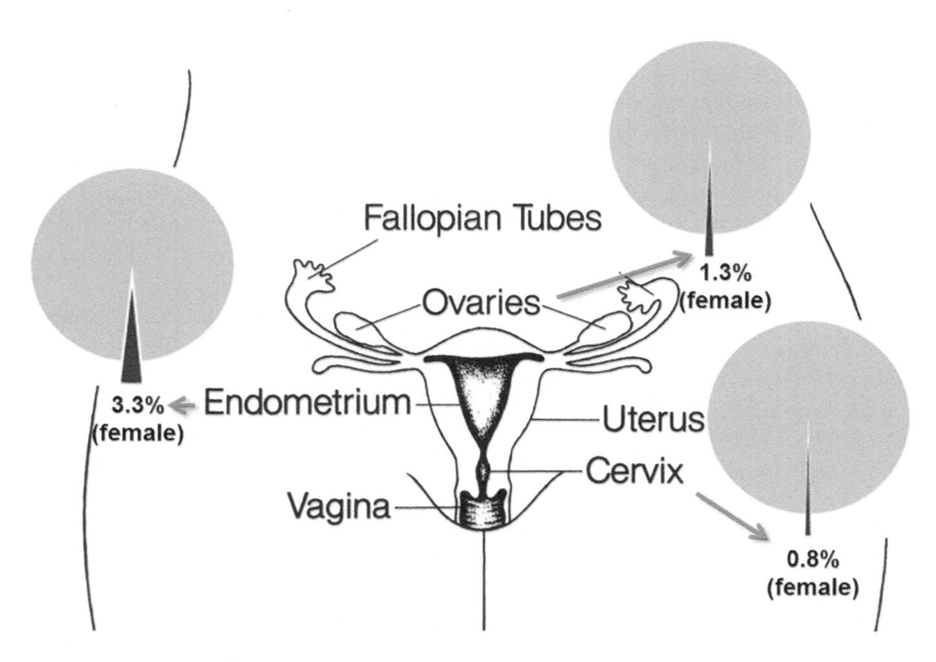

Fig. 7.7 Cancer in the female reproductive tract. Common cancers arise from several organs in the female reproductive tract, including the ovaries, the endometrium that lines the uterus and the uterine cervix. Very rare forms of cancer affect the vagina and fallopian tubes. Illustration from the National Cancer Institute

(Chap. 4). This defect is found in both endometrioid carcinomas as well as in its precursor lesion, CAH.

The most common mutations in endometrial cancers affect the PI3K pathway. Nearly 50 % of endometrioid carcinomas have mutations in *PTEN*. *PTEN* mutations appear to occur early in tumorigenesis, as they are also found in a significant proportion of CAH. Many *PTEN* mutations occur in a region that encodes the phosphatase domain, and result in loss of protein expression. *PIK3CA* mutations are found in over 30 % of endometrioid carcinomas, and often co-exist with a *PTEN* mutation. The functionally related gene *PIK3R1* is also frequently mutated. Mutations in *KRAS*, *TP53*, and *CTNNB1* are also fairly common in endometrioid carcinomas, each occurring at approximate frequencies of 15–20 %.

The two histologically distinguishable forms of endometrial carcinoma show a molecular etiology that is also distinct. *PTEN* mutations are rare in the less-common serous carcinoma, while *TP53* mutations occur at a high frequency in these lesions. Microsatellite instability is very uncommon in serous carcinomas.

Melanoma of the Skin

Melanoma is a common, deadly form of skin cancer that arises from melanocytes, the pigment-producing cells in the skin. The major risk factor for melanoma is exposure to the ultraviolet (UV) component of sunlight. The incidence of melanoma in the US has markedly increased over the past several decades, particularly in the southern latitudes, mirroring an increase in the popularity of tanning and outdoor activities.

Melanocytes arise from embryonic precursors that migrate from the central nervous system into the skin during development. The migratory nature of the melanocyte lineage may in part explain the extreme propensity of melanomas to spread and metastasize.

While melanoma develops in individuals of all ethnic groups, the incidence of melanoma is significantly higher among light-skinned individuals. This increased risk is not the result of a larger number of target cells to be mutated, as light-skinned and dark-skinned individuals have a similar number of melanocytes. Rather, each melanocyte in a dark-skinned individual produces more pigment that confers protection against ultraviolet radiation.

Because they arise in a tissue exposed to a chronic mutagen (sunlight), melanomas typically harbor large numbers of mutations (Chap. 5). The most frequent driver gene in sporadic melanomas is *BRAF*, which functions in the RAS pathway. Activating mutations in *BRAF* have been found in pigmented nevi, as well as in about 50 % of localized and metastatic melanomas. As in other cancers with *BRAF* mutations, the most common mutated allele is V600E. While the genetic alteration that underlies the V600E codon change is not a typical UV signature mutation, the *BRAF* V600E allele is found most commonly in melanomas that occur in sun-exposed areas. In a significant number of melanomas, the RAS pathway is constitutively activated by *NRAS* and, less frequently, *KRAS* mutations. *TP53* mutations are found in about 20 % of melanoma samples.

Germline genetic factors contribute to overall risk. While the majority of melanomas are sporadic, approximately 10 % of cases occur in high risk families, including those affected by the Familial Atypical Multiple Mole Melanoma (FAMMM) syndrome. These families feature a high incidence of pigmented lesions known as atypical nevi (Fig. 7.8). Inactivating germline mutations in *CDKN2A* are the most common cause of FAMMM syndrome. The penetrance of inherited mutant alleles is nearly 70 %. Mutations in *CDKN2A* are also found in sporadic melanoma cases at a frequency of approximately 20 %. Mutations that are somatically acquired often exhibit the UV signature (see Chap. 1), including C → T or CC → TT transitions.

Genetic evidence suggests an important role for the regulation of the $G_1 \rightarrow S$ cell cycle transition in the suppression of melanoma. The *RB1* gene product functions in a common pathway with p16, the product of the *CDKN2A* gene (Chap. 5). Carriers of germline *RB1* mutations who are successfully treated for retinoblastoma in childhood are at an 80-fold risk of developing melanoma later in life. *RB1* mutations have been found in sporadic lesions as well. Another gene that affects cell cycle regulation in concert with *CDKN2A* and *RB1* is *CDK4*, which encodes a cyclin dependent kinase. CDK4 activity, which directly controls the $G_1 \rightarrow S$ cell cycle

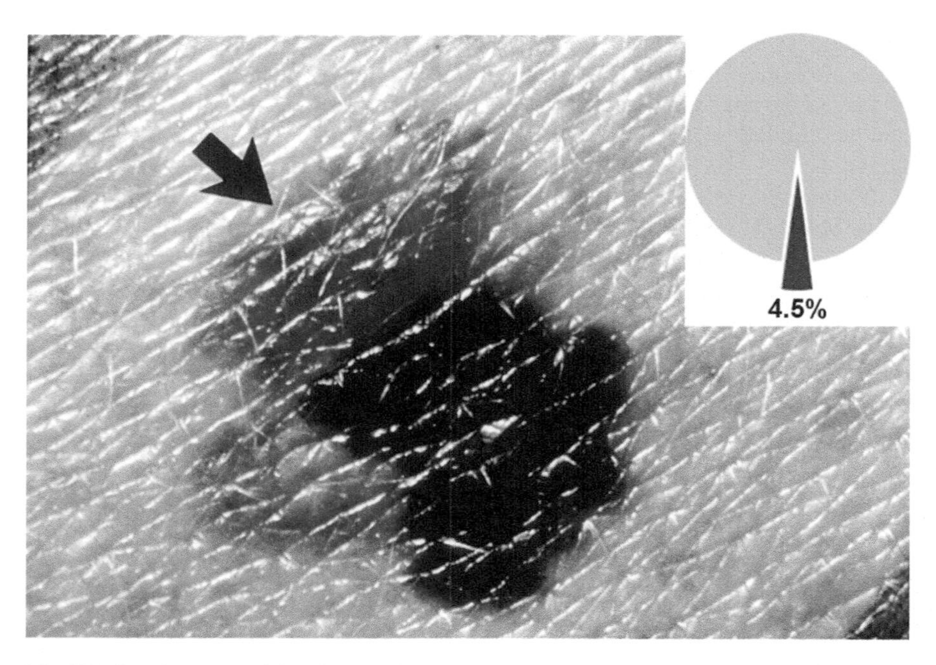

Fig. 7.8 A melanoma arising from a dysplastic nevus. The pink-tan lesion with irregular borders at the upper left (*arrow*) is a dysplastic nevus. Arising from this lesion is an invasive malignant melanoma, with its characteristic blue-black color, notched border, and distorted surface. Image from the National Cancer Institute

transition, is directly inhibited by p16. Analysis of melanoma-prone families without *CDKN2A* mutations has revealed mutations that disrupt the p16 binding site of the *CDK4* encoded protein. As in the case of *CDKN2A*, *CDK4* mutant alleles are highly penetrant. Thus, *CDK4* is another rare example of an oncogene that confers predisposition to cancer when inherited in the germline.

Bladder Cancer

Cancer of the urinary bladder has a fourfold higher incidence in males, in whom it is the fourth most common malignancy. Bladder cancer is strongly associated with local irritation and inflammation caused by environmental toxins in the urine. In the US, tobacco smoking is the most significant risk factor, contributing to about one half of all cases.

Almost all bladder cancers arise from the *urothelium*, a specialized type of epithelium (also known as *transitional epithelium*) that lines the urinary tract (Fig. 7.9). There are two distinct early forms of transitional carcinomas: carcinoma *in situ* and papillary tumors. Carcinoma *in situ* is a flat lesion with a high propensity for progression. It has been demonstrated that 40 % of patients with carcinoma *in situ*

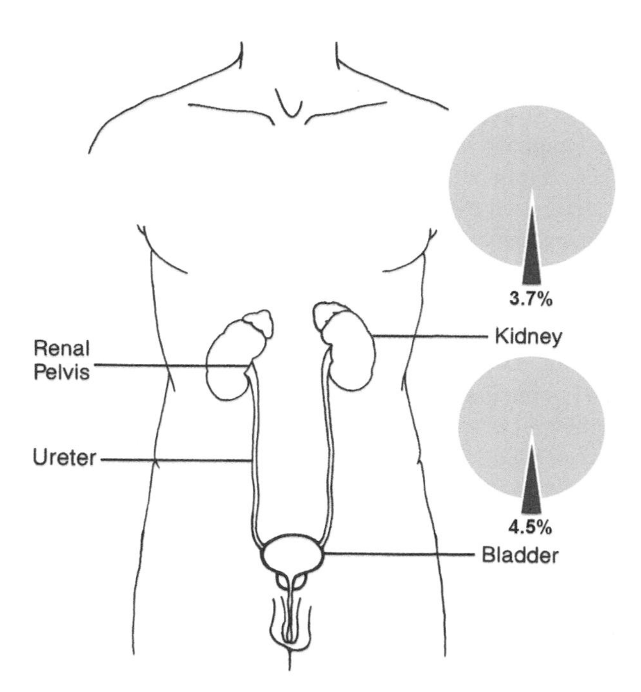

Fig. 7.9 Cancers in the urinary tract. The urinary tract is composed of the kidneys, ureters, the urinary bladder and (in males) the prostate. Illustration from the National Cancer Institute

progress to invasive disease within 5 years. Papillary lesions tend to recur after treatment, but have a less than 20 % risk of progression.

Many bladder cancers appear multifocal at the time of presentation. Alone, this finding would suggest the simultaneous occurrence of multiple independent lesions. Contrary to this interpretation, molecular analyses have revealed that multiple foci are in fact all clonally derived from a single progenitor cell. It would therefore appear that early neoplastic cells within the urothelium are highly mobile.

About 40–50 % of bladder cancers harbor inactivating mutations in *TP53*. Mutations in *PIK3CA*, *RB1*, and *KRAS* are each found in 10–20 % of samples. Deletions of sequences on chromosome 9p that inactivate *CDKN2A* and *CDKN2B* occur at early stage of both flat carcinoma *in situ* and in papillary lesions, and are seen in about one quarter of all advanced lesions. The tumor suppressor *STAG2*, which is required for stable transmission of chromosomes from each cell generation to the next (Chap. 4), is mutated in about 15 % of bladder cancers.

While the majority of bladder cancers are sporadic, a small number of inherited cases occur in the context of HNPCC. Bladder cancer is the fourth most common malignancy in HNPCC patients, and these tumors accordingly exhibit microsatellite instability. Defects in mismatch repair also contribute to sporadic cases, of which approximately 2 % exhibit evidence of microsatellite instability.

Lymphoma

A large and diverse group of malignancies is derived from lymphocytes and their precursors. The lymphoid malignancies that grow as solid tumors are known as lymphomas. These tumor cells frequently migrate to lymph nodes (Fig. 7.10), and are definitively diagnosed by lymph node biopsy. Several forms of lymphoma are closely related to leukemias that also involve lymphoid cells. As a group, the lymphomas account for about 4 % of all cancers and 3 % of all cancer deaths.

There is a bimodal incidence of lymphoma with respect to age at diagnosis. *Hodgkin lymphoma* is a disease of young adulthood with a median age at diagnosis of 38. About 10 % of cases occur in individuals less than 20 years of age. A second peak of Hodgkin lymphoma occurs later in life. The most prevalent lymphomas are non-Hodgkin lymphomas, which are diagnosed at an average age of 67 and account for 90 of all lymphomas.

The *non-Hodgkin lymphomas* can be subdivided by histological and anatomical criteria into numerous subtypes that include (in order of incidence) diffuse large B-cell lymphoma, follicular lymphomas, muscosa-associated lymphoid tissue (MALT) lymphoma, mantle cell lymphoma and Burkitt lymphoma. Of these subtypes, Diffuse Large B-Cell lymphoma and Follicular lymphoma are the most common. Depending on the type, tumors can variably occur in lymph nodes and at a variety of extranodal sites.

The most apparent cytogenetic genetic defects in lymphoma cells are chromosomal translocations. These oncogenic alterations frequently involve highly expressed

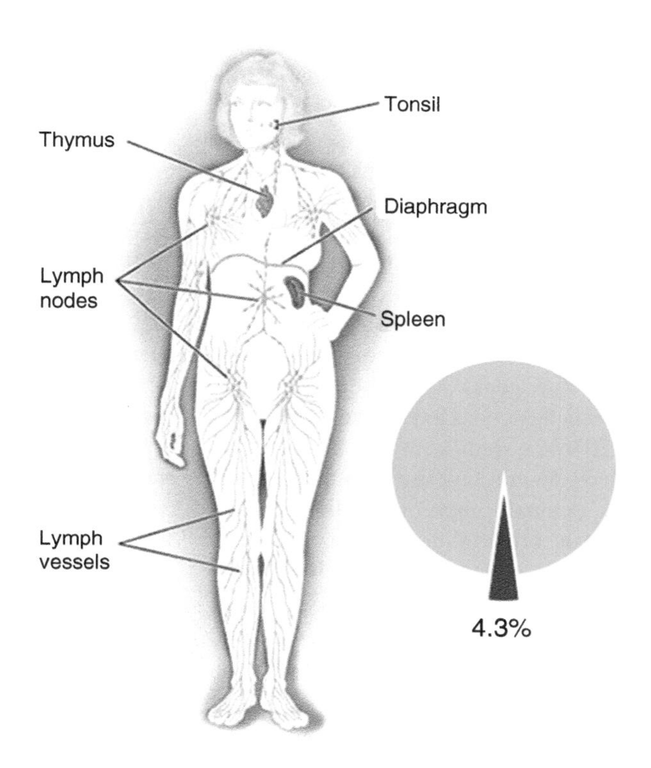

Fig. 7.10 Cancer in the lymphatic system. The diverse tissues of the lymphatic system are located in many parts of the body. Lymphomas can therefore start virtually anywhere. Diagnosis can be facilitated by biopsy of lymph nodes, where malignant cells grow into palpable masses. Illustration from the National Cancer Institute

immunoglobulin loci, and arise as a consequence of a high rate of gene recombination that is intrinsically related to the ontogeny of cells in the lymphoid lineage. These fusion genes are unique to lymphoid cancers and not altered in other tumor types.

Among the genes identified at common breakpoints in follicular lymphomas is *BCL2*, an anti-apoptotic gene on chromosome 18 that is fused to the immunoglobulin heavy chain gene promoter. Approximately 40 % of diffuse large cell lymphomas and 5–10 % of follicular lymphomas harbor translocations that alter the expression of BCL6, a DNA binding protein that represses transcription of specific target genes. In MALT lymphomas, a gene designated *MALT1*, located 5 Megabases away from *BCL2*, is frequently fused to a highly expressed inhibitor of apoptosis, *API2*, on chromosome 11. *MALT1* is required for a variety of inflammatory processes that involve the activation of the pro-proliferative transcription factor NF-κB. MALT lymphomas that occur in the stomach are associated with infection with *Helicobacter pylori*, indicating the role of chronic inflammation in this disease subtype (see Chap. 1). Mantle cell lymphomas have a recurrent translocation between chromosomes 11 and 14 that results in overexpression of *CCND1*, the gene that encodes Cyclin D1. Large B-cell lymphomas frequently harbor deletions involving *CDKN2A* and *CDKN2B*.

In addition to genes located at translocation breakpoints, a number of genes have been found to be somatically mutated by other mechanisms. *TP53* is inactivated by point mutations in approximately 20 % of non-Hodgkin lymphomas. In a small number of cases, constitutive activation of the RAS signaling pathway results from mutations in *BRAF* and *KRAS*.

Burkitt lymphomas are relatively rare outside of Africa, where they are highly endemic. This aggressive form of non-Hodgkin lymphoma is caused by chromosomal translocations that result in the overexpression of *MYC*. In addition, approximately 30 % of Burkitt lymphomas harbor *TP53* mutations. Infection with Epstein Barr virus (EBV) is strongly associated with Burkitt lymphoma, as is infection with the human immunodeficiency virus.

The second major category of lymphomas, Hodgkin lymphomas, feature recurrent gains of sequence on chromosomes 2, 9 and 12, and respective amplification of the oncogenes *REL* (the cellular homolog of the V-REL viral oncogene), *JAK2* (which encodes a tyrosine kinase), and *MDM2*. Infectious mononucleosis caused by EBV is a significant risk factor for Hodgkin lymphoma, and EBV DNA sequences have been found in a significant proportion of Hodgkin lymphoma biopsies.

A small proportion of both non-Hodgkin lymphomas and Hodgkin lymphomas occur in familial clusters. The underlying basis for lymphoma predisposition remains unknown.

Cancers in the Kidney

Cancers in the kidney and renal pelvis account for nearly 4 % of all adult cancers in the US. Males are affected almost twice as frequently as females, and individuals in end-stage renal failure have a risk of cancer that is up to 30-fold that of the general population. Tobacco smoking is a modifiable risk factor. An estimated 1–2 % of all renal cell carcinomas are hereditary in origin.

Renal adenocarcinoma is the predominant form of cancer that occurs in the kidney. This disease occurs in several histological types, the most common of which (80 %) features a type of cell known as the clear cell. A smaller proportion of tumors exhibit a papillary morphology. Both of these tumor types occur in sporadic and hereditary cases.

As in many other types of cancer, the heritable forms of renal carcinoma shed light on the genetic basis of sporadic tumors that are much more common. There are four types of autosomal dominantly inherited renal carcinoma: von Hippel-Lindau (VHL) syndrome, hereditary leiomyomatosis and renal cell cancer (HLRCC), hereditary papillary renal cancer and Birt-Hogg-Dubé syndrome. Similar to the pattern of retinoblastoma, sporadic kidney cancers are typically solitary lesions, while hereditary disease is often multifocal and bilateral. In addition to these dominantly inherited forms of renal carcinoma, there are poorly defined recessive genetic elements that appear to contribute significant to cancer risk. The relative risk of renal carcinoma has been estimated to be 2.5 for a sibling of an affected individual.

The best understood hereditary kidney cancer is VHL. VHL is caused by germline mutations in *VHL,* a 3-exon gene located at 3p26–p25 and cloned in 1993. A variety of inactivating mutations have been found throughout the *VHL* open reading frame, including small insertions and deletions and single base substitutions. As described in Chap. 6, the loss of VHL function causes the widespread development of cysts and an increase in angiogenesis, the proliferation of new blood vessels that can feed tumor growth. Affected individuals are at elevated risk for development of uncommon tumors including pancreatic neuroendocrine tumors and pheochromocytomas, non-malignant hormone-producing tumors that usually occur in the adrenal glands. *VHL* is inactivated in 30–40 % of sporadic clear cell renal carcinomas.

HLRCC is a rare kidney cancer susceptibility syndrome caused by autosomal dominant point mutations in the *FH* gene. *FH* encodes an enzyme called fumarate hydratase, which functions in the citric acid cycle. Mutant FH proteins appear to cause the accumulation of the metabolite fumarate. Fumarate may interfere with oxygen levels in the cell and lead to chronic hypoxia. As described in Chap. 6, hypoxia is a stimulus of the transcription factor HIF1α, which is normally held in check by VHL. The activation of the PI3K pathway causes the downregulation of FH expression.

Hereditary papillary renal cancer is caused by highly penetrant germline mutations that activate the *MET* proto-oncogene, which encodes a receptor tyrosine kinase. *Birt-Hogg-Dubé* syndrome is a cancer predisposition syndrome caused by mutations in the gene *FLCN*, which is involved in nutrient sensing through AMPK in the mammalian target of rapamycin pathway (mTOR, see Chap. 6).

Sporadic renal clear cell carcinomas frequently harbor mutations in *VHL*. Other cancer genes, including *TP53* and the BRCA1-associated protein encoded by *BAP1*, are mutated in relatively smaller numbers of tumors. The cancer genome landscape (Chap. 5) of this disease thus features a single mountain and many small hills.

Thyroid Cancer

Cancers of the thyroid are the most common malignancies of the endocrine system. Unlike many other cancers, rates of incidence of thyroid cancer have markedly increased over the past several decades. Known risk factors include exposure to ionizing radiation, reduced iodine intake, preexisting inflammatory disease and family history. Like most diseases of the thyroid, thyroid cancer has a significantly higher incidence rate in females.

Thyroid cancers arise from epithelial cells that line the thyroid follicles and from parafollicular cells. The prognosis of the disease is closely associated with the extent of differentiation. Well-differentiated thyroid tumors can remain indolent for prolonged periods, and can usually be cured. While most thyroid cancers are highly responsive to therapy, the rare tumors that are undifferentiated and anaplastic are among the most aggressive and lethal of all human cancers.

Papillary carcinomas, the most common thyroid cancer, account for 75–85 % of cases and arise as thyroid nodules (Fig. 7.11). *Follicular cancers* arise from relatively differentiated cell populations that secrete thyroid hormone. A distinct type of tumor

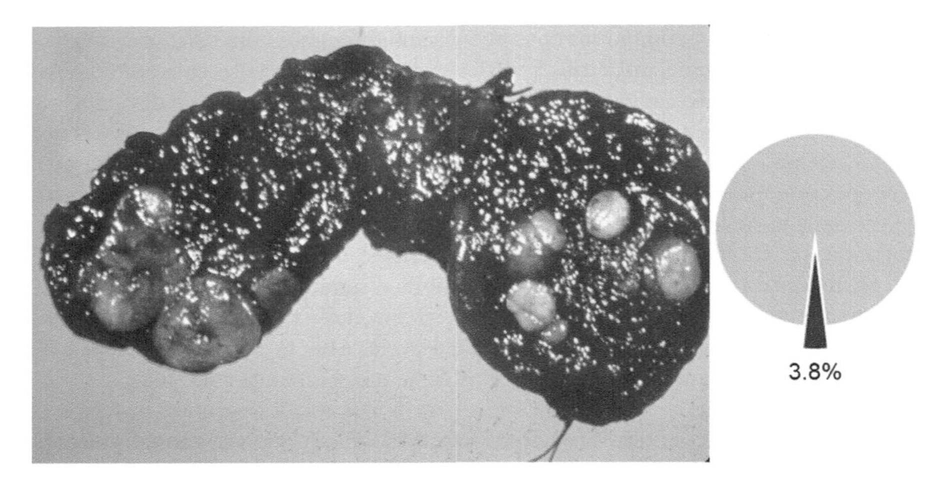

Fig. 7.11 Thyroid cancer nodules. Viewed as a gross specimen, the two lobes of a thryroid gland contain multiple cancerous nodules. Image from the National Cancer Institute

called medullary thyroid carcinoma arises from parafollicular cells that produce the hormone calcitonin, called C-cells, and account for less than 10 % of all cases.

Papillary thyroid cancers are predominantly driven by dysregulation of the RAS pathway. About on half of these tumors harbor a mutation in *BRAF*, usually the activating V600E mutation. Mutations in *NRAS* or *HRAS* are found in an additional 10 % of tumors. These tumors are otherwise genetically diverse, with many mutations occurring at low frequency. Sporadic thyroid cancers attributed to radiation appear to have a distinct molecular etiology. A particularly high incidence of *RET* rearrangements has been observed in childhood thyroid cancers caused by radioactive fallout from the Chernobyl accident, indicating a probable role for radiation-associated chromosome breaks. While the *BRAF* V600E point mutation occurs frequently in thyroid cancers, *BRAF* is altered primarily by translocation in thyroid cancers that are radiation-related.

A positive family history increases risk 3–6 fold, indicating that there is a significant heritable component to thyroid carcinoma. In most of these cases, the genetic etiology remains unknown. A small proportion of heritable thyroid cancers occur in individuals with known cancer predisposition syndromes. Papillary thyroid cancers are part of the spectrum of cancers that occur in individuals with Familial adenomatous polyposis (FAP) and Cowden syndrome. Up to 25 % of medullary thyroid cancers occur in the context of multiple endocrine neoplasia type 2 (MEN2).

Leukemia

The leukemias are a diverse group of cancers that arise in the blood and blood-forming tissues. Over 300,000 people in the US have a current or past diagnosis of leukemia. While leukemia is the leading form of pediatric cancer, leukemia affects many more adults than children.

Leukemias arise in blood-forming tissues such as the bone marrow, from cells in the lymphoid or the myeloid lineage. Both lymphocytic and myeloid leukemias can present in acute and chronic forms. Acute myeloid leukemia (AML; Fig. 7.12) and chronic lymphocytic leukemia (CLL) are the most common leukemias in adults. Acute lymphocytic leukemia (ALL) is the most common pediatric cancer. Additional types of leukemia arise from cells at various stages of hematological development.

Chromosomal translocations are found in over 50 % of leukemias in both in children and adults. As described in Chap. 2, translocations can activate proto-oncogenes near breakpoints by fusing together the coding sequences of two genes that are normally unrelated, or by placing a gene under the transcriptional control of an unrelated gene that is expressed at high levels.

A classic example of oncogene activation by translocation is the translocation between chromosomes 9 and 22 that creates the Philadelphia chromosome, originally observed in chronic myelocytic leukemia (CML) and subsequently detected in ALL (Chap. 2). This translocation event creates a hybrid gene that contains downstream elements of *ABL*, which encodes a tyrosine kinase, fused with upstream elements of *BCR*, a gene that is highly expressed.

Recurrent translocations involving chromosome 11 have been observed in aggressive forms of both AML and ALL. The gene at the common breakpoint of these translocations is designated *MLL*, for mixed lineage leukemia. Different trans-

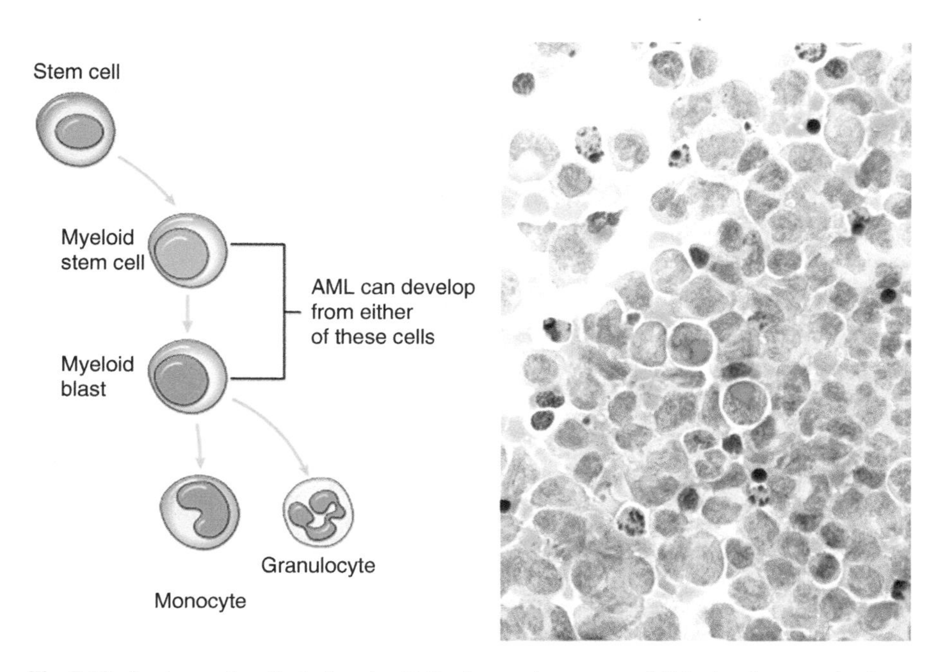

Fig. 7.12 Acute myelocytic leukemia. AML, the most common adult leukemia, can arise from either the lineage-committed myeloid stem cell or the myeloid blast cell (*left panel*, from Cancer Research UK). AML cells obtained from cardiac fluid, stained with esterase, at 400× magnification (*right panel*, from the National Cancer Institute)

location events activate *MLL* activity by creating in-frame fusion proteins. *MLL* encodes a protein with intrinsic methyltransferase activity that, by catalyzing the methylation of cytosine bases (Chap. 1), regulates the expression of known mediators of development. Another common breakpoint gene is *TCL1*, first identified in a T-cell leukemia. Translocations involving chromosome 14q frequently place the *TCL1* locus in the vicinity of a highly expressed T-cell receptor gene. The protein encoded by *TCL1* has been shown to directly bind AKT within its pleckstrin homology domain, and thus activate the PI3K/AKT pathway (Chap. 6).

About one quarter of AML samples harbor mutations in the receptor tyrosine kinase encoded by *FLT3*. A similar proportion of leukemias inactivate the tumor suppressor *NPM1*, which encodes a protein called nucleophosmin. Nucleophosmin performs multiple functions in the cell nucleus in response to cell stress, and mediates cell survival. *IDH1*, *IDH2*, *DNMT3A*, *NRAS* and *TP53* are each mutated in 5–25 % of AML cases.

The environmental risk factors for the development of leukemia tend to be those that promote chromosome breakage. Ionizing radiation exposure is notable in this regard. The survivors of the atomic bombs detonated in Japan at the end of World War II, as well as early radiation scientists who worked without effective shielding, exhibited a striking increase in leukemia incidence.

While most leukemias are sporadic and commonly caused by translocations and more subtle mutations that are somatically acquired, a small proportion of leukemias arise in a manner that is clearly hereditary. Individuals affected by Fanconi anemia, ataxia telangiectasia, Li-Fraumeni syndrome and HNPCC are at significantly greater risk of leukemia. Individuals with Down syndrome, who harbor constitutional trisomy 21, have a significantly increased risk of AML.

Cancer in the Pancreas

Cancer of the pancreas is the fifth leading cause of cancer death in the US. It is a highly aggressive and lethal form of cancer, with a mortality rate that approaches the incidence. Known risk factors for pancreatic cancer include cigarette smoking and obesity. Men have a higher risk of developing pancreatic cancer, as do individuals with a family history of the disease.

The majority of cancers of the pancreas are adenocarcinomas that arise in the epithelia of the pancreatic ducts. The earliest lesions are known as *pancreatic intraepithelial neoplasia* (PanINs). PanINs are precursors of more advanced lesions in the epithelia of the pancreatic duct in a similar way that adenomas progress to invasive carcinomas in the colorectal epithelia. Because early pancreatic tumors tend to be associated with vague symptoms or are asymptomatic, most pancreatic cancers are advanced at the time of diagnosis. The pancreas is located deep in the abdominal cavity, in an anatomical region known as the retroperitoneal space (Fig. 7.13). Symptoms of bulky, advanced cancers are related to the obstruction of neighboring ducts and tracts.

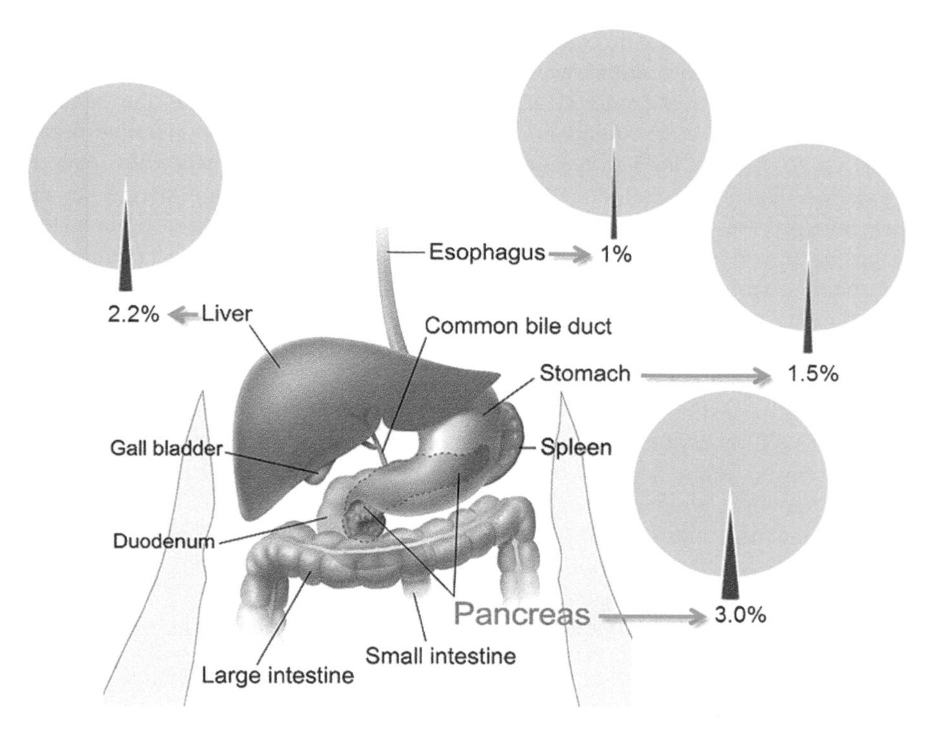

Fig. 7.13 Cancers in the upper digestive tract. Cancers in the pancreas represent about 3 % of all cancers in the US. Cancer can also arise in the esophagus, stomach and liver. Illustration from the National Cancer Institute

Several genetic alterations are found at very high frequencies in pancreatic adenocarcinomas. Activation of *KRAS* by point mutation of codon 12 occurs in a large proportion of these cancers. Some of the tumors that retain wild type *KRAS* alleles have activating mutations in *BRAF*. One third of pancreatic adenocarcinomas inactivate *TP53*. Deletions involving *CDKN2A* and *CDKN2B* are found in nearly 30 % of samples. Inactivation of *SMAD4* and the tumor suppressors encoded by the ARID gene family are also significant features of the pancreatic cancer landscape. This spectrum of mutations highlight the importance of the RAS, TGF-β/SMAD, p53, cell cycle regulatory and chromatin modulation pathways in the evolution of pancreatic adenocarcinomas.

As is the case with several common types of cancer, pancreatic cancer can arise in the setting of chronic inflammation (Chap. 1). An inflammatory disease known as *hereditary pancreatitis* predisposes affected individuals to pancreatic cancer. Many cases of hereditary pancreatitis have been attributed to germline mutations in the *PRSS1* gene, which encodes a protease proenzyme called *cationic trypsinogen*. Missense mutations in *PRSS1* cause the encoded protein to be inappropriately activated, leading to auto-digestion of tissues in the pancreas, which triggers a chronic inflammatory response.

Up to 10 % of pancreatic cancers have an inherited genetic component. In addition to hereditary pancreatitis, several known cancer syndromes predispose affected individuals to pancreatic cancer. A subset of individuals affected by the Familial Atypical Multiple Mole Melanoma (FAMMM) syndrome harbor germline mutations in *CDKN2A* and has a significantly increased risk of pancreatic cancer. Pancreatic cancer is also among the spectrum of cancers that occur as part of hereditary nonpolyposis colorectal cancer (HNPCC). Peutz-Jeghers syndrome, ataxia telangiectasia, von Hippel-Lindau syndrome and the familial breast cancer syndrome caused by germline mutations in *BRCA2*. The *PALB2* gene, which encodes the protein binding partner of BRCA2, is involved in about 3 % of familial pancreatic cancers. About 20 % of familial pancreatic cancers remain genetically undefined.

A small minority of pancreatic tumors arise in non-epithelial cell populations and are clinically distinct. Most of these are pancreatic neuroendocrine tumors (PanNETs). Tumors of this type develop in cell lineages that integrate the endocrine and nervous systems. Some of these tumors produce hormones such as gastrin or insulin. PanNETs are a frequent component of MEN1 syndrome (Chap. 3), caused by germline mutations in *MEN1*. *MEN1* mutations are also found in a large proportion of sporadic (non-familial) tumors. The encoded protein, menin, is involved in chromatin remodeling. Frequent somatic mutations in *DAXX* and *ATRX* also cause aberrant chromatin remodeling in these lesions. About 15 % of PanNETs exhibit mutations that affect the mTOR pathway.

Ovarian Cancer

Ovarian cancer is the fifth leading cause of cancer deaths among women in the US. Tumors are rarely detected at an early, curable stage; most ovarian cancers are spread throughout the pelvis at the time of diagnosis. Most ovarian cancers are sporadic, but a significant number are associated with known familial cancer syndromes. A major risk factor is cumulative ovulatory activity, which in many individuals is increased by early onset of menarche and nulliparity.

Ovarian cancers are a heterogeneous group of histologically distinct tumors. The most common ovarian cancers are *ovarian carcinomas*, which arise among the epithelial cells on the surface of the ovary. Histological subtypes include serous, clear cell, endometrioid and mucinous. The precise cellular origin of some ovarian cancers remains to be definitively determined.

The subtypes of ovarian tumors arise from distinct precursor lesions and generally exhibit different genetic alterations. Molecular analysis has shown that low- and high-grade serous carcinomas probably arise via alterations in different pathways, the former involving mutations in *KRAS* and *BRAF* and the latter involving mutations of *TP53*. *TP53* is mutated in approximately one half percent of serous and endometrioid carcinomas, but less often in mucinous and clear cell carcinomas. These tumors exhibit evidence of extensive gene amplification, frequently involving the *MYC* locus.

Mucinous ovarian tumors, which are believed to arise from precursor adenomas, exhibit a high frequency of *KRAS* mutations. Endometrioid carcinomas arise in regions of endometriosis, an inflammatory lesion that resembles the lining of the uterine endometrium. These cancers harbor frequent mutations in *CTNNB1* that constitutively activate the WNT/APC pathway. Endometrioid tumors with dysregulated WNT/APC signaling frequently have concurrent mutations that dysregulate PI3K signaling, most often in *PTEN* but also in *PIK3CA*.

A rare and aggressive form of ovarian cancer known as *small cell carcinoma of the ovary* is frequently caused by somatic mutations in *SMARCA4*, which encodes a component of the SWI/SNF chromatin remodeling complex (Chap. 6). The *SMARCA4* mutation rate is greater than 90 % in these tumors; mutations in *JAK3* and *NOTCH2* have also been detected.

Up to 25 % of all ovarian cancers are estimated to occur in individuals with an inherited predisposition. Familial ovarian cancer is a significant component of familial breast cancer, associated with germline mutations in *BRCA1* and *BRCA2* (Chap. 3) and of HNPCC, which is caused by alterations in mismatch repair genes (Chap. 4). Women with HNPCC have a 12 % lifetime risk of developing ovarian cancer.

Cancers of the Oral Cavity and Pharynx

Oral and pharyngeal cancers, including those of the lip, tongue, mouth and pharynx, are relatively uncommon in the US, but highly prevalent around the world. In some countries, up to 40 % of all cancers occur in the oral cavity and pharynx. Men are affected more often than women. In the US, the major risk factors are smokeless tobacco and alcohol consumption. A distinct form of squamous cell cancer is caused by a sexually transmitted virus.

The most common cancers of the oral cavity and pharynx are head and neck squamous cell carcinomas (HNSCC). These cancers typically arise in patients with preexisting dysplasia, in the form of ulcers and plaques. Most early lesions are asymptomatic in their early stages. Developing tumors often grow laterally, sometimes becoming invasive and spreading to regional lymph nodes. Blood borne metastasis is uncommon.

TP53 mutations are highly common in cancers throughout the head and neck, occurring in about two thirds of all samples. The hotspots at which the *TP53* gene is mutated in head and neck cancers overlap, but are partially distinct from, those found in the lung and bladder cancers of cigarette smokers. Interestingly, the $G \rightarrow T$ transversions associated with benzo[a] pyrene exposure in lung cancers (Chap. 1) are not commonly found in oropharyngeal cancers even though the oral and pharyngeal mucosae are exposed to the same agent. The occurrence of an inactivating mutation in *TP53* is a negative prognostic sign.

Mutations in *PIK3CA* and *NOTCH1* are found in up to 10 % of tumor samples. *HRAS* is activated in about 10 % of US cases of HNSCC, while other members of

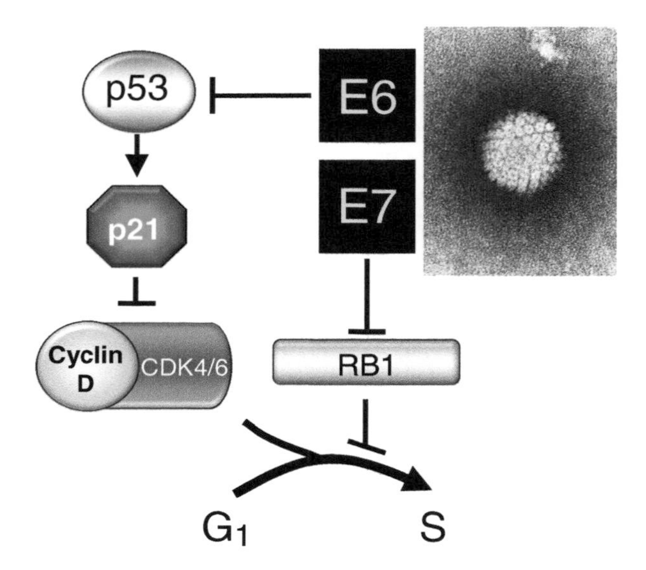

Fig. 7.14 Human Papilloma Virus promotes cell cycle progression. HPV-encoded E6 and E7 proteins bind and functionally inhibit p53 and RB1, respectively, leading to loss of $G_1 \rightarrow S$ checkpoint control in chronically infected cells. The electron micrograph of an HPV particle is from the National Cancer Institute

the RAS family appear to be mutated at higher numbers in populations outside of the US.

An important risk factor for the development of HNSCC is infection with high-risk serotypes of *human papillomaviruses* (HPV). These viruses, transmitted by sexual activity, are small DNA-based viruses with a circular genome that is roughly 8 kilobases in size. Viral DNA sequences are found in over 90 % of HPV related cancers, which include HPV-associated HNSCC, cancer of the uterine cervix (see below), vulvar cancer, penile cancer and anal cancer. HPV variants are distinguished by their antigenicity and assigned a serotype. Most serotypes are associated with benign conditions such as warts, but the high-risk serotypes including HPV-16 and -18 are strongly carcinogenic. Most HPV infections are rapidly eliminated by the immune system and only a small proportion of HPV-infected individuals eventually develop cancer. More than one half of all HNSCC are caused by chronic infection with HPV.

Many of the viruses linked to cancer cause chronic inflammation. HPV-associated cancers are different in that they express viral oncoproteins that directly influence a cancer gene pathway (Fig. 7.14). Two small viral open reading frames designated E6 and E7 promote tumorigenesis. (The designation 'E' for 'early'denotes that these genes are expressed at an early stage of the viral replication cycle.) DNA containing E6 and E7 genes from high-risk serotypes can induce cancer-related phenotypes when experimentally transferred to cultured normal cells. Homologous DNA sequences from low-risk serotypes do not have this ability. Unlike the retroviral oncogenes described in Chap. 2, the E6 and E7 oncogenes of HPV, a DNA tumor virus, have no known cellular homologs.

The E6 protein encoded by HPV binds to p53. Upon binding, HPV E6 recruits a cellular ubiquitin ligase, the E6-associated protein (E6-AP). These three proteins form a complex that functions to target p53 for degradation by the proteasome. Thus, HPV E6 facilitates the degradation of p53 and the consequent loss of p53 function in a fashion similar to the oncogene product MDM2 (Chap. 3). In addition, the HPV E7 protein has been shown to bind to and inactivate RB1. The simultaneous inactivation of two tumor suppressor genes by a cancer-causing virus strongly underscores the functional importance of these genes in maintaining tissue homeostasis within the epithelia of the cervix. The integrated virus benefits from the loss of growth control of its cellular host.

As might be expected, HPV-associated HNSCC typically retain wild type *TP53* alleles. These cancers are less strongly associated with alcohol and tobacco use, and are generally more responsive to therapy. Thus, at both the molecular and clinical levels, HPV-positive and HPV–negative HNSCC can be considered as two distinct diseases.

Liver Cancer

Relatively uncommon in the US, primary liver cancer is a significant public health concern in much of the world. The highest incidence of this disease is found in southern China and sub-Saharan Africa, where it is responsible for over one million deaths each year, or about 10 % of deaths from all causes. About 35,000 new cases of liver cancer are diagnosed in the US each year.

Three quarters of liver cancers arise in the predominant epithelial cells in the liver, the *hepatocytes*. These tumors are referred to *hepatocellular carcinomas* (HCC). Less frequently, cancers can arise in the bile duct (choloangiocarcinomas), blood vessels (mesenchymal tumors) and immune cells (lymphomas). Cancers that originate at extra-hepatic sites, predominantly in the colon, often metastasize to the liver; these secondary tumors are not called liver cancers.

The major risk factors are chronic infection by the hepatitis B virus (HBV) and hepatitis C virus (HCV), contamination of food with aflatoxin B1 (Chap. 1), and excessive consumption of alcohol. More than twice as many men as women are affected by liver cancer.

The majority of HCCs feature the functional inactivation of p53-dependent transcription. There are several mechanisms by which loss of p53 function occurs. Many liver cancers harbor mutations in *TP53*; the proportion depends on the etiology. The best known example of toxin-specific mutagenesis is caused by the dietary toxin aflatoxin B1, which frequently contaminates corn, rice and peanuts. Aflatoxin B1 causes G→T transversions at *TP53* codon 249, a site rarely mutated in other cancer types (Chap. 1). In areas of low aflatoxin B1 intake, a distinct spectrum of *TP53* mutations is observed. In HBV-associated HCC, the p53 protein interacts with the product of a viral oncogene known as gene X, which encodes a protein called HBx. HBx is expressed as a result of the frequent integration of the HBV genome into the DNA of the host cells, and directly binds a number of cellular proteins, including p53. HBx inhibits the association of p53 with its target sequences in the genome, thus repressing p53-mediated transcription and promoting cell cycle progression. In addition, HBV infection causes chronic inflammation, which is a more general mediator of malignant transformation. In contrast to HBV, the genome of HCV does not encode a functional homolog of HBx. It therefore appears that the risk of HCC caused by HCV infection is entirely attributable to the effects of chronic inflammation.

Besides *TP53*, hepatocellular carcinomas recurrently harbor activating mutations in *CTNNB1*, which encodes the activator of WNT signaling β-catenin. Intrahepatic cholangiocarcinomas frequently harbor mutations in *TP53, KRAS, BAP1, IDH1*, and *ARID1A*, a chromatin remodeling protein in the SWI/SNF complex.

There are no recognized familial forms of liver cancer, but several rare genetic diseases can increase cancer risk. These include hemochromatosis (an iron overload disease), Wilson disease (a copper overload disease), porphyria (a heme-pigment overload disease) and α1-antitrypsin deficiency.

Cancer of the Uterine Cervix

Carcinoma of the uterine cervix, commonly referred to as cervical cancer, ranks fourth as a cause of cancer death in women worldwide. In the US, the incidence of cervical cancer has dropped considerably over the past several decades. This decline has been largely attributed to effective screening and treatment of precursor lesions. Among women with inadequate access to health care, particularly those in the developing world, cervical cancer remains highly prevalent.

More than 90 % of cervical cancers can be attributed to chronic infection with high-risk serotypes of human papillomavirus (HPV). Screening for HPV infection and immunizing against HPV are projected to contribute to a continued decrease in the incidence of cancers of the cervix, as well as the HPV-associated tumors in the head and neck, anus, vulva and penis.

Most cervical cancers are squamous carcinomas that arise in a region between two histologically distinct types of cervical epithelium, a region known as the *transition zone*. Disorganized lesions known as low-grade squamous intraepithelial lesions and high-grade squamous intraepithelial lesions are confined to the epithelia. The high-grade lesions are precursors that eventually develop into invasive squamous cell carcinomas.

The most common mutations in cervical squamous cell carcinomas occur in *PIK3CA*, at a frequency of about 17 %. Another 20 % of tumors harbor amplifications involving the *PIK3CA* locus. Smaller proportions of tumors harbor mutations in *PTEN, FBXW7* and in the chromatid remodeling gene *ARID1A*.

Stomach Cancer

Stomach cancer was once the leading cause of cancers deaths in the US, but its incidence in the US and other developed countries has decreased significantly over the past several decades. This decline can be attributed to improvements in living conditions, particularly the advent of refrigeration for food storage. This disease remains a leading cause of cancer death in many developing countries, and ranks just below lung cancer as the second most common cause of total cancer deaths worldwide.

Environmental factors play a significant role in stomach cancer risk. Stomach cancers are strongly associated with chronic inflammation (Chap. 1). An important etiologic agent, involved in about 60 % of cases, is the bacterium *Helicobacter pylori*, which causes ulcerative disease. Stomach cancer is particularly prevalent in developing countries with a high incidence of *H. pylori* infection that occurs early in life. The inflammatory lesion *chronic atrophic gastritis* is a precursor to invasive cancers. Other disease states that involve both inflammation of the gastric mucosae and increased cancer risk are pernicious anemia and Epstein Barr Virus infection.

The most common cancer in the stomach is *gastric adenocarcinoma*, which arises from the glands of the gastric epithelium. Two histologically distinct forms of gastric adenocarcinoma have been identified: an intestinal type that forms gland-like structures, and a diffuse form that is infiltrative in nature. The intestinal form arises most typically in older individuals from precursor lesions, and spreads via bloodstream to the liver. In contrast, the diffuse form of gastric adenocarcinoma tends occur in all age groups, has no identifiable precursor lesions and spreads mainly into contiguous tissues. Most gastric adenocarcinomas present as advanced lesions, and therefore have a high mortality rate. The intestinal form is more closely associated with environmental agents, and cancers of this type appear to acquire a distinct pattern of genetic alterations. The diffuse form has been more closely linked to heritable factors, as will be described below.

Mutations in *TP53* have been detected in approximately one-third of sporadic gastric carcinomas. Chromatin remodeling is dysregulated in about 20 % of tumors by inactivation of *ARID1A*. About 15 % of tumors harbor inactivating mutations in *CDH1*. *CDH1* encodes E-cadherin, an important mediator of cell-cell adhesion (Chap. 6).

Approximately 10 % of stomach cancers occur in familial clusters, and 1–3 % have a clearly defined pattern of inheritance. The best-defined familial stomach cancer syndrome is *hereditary diffuse gastric cancer* (HDGC). About 30 % of families with HDGC carry germline mutations in *CDH1*. Most frequently, premature termination codons truncate the *CDH1* open reading frame. The penetrance of mutant *CDH1* alleles is high. In the Maori kindred in whom the disease was first identified, more than 25 individuals have died of stomach cancer as early as 14 years of age. Affected women are also at significantly increased risk of lobular breast cancer. *CDH1* therefore exhibits the characteristics of a classic tumor suppressor gene: inactivating mutations are found in a significant proportion of sporadic tumors and also in the germline of cancer-predisposed individuals.

Stomach cancer is a significant component of the hereditary nonpolyposis colorectal cancer (HNPCC) disease spectrum. Accordingly, many stomach cancers exhibit evidence of microsatellite instability.

Brain Tumors

In the US, more than 20,000 individuals are diagnosed with primary brain cancer each year. Brain cancers occur in all age groups; greater than 20 % of brain tumors occur in individuals younger than 34 years.

Most of the malignant tumors that occur within the central nervous system are not derived from neurons, but rather from supportive tissues known as the *neuroglia*. Several types of glial cells can develop into tumors. The most common type of glial cell tumor, or *glioma*, develops from a star-shaped brain cell called an astrocyte and is accordingly called an *astrocytoma*. Astrocytomas can occur in all areas of the brain and spinal cord of children and adults (Fig. 7.15), and can be classified in four distinct grades. The most malignant form of astrocytoma is the grade IV tumor, also known as the *glioblastoma multiforme* (GBM). GBM are the most common primary brain cancers in adults, and among the most lethal cancers of any type.

Low grade gliomas frequently (30–40 %) harbor activating mutations in *IDH1* and inactivating mutations in *TP53*. Smaller proportions (5–20 %) of these tumors harbor mutations in *NOTCH1* and *PIK3CA*.

As the name multiforme implies, GBMs are morphologically heterogeneous. GBM appears to arise via two distinct pathways. Some GBMs rapidly arise in older individuals, often in the cerebral hemispheres, in the absence of any precursor lesion. These tumors are known as primary, or *de novo* GBMs. In contrast, secondary, or progressive, GBMs arise as lower grade gliomas and slowly progress to more aggressive cancers. The two categories of GBM harbor distinct but overlapping patterns of genetic alterations. About one half of primary GBMs harbor deletions involving *CDKN2A* and *CDKN2B*; amplification of *EGFR* occurs in over 40 % of samples. Subtle mutations in *TP53* and *PTEN* occur in about 10 % of these tumors. Ten percent of primary GBMs harbor mutations in either *PIK3CA* or *PIK3R1*. As one would predict, secondary GBMs harbor the mutations found in the low grade gliomas, including *IDH1* and *TP53* mutations, particularly those that alter codon 273, and activating point mutations in *PIK3CA*.

Most GBMs are sporadic and therefore arise as a result of somatically-acquired mutations. In small numbers of cases, GBMs occur as a component of familial adenomatous polyposis, Li-Fraumeni syndrome, and central neurofibromatosis (Chap. 3).

Medulloblastoma, the most common primary malignant brain tumor among children, arises in the cerebellum (Fig. 7.15). At the molecular level, these tumors can be categorized into 4 distinct subtypes, based on their patterns of genetic alteration and signaling pathway activation. Group 1 tumors are characterized by active WNT/APC signaling, and frequently harbor mutations in *CTNBB1*. Group 2 tumors

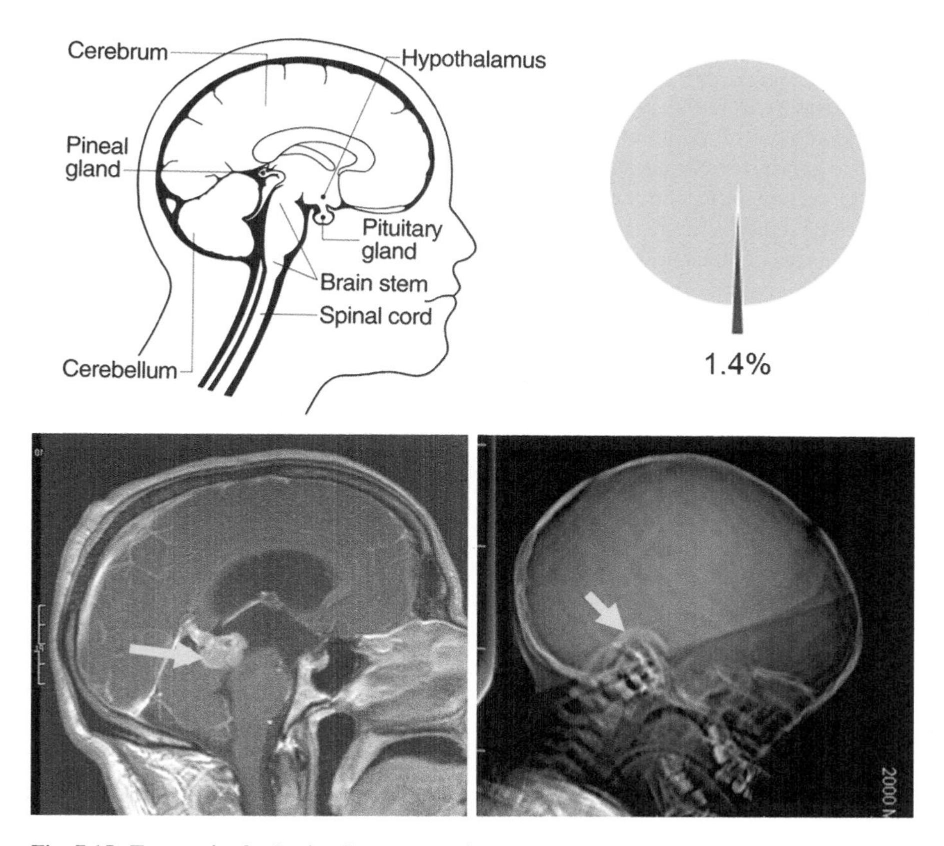

Fig. 7.15 Tumors in the brain. Cancer can arise in various tissues within the brain. Computed tomography (CT) scans showing a low grade astrocytoma of the midbrain (*left*) and a medulloblastoma in a pediatric patient, with accompanying hydrocephalus (*right*). Tumors are indicated by *arrows*. Images from Wikimedia Commons, uploaded by MBq and Reytan. Illustration from the National Cancer Institute

exhibit molecular evidence of active hedgehog signaling, and many of these tumors accordingly harbor mutations in *PTCH1*. *TP53* is also mutated at a moderate frequency in this subtype. Group 3 medulloblastomas harbor mutations that affect chromatin remodeling, including *SMARCA4*. Group 4 tumors appear to be driven by loss of histone methyltransferase activity, caused by recurrent mutations in genes such as *MLL*. Tumors in groups 3 and 4 typically harbor large numbers of large deletions and amplifications that affect many loci. These tumors tend to respond poorly to standard therapy.

The heritable predisposition to medulloblastoma is closely reflected in the patterns of mutation found in sporadic tumors. Group 1 medulloblastomas are promoted by activation of the WNT pathway, and are accordingly a component of familial adenomatous polyposis, caused by *APC* mutations. The Group 2 medulloblastomas, which are driven by canonical hedgehog pathway activation, are an important component of basal call nevus syndrome (BCNS; also known as Gorlin syndrome; see Chap. 3). This syndrome is caused by germline mutations in the tumor suppressor *PTCH1* that cause constitutive hedgehog pathway activity. Individuals with Li-Fraumeni syndrome, who harbor germline mutations in *TP53*, are also at risk for Group 2 medulloblastomas.

The second most common adult brain cancer is the *meningioma*, derived from glial cells in the meningeal coverings of the brain and spinal cord. Meningiomas are a component of the neurofibromatosis type 2 cancer syndrome (Chap. 3); sporadic tumors frequently harbor somatically-acquired mutations in the *NF2* gene.

Further Reading

Agrawal N et al (2011) Exome sequencing of head and neck squamous cell carcinoma reveals inactivating mutations in NOTCH1. Science 333:1154–1157

Ahn SM et al (2014) Genomic portrait of resectable hepatocellular carcinomas: implications of RB1 and FGF19 aberrations for patient stratification. Hepatology 60:1972–1982

Brennan CW et al (2013) The somatic genomic landscape of glioblastoma. Cell 155:462–477

Cancer Genome Atlas Research Network (2012a) Comprehensive molecular portraits of human breast tumors. Nature 490:61–70

Cancer Genome Atlas Research Network (2012b) Integrated genomic analyses of ovarian carcinoma. Nature 474:609–615

Cancer Genome Atlas Research Network (2013a) Genomic and epigenomic landscapes of adult de novo acute myeloid leukemia. N Engl J Med 368:2059–2074

Cancer Genome Atlas Research Network (2013b) Comprehensive molecular characterization of clear cell renal cell carcinoma. Nature 499:43–49

Cancer Genome Atlas Research Network (2014) Comprehensive molecular profiling of lung adenocarcinoma. Nature 511:543–550

de Snoo FA, Hayward NK (2005) Cutaneous melanoma susceptibility and progression genes. Cancer Lett 230:153–186

Ellenson LH, Wu TC (2004) Focus on endometrial and cervical cancer. Cancer Cell 5:533–538

El-Rifai W, Powell SM (2002) Molecular biology of gastric cancer. Semin Radiat Oncol 12:128–140

Farazi PA, DePinho RA (2006) Hepatocellular carcinoma pathogenesis: from genes to environment. Nat Rev Cancer 6:674–687

Gao JJ et al (2013) Integrative analysis of complex cancer genomics and clinical profiles using the cBioPortal. Sci Signal 6:l1

Grasso CS et al (2012) The mutational landscape of lethal castration-resistant prostate cancer. Nature 487:239–243

Haluska FG et al (2006) Genetic alterations in signaling pathways in melanoma. Clin Cancer Res 12:2301s–2307s

Hussain SP, Schwank J, Staib F, Wang XW, Harris CC (2007) TP53 mutations and hepatocellular carcinoma: insights into the etiology and pathogenesis of liver cancer. Oncogene 26:2166–2176

Iyer G et al (2013) Prevalence and co-occurrence of actionable genomic alterations in high-grade bladder cancer. J Clin Oncol 31:3133–3140

Jones S et al (2008) Core signaling pathways in human pancreatic cancers revealed by global genomic analyses. Science 321:1801–1806

Kangelaris KN, Gruber SB (2007) Clinical implications of founder and recurrent CDH1 mutations in hereditary diffuse gastric cancer. JAMA 297:2410–2411

Kondo T, Ezzat S, Asa SL (2006) Pathogenetic mechanisms in thyroid follicular-cell neoplasia. Nat Rev Cancer 6:292–306
Linehan WM, Walther MM, Zbar B (2003) The genetic basis of cancer of the kidney. J Urol 170:2163–2172
Munger K et al (2004) Mechanisms of human papillomavirus-induced oncogenesis. J Virol 78:11451–11460
Northcott PA et al (2011) Medulloblastoma comprises four distinct molecular variants. JCO 29:1408–1414
Ohgaki H, Kleihues P (2007) Genetic pathways to primary and secondary glioblastoma. Am J Pathol 170:1445–1453
Rudin CM et al (2012) Comprehensive genomic analysis identifies SOX2 as a frequently amplified gene in small-cell lung cancer. Nat Genet 44:1111–1116
Seshagiri S et al (2012) Recurrent R-spondin fusions in colon cancer. Nature 488:660–664
Sjoblom T et al (2006) The consensus coding sequences of human breast and colorectal cancers. Science 314:268–274
Wang K et al (2014) Whole-genome sequencing and comprehensive molecular profiling identify new driver mutations in gastric cancer. Nat Genet 46:573–582
Warnakulasuriya KA, Ralhan R (2007) Clinical, pathological, cellular and molecular lesions caused by oral smokeless tobacco – a review. J Oral Pathol Med 36:63–77
Wood LD et al (2007) The genomic landscapes of human breast and colorectal cancers. Science 318:1108–1113

Chapter 8
Cancer Genetics in the Clinic

The Uses of Genetic Information

The cancer gene theory has provided an intellectual framework for understanding how cancers arise and how they grow. We can now appreciate how somatic mutations promote the evolutionary growth of neoplasia, and how germline mutations can affect cancer risk. These insights rank among the great accomplishments of modern science. Most importantly, the cancer gene theory guides the most promising efforts to prevent, diagnose, treat and cure cancer.

The clinical uses of genetic information in oncology are many and varied. This final chapter will briefly highlight some of the practical applications of cancer genetics:

Genetic testing for risk assessment. For some individuals, inherited cancer genes can significantly increase the lifetime risk of developing cancer. The identification of cancer genes in the germline can be used to quantify cancer risk and to implement a customized plan for surveillance or prophylaxis.

Early detection. The most treatable cancers are those that are diagnosed at an early stage. Molecular genetic methods have the potential to detect cancer with high sensitivity and high specificity. Cancer cells and DNA from cancer cells can be detected in blood and other bodily fluids, providing opportunities for early diagnosis.

Diagnosis and prognosis. Many types of cancer have a course that varies from patient to patient, making prognosis difficult. Because cancer genes dictate the aberrant phenotypes of cancer cells, genetic analysis can therefore be used to more precisely categorize tumors, and to provide information on their capacity to grow and spread.

Enhancing responses to conventional forms of therapy. Most first-line cancer therapies predate the genomic age. Cytotoxic drugs and radiation were used against cancers before there was knowledge of cancer genes and their phenotypes. Genetic information can be used to predict how tumors will respond, and also to

F. Bunz, *Principles of Cancer Genetics*, DOI 10.1007/978-94-017-7484-0_8

shape strategies for most effectively using conventional agents and more targeted drugs in combination.

Targeted therapies, rational combinations. Cancer genes represent the essential difference between cancer cells and their normal neighbors. Insights into cancer genes and the pathways they control therefore demarcate prospective molecular targets, against which highly specific therapies can be designed. Cancer genes dictate mechanisms of disease response and also mediate recurrence.

Elements of Cancer Risk: Carcinogens and Genes

All humans are at risk of developing cancer. This basal level of risk is due to the stochastic accumulation of somatic mutations. As outlined in Chap. 1, there is compelling evidence to suggest that a substantial proportion of all cancers can be attributed to the unavoidable mutations that arise as a result of normal cell division. This is the element of risk that we all share.

However, cancers are not evenly distributed throughout the entire human population. Many individuals have an increased risk of developing cancer. For many common cancers, the rate of incidence is clearly higher in some identifiable groups of people than in others. These differences in risk are attributable to variations in the cumulative exposure to carcinogens and also to genetic inheritance. In some cases, these two factors can be synergistic. The development of sun-related skin cancers in individuals affected by xeroderma pigmentosum (Chap. 4) is an extreme case that exemplifies the interplay between genes and the environment.

Carcinogen exposure is largely a function of lifestyle and geographic location. The risk of lung cancer is much higher for individuals who smoke. Liver cancer has a much higher incidence among groups of individuals who live in areas where aflatoxin B1 contaminates the food supply and where the hepatitis B virus is endemic. There are many other examples in which the prevalence of cancer is linearly related to exposure to a known carcinogen. In addition, there are probably numerous environmental factors that contribute to cancer risk in subtle ways that remain incompletely understood.

While non-genetic factors are clearly important, the composition of one's genetic inheritance can also increase cancer risk. This conclusion is based upon a large body of epidemiological evidence. While most human cancers occur sporadically, a small percentage of all cancers cluster in families. These apparent familial clusters can occur solely by chance, most often in cases in which the type of cancer is a common one. For example, about one in seven American men develop prostate cancer. Because the basal risk of prostate cancer is so high, several cases of prostate cancer in a large family would not necessarily imply that those cases reflect an increased risk. However, when clusters are statistically non-random, familial cases may reflect underlying germline cancer genes.

An estimated 5–10 % of all cancers can be attributed to a heritable mutation in a cancer gene. In most cases, such genes are tumor suppressors (Chap. 3). Individuals that inherit mutated, inactivated tumor suppressor alleles tend to develop benign and/or malignant tumors at a young age, and in many cases develop more than one primary tumor.

A familial cluster of cancer could also conceivably result from the cumulative effect of multiple low-penetrance cancer genes. Because low-penetrance cancer genes are inherently more difficult to identify and to assess, fewer of these genes have been characterized extensively.

Identifying Carriers of Germline Cancer Genes

A known set of germline cancer genes confers quantifiable risks of developing cancer. The best understood are those that have been associated with a clinically-defined cancer predisposition syndrome. Testing for these alleles, and discovering new alleles that quantifiably impact the attributable risk, are important goals of cancer prevention efforts. There are at least two essential questions regarding genetic testing. Which alleles provide useful information? Who should be tested? The answers to these questions are often not simple. Particularly difficult are the cases in which a germline mutation confers a risk that is only minimally elevated or not yet quantified.

It is useful to outline the benefits to individuals and families of identifying a germline allele that confers an increased risk of cancer. Carriers of well-characterized cancer genes have a significantly increased absolute risk of developing specific types of cancer. In these cases, a positive genetic test constitutes an early warning that may prompt close monitoring of that patient and additional testing of close relatives. Depending on the gene and the level of risk, some carriers may have latent tumors that warrant immediate therapy. For most types of cancer, there is a much higher probability that treatment will be successful if it can be delivered before the onset of symptomatic disease.

Chemopreventive drugs can partially ameliorate the risk of some types of cancer. In other cases, prophylactic surgery may be an option. For example, a diagnosis of classical familial adenomatous polyposis implies a certainty that a person will eventually develop colorectal cancer. Family members who carry high-penetrance *APC* mutations often elect to undergo a total colectomy (surgical removal of the colon), greatly reducing their risk of cancer. Similarly, the high risk of breast and ovarian cancer conferred by germline mutations in *BRCA1* and *BRCA2* can be lowered by prophylactic surgery to preemptively remove the tissues from which tumors may arise.

At the other extreme, there are diseases in which definitive genetic information has little impact on the medical management of carriers. In such cases, the benefit to patients may be less clear. A classic example is Huntington's disease, a degenerative neurological disorder caused by the autosomal dominant inheritance of mutations in the gene *HTT*. *HTT* mutations have very high penetrance and genetic testing therefore provides a powerful estimate of disease risk. The problem with *HTT* mutation testing is that despite advances in analytical technology, there unfortunately remains nothing that can be done to prevent Huntington's disease and little that can alter its progressive course. Whether to test becomes a decision highly based on personal preference. As aptly stated by the blind seer Tiresias in *Oedipus the King* by Sophocles: 'It is but sorrow to be wise when wisdom profits not'. The ability to test for a genetic condition for which there is no impactful intervention can present a dilemma.

Cancer risk factors are perhaps best discussed in the context of how they might be used to affect patient management. A mutation that could prompt a specific change in screening intervals, a recommendation for a risk-modifying change in habits, or indicate the need for a more focused test is often said to be *actionable*. (In the context of a tumor biopsy, an actionable mutation is one that would suggest a preferred form of therapy. This is discussed in a later section.) For most types of cancer, some form of intervention is available for the early stages of disease. Therefore, there is a generally a benefit to detecting actionable germline cancer genes that identify individuals who have an elevated risk. The magnitude of that benefit depends on the type of cancer and the extent to which early intervention changes the outcome.

Current methods of automated genomic DNA sequencing have dramatically reduced the unit cost of DNA sequencing (Fig. 8.1). When an exome or whole genome is sequenced, each short segment of DNA is analyzed not just once but hundreds of times to ensure a level of sensitivity that can reliably capture the sequence of all bases in both alleles. The increased volume of DNA sequence data has been accompanied by a corresponding increase in the computational

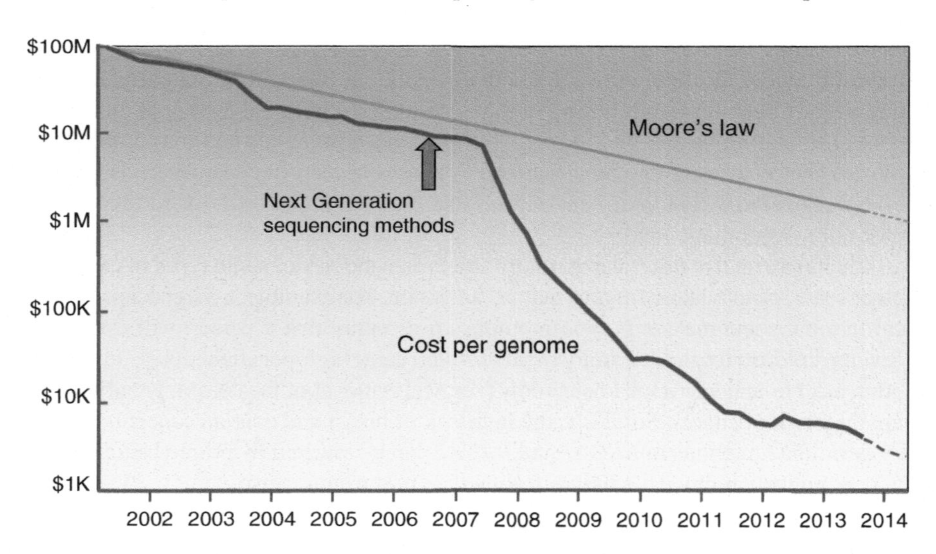

Fig. 8.1 The rapidly decreasing cost of human genome sequencing. The cost of DNA sequencing declined in the years immediately following the completion of the Human Genome Project. The rate of decline initially followed Moore's law, which accurately predicted the rate of decline in computing costs. A more dramatic decline was precipitated by the commercial introduction of new, high-throughput DNA analysis technologies that are collectively known as Next Generation Sequencing. Data from the National Human Genome Research Institute

infrastructure that is required to organize, interpret and store many terabytes of information. Ultimately, the identification of a germline cancer gene necessitates a discussion between the patient and a appropriately trained physician or genetic counselor as to the meaning of the result and the need for follow up studies or interventions. The complete costs of genetic testing are therefore not completely reflected by the unit cost of DNA sequence acquisition.

The allele frequencies of actionable cancer genes are low. Even the more prevalent cancer genes, such as mutant alleles of *ATM*, are present in less than 1 % of individuals in the general population. The low frequency of known cancer genes in the general population necessitates the testing of many non-carriers for every carrier who is ultimately identified. Applied to the general population, efforts to identify germline cancer genes that significantly increase cancer risk would be predicted to have a fairly low yield.

Importantly, not all mutations in cancer genes are actionable. As described in Chap. 5, cancer genes are defined by the occurrence of somatic driver mutations. However, passenger mutations also occur in known cancer genes. The dichotomy between drivers and passengers is applicable to germline cancer genes as well. It is not always straightforward to determine if a detected mutation has any relevance to cancer risk, particularly when the mutation is found in the germline of an individual who is asymptomatic and has no remarkable family history. In large-scale studies of genetically diverse human populations, allelic variants are frequently encountered that have never before been observed. While such alleles may be worthy of further study, their immediate utility is usually minimal. Unless a newly discovered germline mutation truncates an open reading frame or would be predicted to have a profound effect on the function of an encoded protein, it could be very difficult or impossible to use that information to estimate cancer risk. Such a finding would be designated as a *variant of uncertain significance* (VUS). In routine genetic screens, the cumulative frequency of VUSs will typically exceed the yield of alleles that confer a known risk.

Ideally, genetic testing provides a measure of relief when the results are negative (no mutations in known cancer genes). And a positive result (a cancer gene that confers a known risk) will prompt measures to monitor an individual closely or perform prophylactic surgery that will dramatically decrease the risk of cancer. However, the finding of a VUS in a genetic test presents a dilemma. In the strictest sense, a VUS might not be quite considered 'normal', but neither does it meet the standard of a positive test if is not actionable. A VUS could be a completely incidental finding with no relation to cancer risk, or it could represent a mutation that confers an attributable risk that has yet to be quantified. In consideration of these possible scenarios, a VUS can be a source of anxiety.

The true costs and predicted low yield of cancer gene screening and the uncertainty surrounding VUSs are important factors when considering the widespread application of genetic testing to the general population. Even in wealthy nations, the monetary resources dedicated to health care are finite. Money dedicated to large scale screening efforts could be otherwise be used for direct patient care, or invested in programs designed to improve cancer prevention, education and research.

Large-scale genetic testing is only feasible if it *lowers* the overall cost of health care, reduces the burden of cancer, and decreases anxiety among the individuals tested.

The discovery of *BRCA1* and *BRCA2* in the 1990s made it newly possible to definitively test for breast cancer susceptibility. Collectively, mutations in the BRCA genes occur in the general population of the US at a frequency of roughly 1 in 800 individuals. However, due to founder effects, some ethnically-defined subpopulations harbor mutant BRCA genes at a much higher frequency. An important example is the Jewish community with ethnic roots in Central or Eastern Europe, a group known as the Ashkenazim. A high proportion of *BRCA1* or *BRCA2* mutations are found in women of Ashkenazi Jewish ancestry who have breast cancer. Among Ashkenazi Jewish women, founder effects have resulted in a high frequency of three characteristic breast cancer mutations, two in *BRCA1* (185delC and 5382insC) and one in *BRCA2* (6174delT). About 1 in 40 individuals of Ashkenazi Jewish ancestry harbors one of these mutations. If a Jewish woman does not carry one of these founder mutations, her risk of breast cancer will probably be similar that that of the general population.

As illustrated by the case of familial breast cancer, screening efforts focused on high-risk populations, in which cancer gene allele frequencies are known to be relatively high, can significantly increase the yield of actionable alleles identified. Individuals with an extensive family history of cancer or those from certain subpopulations known to harbor specific, quantifiable genetic risk factors are much more likely to benefit from testing.

The employment of defined gene panels instead of whole exome or genome sequencing can lower the costs of genetic testing by simplifying interpretation. Such panels, currently marketed by several companies and university-affiliated medical centers, can be composed of as few as three and as many as 100 genes that have been conclusively associated with cancer risk. *ATM, BRCA1, BRCA2, CDH1, CDKN2A, CHEK2, PALB2, PTEN, STK11* and *TP53* are some of the genes that are commonly included in such screening panels.

Cancer Genes as Biomarkers of Early Stage Malignancies

Cancer prevention is an important component of global efforts to reduce the burden of cancer. While lowering the levels of environmental mutagens and encouraging risk-modifying lifestyle changes can greatly impact the incidence of certain types of cancer, even the most highly effective preventive strategies will not totally eliminate all cancers from occurring. As described in Chap. 1, a large proportion of somatic mutations result from stochastic processes that are independent of environmental toxins or hereditary risk factors. In an idealized world with no environmental carcinogens and total knowledge of every individual's genome, cancers would still arise as a result of the unavoidable consequences of cell division.

Early detection will be an increasingly important approach to reducing cancer morbidity and mortality. Cancers that are detected at early stages are most likely to respond to curative therapies. For the types of tumors that grow in a stepwise manner, early lesions have not yet acquired all of the genetic alterations that give rise to invasive, metastatic growth. Such lesions are typically cured by surgical resection alone, entirely eliminating the risk of progression. In the colon for example, smaller, noninvasive colorectal tumors such as adenomas can simply be removed during colonoscopy before they develop into advanced tumors that invade the surrounding wall and spread to local lymph nodes. Even highly malignant tumors, such as melanomas of the skin can often be cured if they are recognized and excised at an early stage, when they are still small and thin.

In contrast, cancers that arise in relatively inaccessible organs, such as the pancreas and ovary, are not easily detected in routine examinations or screens. More typically, these internal cancers are diagnosed at advanced stages, when they have already spread beyond their primary site. The mortality rates for these difficult-to-detect tumors are accordingly much higher. Effective strategies to reliably detect these types of malignancies at earlier stages could substantially decrease the rates of cancer death.

Cancer cells leave detectable components in circulating blood. Proteins such as carcinoma antigen-125 (CA-125), carcinoembryonic antigen (CEA), and prostate-specific antigen (PSA) are secreted or otherwise derived from ovarian, colorectal and prostate cancer cells, respectively, and subsequently appear in the serum fraction of blood. These proteins are known as cancer *biomarkers*. A *biomarker*, a portmanteau of the phrase 'biological marker', is by definition an objective and quantifiable characteristic of a biological process. The protein biomarkers used in oncology generally reflect underlying processes involving cell growth or inflammation, and have accordingly been shown to be expressed at measurable levels in the blood of individuals with cancer. However, the protein biomarkers most commonly in use are tissue specific, but not specific to the altered processes of cancer cells; these biomarkers are expressed by non-cancer cells under a variety of conditions. This lack of specificity limits their utility as primary diagnostic tools. Most often, protein biomarkers are used to assess the effects of anticancer therapy or as a means of monitoring cancer survivors for early signs of recurrence.

As described throughout this text, cancer genes are intimately related to the evolutionary development of cancer in all of its forms. Accordingly, the unique DNA sequences of cancer genes can be used as highly specific biomarkers for growing tumors. Such biomarkers have the potential to detect precursor lesions that have a high potential of developing into cancers, or to detect cancers before they become symptomatic.

Cancer cells are continuously sloughed from the surfaces of growing tumors into various bodily fluids and tissue spaces, including the blood. This tendency to continuously grow and spread beyond the confines of the primary mass is a reflection of the phenotypic qualities that ultimately make tumor cells so dangerous. However, the detached cells and the DNA they carry into the bloodstream can represent a powerful opportunity to detect pre-cancerous lesions and early cancers that arise at sites that are otherwise relatively inaccessible, during the crucial period before symptoms arise. Tests based on specific DNA sequences are as specific as the mutations that caused the cancers to grow.

There are two major sources of tumor DNA in the bloodstream. Circulating tumor cells can remain intact, and in some cases viable. These cells can be purified and genetically analyzed. Alternatively, cell-free circulating tumor DNAs (ctDNA) are small DNA fragments that are not associated with intact cells or cell fragments. In practice, ctDNA appears to be present at significantly higher levels than CTCs, and is therefore more readily detectable.

The genetically normal cells that are invariably present in clinical samples greatly outnumber the cancer cells that are the object of detection. This imbalance is especially true in the blood, which normally has 4,500–10,500 white blood cells per microliter. The detection of rare cancer DNAs against a numerically overwhelming background of normal DNA presents a technical challenge that has been addressed by a variety of strategies for the parallel evaluation large numbers of normal and mutant DNAs (Fig. 8.2).

The assessment of ctDNAs in blood samples, an approach that has been termed the 'liquid biopsy', has been applied experimentally in the detection of several common types of cancer. Early results have demonstrated the promise and the potential limitations of using driver genes as biomarkers for cancer detection. Most common types of cancer release detectable levels of ctDNA. Liquid biopsies for driver mutations are highly specific; the mutations detected in ctDNA reflect the mutations that occur in the primary tumor biopsy. As one might predict, metastatic cancers generally appear to be more detectable than small tumors. However, an exploratory survey by a team at Johns Hopkins has suggested that nearly one-half of all patients with the earliest stage of cancer, an interval when cancer is nearly always curable, have ctDNA that is detectable by liquid biopsy. Notably, cancers in the central nervous system were particularly difficult to detect in the blood, possibly because of the obstacle presented by the blood-brain barrier.

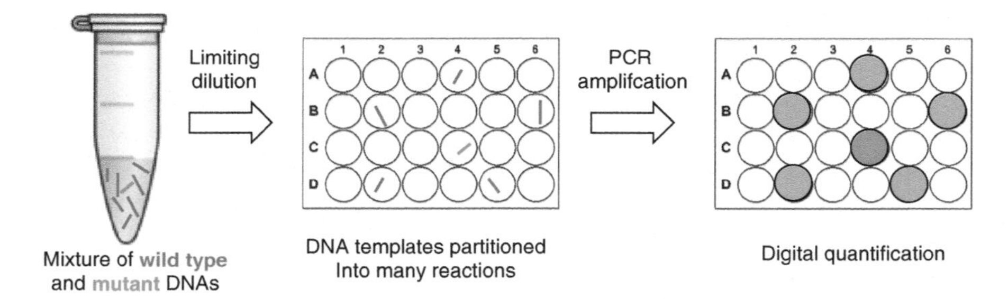

Fig. 8.2 Digital PCR. The deep analysis of complex DNA samples requires a method suitable for the assessment of many molecules in parallel. A simple method known as digital PCR relies on separating the normal alleles (*blue*) and numerically rare mutant alleles (*red*) into separate reactions by limiting dilution of the DNA templates. Parallel amplification of many reactions in which templates are limiting provides a digitized sampling of the original mixture. A small number of wells are shown to demonstrate the principle. In practice, many thousands of templates would be sampled. Next Generation DNA sequencing methods similarly incorporate parallel approaches that allow the detection of rare mutants against a background of non-mutated DNAs

Driver genes can be detected in various types of clinical samples, in addition to blood. A promising application of gene-based diagnosis is the analysis of fluid collected during the routine evaluation of the female reproductive tract. One of the most effective cancer screens is the Papanicolaou test, more commonly known as the Pap smear. Originally based on the abnormal appearance of precancerous and cancerous cells scraped from the uterine cervix, the traditional Pap smear had been modified to facilitate the genetic analysis of endocervical fluid for the presence of human papillomaviruses, the causative agent of cervical cancer (see Chap. 7). This method has allowed the early detection of curable cervical tumors and thereby reduced the incidence and mortality of cervical cancer in screened populations by more than 75 %.

Interestingly, the team from Johns Hopkins found that endocervical fluid collected for the Pap test also contains genetic evidence of cancers that develop higher in the reproductive tract, in the endometrium and ovaries. Endometrial cancer is among the most common cancers in women. While relatively rare, ovarian cancer is typically detected at a late stage and is associated with a high rate of mortality. A molecular Pap smear that could sensitively and specifically detect these cancers would be a major positive development. A 12-gene screening panel that includes *APC, AKT1, BRAF, CTNNB1, EGFR, FBXW7, KRAS, NRAS, PIK3CA, PPP2R1A, PTEN*, and *TP53* would be predicted to capture at least one mutation in more than 90 % of endometrial and ovarian cancers.

The potential power of molecular approaches to detect early stage cancers is underscored by the occasional detection of an undiagnosed, asymptomatic cancer (known as an *occult malignancy*) by a blood test administered for an unrelated purpose. Molecular genetic analysis is frequently employed in the obstetric setting, as a prenatal screening tool to evaluate the risk of aneuploidies in the developing fetus. Noninvasive prenatal testing involves a high-throughput approach to sequence and thereby count alleles in the circulating placental DNA in the pregnant mother. This type of genetic screen can detect aneuploidy with a sensitivity of >95 %. In a small number of subjects, the sequencing of cell-free DNA reveals that more than one aneuploidy is present. Fetal aneuploidies involve only a single chromosome; the detection of copy number gains and losses among multiple chromosomes is a strong indication that more highly aneuploid cells have disseminated from an occult malignancy. The incidence of cancer during pregnancy is about 1 in 1,000 gestations. The incidental finding of an occult malignancy prompts further studies to establish a definitive diagnosis, and in many cases allows a cancer to be treated at a stage in which it is still curable.

Cancer Genes as Biomarkers for Diagnosis, Prognosis and Recurrence

In oncology, biomarkers can be used to screen for cancer at the earliest stages. Biomarkers can also be used to refine a diagnosis, to inform prognosis and to monitor recurrence. There are many types of biomarkers that can be used for these diverse purposes, including tumor-associated proteins, gene expression profiles, and driver mutations in cancer genes.

The detection of a tumor immediately raises several critical questions. What type of cancer is this? What is the most probable future course of this cancer? Oncologists assess many different parameters of a newly discovered tumor, including size, location and spread, cellular composition and cellular appearance, as they attempt to predict the future course of the disease and plan an optimal course of treatment. In general, new tumors are compared with the previously documented tumors that they most resemble. Following detailed analysis and evaluation by highly experienced physicians, uncertainties often remain. Tumors that appear similar can subsequently exhibit very different clinical courses that result in different outcomes. In many instances, there is simply not enough histological or morphological information available to make useful predictions. Biomarkers provide a potential means of reducing the level of uncertainty.

The genetic etiology of a cancer can define a cancer type. A classic example is chronic myelogenous leukemia (CML), in which the observation of the Philadelphia chromosome is diagnostic (Chap. 2). The hybrid *BCR-ABL* oncogene can be detected in 95 % of CML patients. The proportion of Philadelphia chromosome-positive cells present in the blood and bone marrow is directly proportional to the total expression of *BCR-ABL*. Therefore, the response of CML to therapy can be monitored by assessing the levels of *BCR-ABL* genomic DNAs or *BCR-ABL* RNA transcripts.

Genetic tools can be used to determine the identity or origin of a cancer, if the primary site is not apparent. In some instances there is a need to determine if a tumor is a primary lesion or one that has metastasized from another site. If two tumors have the same spectrum of driver mutations, they are probably related. If driver mutations differ, they can be conclusively identified as distinct primary tumors. In unusual cases (3–5 %) the primary lesion may be undetectable because it is very small or has regressed. The patient is then said to have *cancer of unknown primary origin*. The evaluation of driver mutations has not yet been shown to be useful in identifying the primary tissue source of such lesions, but gene expression profile-based approaches to diagnosis have been proposed.

Genetic information has the potential to significantly factor into disease prognosis. Again, an illustrative example provided by the *TP53* gene. In several common cancers, somatic *TP53* mutations correlate with progression to the advanced stages of disease, and the detection of these mutations accordingly portends an unfavorable outcome. A good example of a disease that is progressively linked to *TP53* loss is *Barrett's esophagus*. Barrett's esophagus is an established precursor of esophageal adenocarcinoma. Whereas most cases of Barrett's esophagus do not progress to cancer, patients that do progress have a poor prognosis. Mutated *TP53* is frequently observed in esophageal adenocarcinomas, but is uncommon in earlier precursor lesions. As in colorectal cancer, loss of *TP53* occurs when esophageal neoplasia begin to invade surrounding tissues. Mutant *TP53* has been proposed as a prospective biomarker to identify the individuals in whom Barrett's esophagus is most likely to progress. The absence of a detectable *TP53* mutation cannot rule out progression of Barrett's esophagus, but individuals identified by a positive molecular diagnosis could potentially benefit from close surveillance. While the detection of mutant *TP53* as a predictive biomarker is theoretically attractive, it has not been proven sufficiently predictive for routine clinical use.

Another disease that has been highly studied in this regard is breast cancer. About one quarter of invasive breast cancers harbor mutations in *TP53*. In numerous studies, *TP53* mutations have been shown to predict an unfavorable prognosis. The predictive value of a *TP53* mutation appears to be independent of other prognostic factors such as tumor size, lymph node status and expression of the estrogen receptor. Mutations that alter the DNA binding domain of p53, and thus effect transcriptional transactivation, appear to be associated with worse prognosis that the rare mutations that occur outside this domain.

A challenge often faced during the course of cancer treatment is the recurrence of disease after surgery and chemotherapy. Cancers of the oral cavity and pharynx, for example, exhibit a high recurrence rate after surgical excision. Recurrence can be attributed to a small number of cancer cells that remain on the margins of the excised region. The squamous cell cancers in the head and neck frequently contain *TP53* mutations. In such cases, the detection of frequently-observed mutated *TP53* alleles in clinical specimens such as oral swabs would have the potential to improve detection of residual cancer cells.

The relative expression of genes associated with cell proliferation has been used to predict the likelihood of local breast cancer recurrence, or to predict the relative benefit of chemotherapy for more invasive disease. Commercially-available tests can quantitatively measure the expression of 12–21 genes in tumor biopsy samples. This information is then used to generate a score that predicts the likelihood of disease recurrence at 10 years. While the gene expression profiles assessed by these tests are reflective of the alteration of cancer gene pathways in evolving breast tumors, these assays do not examine cancer gene mutations directly. Similar expression-based predictive tests have recently been developed for colorectal and prostate cancers.

The specific genetic alterations in a tumor can in some cases provide useful information regarding the probability of recurrence. Inactivating *TP53* mutations in head and neck squamous cell cancers have been shown to be tightly associated with recurrence and with decreased longer-term survival. A second biomarker that is informative for this disease is a region of recurrent allelic loss on the short are of chromosome 3 (designated chr3p). Notably, the combination of chr3p loss and *TP53* inactivation was associated with a survival time of less than 2 years, compared with >5 years for head and neck squamous cell tumors with *TP53* mutation alone. Thus the genetic analysis of *TP53* and chr3p has enabled a new multi-tiered classification of tumors at this site.

Conventional Anticancer Therapies Inhibit Cell Growth

Most of the anticancer therapies currently in use predate the cancer gene theory. Well before the first report of a mutation in a RAS gene in 1982, cancer was understood to involve the dysregulation of cell proliferation. Ionizing radiation and chemotherapeutic drugs that are widely used in the treatment of cancer were adopted in the clinic not because they necessarily discriminate between the genomes of normal cells and cancer cells, but because they are potent inhibitors of cell growth. These types of agents have been collectively referred to as *conventional cancer therapies*, to distinguish them from *targeted therapies* that were designed to specifically exploit known molecular attributes of cancer cells. In some respects, this designation does not do these agents justice. Conventional forms of therapy have had a profound impact on many types of cancer, often achieving lengthy remissions or cures of diseases that were once uniformly lethal. These agents do in fact engage specific targets and these interactions often allow cancer cells to be selectively killed, but in many cases the mechanistic basis for efficacy is not well understood.

Conventional therapeutic agents can be applied as a primary mode of therapy, but are often used as *adjuvant therapy*. Adjuvant therapies are those that are applied after an initial treatment, usually surgery. Sometimes conventional therapy is applied to shrink the tumor before the main mode of treatment (usually surgery) and in this context is called *neoadjuvant therapy*.

Many anticancer agents that inhibit cell growth work by one of two general mechanisms and can be thus categorized:

DNA damaging agents. Double- and single-strand DNA breaks are sensed by the DNA damage signaling and repair network (Chap. 6). By causing the activation of multiple downstream pathways, DNA damage has growth inhibitory affects such as cell cycle arrest and apoptosis. DNA damaging agents include ionizing radiation and drugs that similarly induce DNA breakage, sometimes known as *radiomimetics*.

DNA synthesis inhibitors. Because proliferating cell populations replicate their genomic DNA once per cell cycle, inhibition of DNA replication effectively halts cell growth. There are at least two ways in which DNA synthesis can be pharmacologically inhibited. *Nucleotide analogs* either terminate nascent DNA strands or competitively inhibit DNA polymerases, whereas *antimetabolites* inhibit the enzymes that catalyze the synthesis of nucleotides and thereby cause them to be depleted. Effective targets of antimetabolites include the enzymes *ribonucleotide reductase* and *thymidylate synthase*. By either of these approaches, inhibition of DNA synthesis can lead to the accumulation of DNA strand breaks. Thus, DNA synthesis inhibitors indirectly trigger the DNA damage signaling and repair network.

Anticancer therapy based solely on growth inhibition is often highly successful. The reason behind this success is not obvious. The cells that compose most tumors do not necessarily proliferate at a higher rate than those in normal regenerative tissue compartments, and in fact tumor cells may proliferate at a lower rate (Chap. 1). Furthermore, the effects of DNA damaging agents and DNA synthesis inhibitors on DNA are not fundamentally different in normal and tumor cells, nor do these agents directly interact with cancer genes or the proteins they encode. Yet, despite their non-specificity for cancer gene mutations, these widely used drugs can be highly effective in killing tumor cells and reducing the burden of cancer.

DNA damaging agents and DNA synthesis inhibitors cause chromosome breaks and DNA replication intermediates, respectively, in cancer cells and normal cells alike. As observed by Paracelsus, an early toxicologist who lived in the sixteenth century, "the dose makes the poison". In modern oncology, the most widely employed anti-cancer agents are poisonous to all cells at high doses, but at lower doses these drugs can selectively kill cancer cells. How might this work?

The critical difference appears to lie in the cellular responses to the insult of DNA damage. The genetically programmed responses of cancer cells to DNA strand breaks and aberrant chromosome structures are often defective (Chap. 6). The tumor suppressor p53, for example, is a common node in signaling pathways that monitor chromosome integrity. Loss of p53 function, acquired during tumorigenesis, can decrease a cell's capacity to undergo growth arrest and to trigger apoptosis in response to DNA damage and DNA replication intermediates. Analysis of cultured p53-deficient cancer cells exposed to common therapeutic agents has revealed that failure to normally arrest cell cycle progression in the presence of damaged DNA can cause aberrant cell division, leading to cell death. The genetic alterations that liberate cancer cells from the normal restraints on growth can apparently leave them uniquely vulnerable to conventional therapeutic agents.

Exploiting the Loss of DNA Repair Pathways: Synthetic Lethality

The mainstays of cancer therapy are agents that damage DNA. DNA damage can occur directly, by agents that break the covalent bonds within and between bases, or indirectly, by agents that interrupt DNA replication or destabilize DNA replication forks. Normal cells possess numerous intricate mechanisms for repairing single-strand and double-strand DNA breaks, DNA adducts, misincorporated bases and DNA crosslinks. Germline or somatic mutations that cause even subtle defects in the DNA repair machinery are strongly associated with cancer.

A defect in DNA repair can be a two-edged sword. In a developing neoplasm, a repair defect can cause an increase in the rate of mutation and therefore a loss of genomic stability that drives tumorigenesis. However, the resulting cancer can be preferentially sensitive to specific forms of DNA damage. The sword of DNA repair thus cuts both ways, as all cells ultimately require DNA repair to remain alive.

The partially disabled DNA repair pathways in some cancers can render them more dependent their remaining DNA repair pathways, which allow them to retain their viability. In some cases, these unique dependencies can be exploited. The best example of this concept is provided by the breast cancers that arise in women who are heterozygous for mutations in either *BRCA1* or *BRCA2*. The proteins encoded by the BRCA genes, as well as *PALB2,* are central participants in a basic cellular process called *homologous recombination*, which is required for gene conversion and is also used in the repair of double-strand DNA breaks. Breast cancer cells that spontaneously undergo loss of heterozygosity (LOH) at a *BRCA1* or *BRCA2* locus will be deficient in homologous recombination and therefore completely incapable of repairing double-strand DNA breaks.

An effective therapeutic strategy to exploit homologous recombination-deficiency is to selectively create double-strand DNA breaks in cancer cells (Fig. 8.3). In untreated cell populations, double-strand breaks occur very infrequently. In stark contrast, single-strand DNA breaks occur spontaneously and in high numbers. Under normal conditions, these lesions are relatively innocuous; it has been estimated that the average cell may repair 10,000 single-strand breaks every day. An important cellular mechanism for the ongoing repair of single-strand breaks is the base excision repair (BER) pathway. Blockade of BER causes single-strand DNA breaks to accumulate. Unrepaired, these single-strand breaks potentially become problematic during S-phase. When the two DNA strands are separated during replicative synthesis, single-strand breaks can be converted into double-strand breaks. Normally, a double-strand break that arises during S-phase would be resolved by homologous recombination that causes gene conversion with the

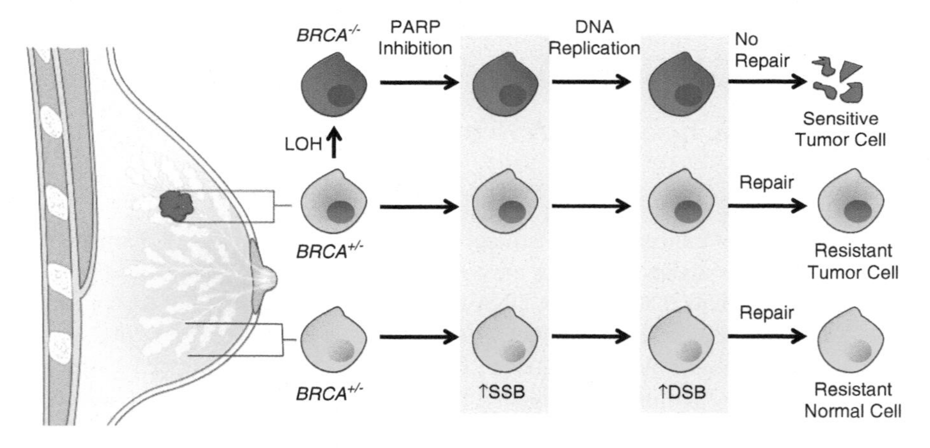

Fig. 8.3 Synthetic lethality of BRCA-deficient cancer **cells treated with a PARP inhibitor**. Breast cancers arise at an elevated rate in women who harbor heterozygous mutations ($BRCA^{+/-}$) in either *BRCA1* or *BRCA2*. Many tumor cells undergo loss of heterozygosity at the relevant locus and thereby become completely BRCA-deficient ($BRCA^{-/-}$). Systemic treatment with a PARP inhibitor results in the transient accumulation of single-strand breaks (*SSB*) in all cells. During DNA replication, unrepaired SSB are converted to double-strand breaks (*DSB*). Normal cells and tumor cells that retain *BRCA* heterozygosity are capable of repairing DSB via the pathway of homologous recombination. BRCA-deficient cells lack this capability, and will accumulate lethal levels of DSBs. Breast tumor image from Cancer Research UK

remaining unbroken allele. Cells with deficiency in one of the BRCA genes are incapable of orchestrating this complex form of DNA repair.

In an approach originally devised by Alan Ashworth and colleagues, spontaneously occurring single-strand DNA breaks can be stabilized by inhibiting a class of enzyme called poly (ADP) ribose polymerase, or PARP. More than ten PARP family members are encoded in the human genome, the best understood and most abundant of these is PARP1. The PARPs bind to DNA strand nicks and breaks and catalyze the addition of a polymeric modification called poly (ADP) ribose to neighboring proteins, including histones. The covalent addition of a poly (ADP) ribose chain to these proteins modifies some of their activities and, critically, causes the recruitment of additional proteins required for the subsequent steps of BER. The blockade of BER caused by PARP inhibition causes single-strand breaks to accumulate. When proliferating cells enter S-phase, many of the single-strand breaks are converted to double-strand breaks. Normal cells that retain BRCA activity can effectively repair these lesions and remain viable. Breast cancer cells deficient in BRCA activity accumulate highly deleterious double-strand breaks and die.

PARP inhibitors as a class are a new category of anti-cancer agents that were developed on the basis of their ability to inhibit a critical step in the BER pathway. The PARP inhibitor olaparib (marketed as Lynparza) was approved in December 2014 for use as a single agent, and several others are in various stages of development. As anticipated, PARP inhibitors appear to be most effective against the 5 % of breast and 10 % of cancers that have defects in one of the BRCA genes or in another gene in the homologous recombination pathway. The broader utility of PARP inhibitors against BRCA-proficient breast cancer, and in prostate, colorectal and lung cancer are under investigation.

In genetic models, two mutated genes are said to be synthetically lethal if both mutations together cause cell death, whereas a mutation in either one does not impact viability. *Synthetic lethality* is therefore an outcome that indicates that two genes function together to carry out an essential function. In the clinical setting, a variation on synthetic lethality can be achieved by employing a drug against one pathway that has an enhanced effect when a second pathway is altered by a mutation. The pharmacologic inhibition of PARP in cancers with an underlying mutation in one of the BRCA genes is an example of this strategy in action. The emerging concept of synthetic lethality is shaping new efforts to exploit the phenotypic deficiencies caused by cancer gene mutations.

On the Horizon: Achieving Synthetic Lethality in *TP53*-Mutant Cancers

The successful treatment of BRCA-defective breast cancers with PARP inhibitors provides a useful paradigm for devising new therapies for cancers with more common mutations. Inactivating mutations in *TP53* occur at a high frequency in many types of cancer, including some that are highly aggressive and difficult to effectively treat. A general means of effectively exploiting this widespread cellular defect would be broadly useful, and has accordingly been the focus of intensive research. While this goal remains elusive, substantial progress has been made.

The p53 protein is stabilized by DNA damage, and is accordingly activated by radiotherapy as well as many of the agents routinely used for chemotherapy. Among the most experimentally obvious effects of p53 activation is the arrest of the cell cycle at distinct intervals known as checkpoints. As described in Chap. 6, the checkpoint activators induced by p53 control two important cell cycle transitions. One is the transition from G_1-phase to S-phase, which defines the onset of DNA replication. The second p53-dependent checkpoint controls the entry into mitosis from G_2-phase. Cancer cells that compose *TP53*-mutant tumors are accordingly checkpoint-deficient. These cells are unable to properly control the initiation of DNA replication and the entry into mitosis when they encounter DNA damage.

Based on this basic function of p53, an approach to enhancing the selectivity of DNA damaging agents can be envisioned (Fig. 8.4). *TP53*-mutant tumor cells with defective checkpoint function would theoretically be sensitized to the perturbation of survival pathways that are specific to S-phase and mitosis. Intensive investigation of the basic mechanisms of cell cycle progression has revealed several prospective targets. ATR, a protein kinase that is activated by stalled DNA replication forks, plays a central role in determining whether a damaged cell dies or survives. In mitosis, a protein kinase called polo-like kinase 1, encoded by *PLK1*, phosphorylates numerous substrates during mitosis that collectively contribute to successful chromosome segregation into daughter cells. Small molecules that can avidly and specifically bind and inhibit these enzymes have been developed, and are currently being tested.

The combination of these targeted inhibitors with a conventional DNA damaging therapeutic could, in theory, preferentially kill cancer cells with *TP53* mutations. In response to DNA damage, normal proliferating stem cells would be safely arrested prior to S-phase or mitosis, and would be relatively unaffected by the targeting of S-phase and M-phase-specific survival factors. *TP53*-mutant cells would enter S-phase and mitosis, where they would be vulnerable. Thus, such synthetic lethal combinations could broaden the therapeutic window of a conventional agent already in use, rendering it safer and more effective. Whether such regimens would be effective in the clinic remains to be definitively determined.

Molecularly Targeted Therapy: *BCR-ABL* and Imatinib

While some types of cancer are exquisitely sensitive to commonly-employed forms of anticancer therapy – and are therefore curable or treatable – many advanced cancers remain highly refractory to DNA damaging agents and DNA synthesis inhibitors. New therapeutic strategies are desperately needed. Among the many

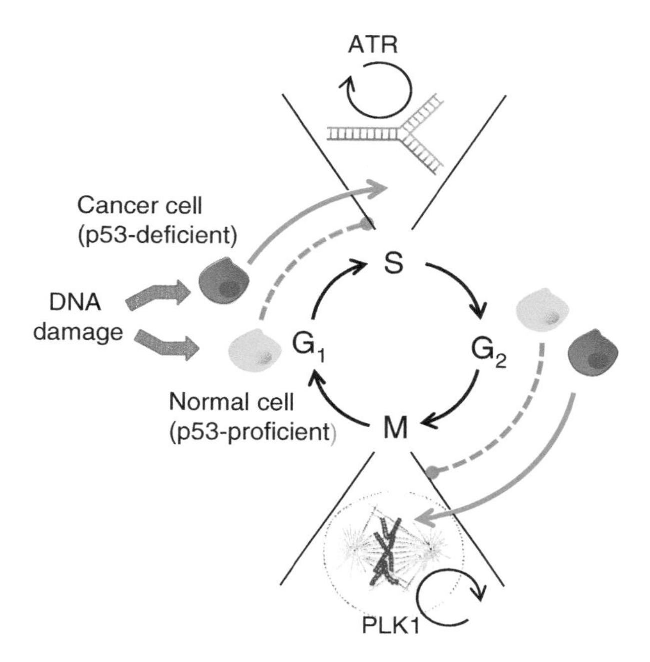

Fig. 8.4 Checkpoint defects in p53-deficient cancer cells present opportunities for synthetic lethality. Normal proliferating cell undergo a p53-dependent growth arrest at the G_1-S and G_2-M boundaries after treatment with DNA damaging agents. Cancer cells that harbor *TP53* mutations fail to arrest at these checkpoints and, depending on where in the cell cycle they were at the time of treatment, aberrantly enter S-phase or mitosis. Specific regulators that monitor the progress of these cell cycle phases are mediators of cell survival. These include the ATR kinase, which monitors the progress of DNA replication forks during S-phase and PLK1, which mediates the transition to anaphase during mitosis. Both of these enzymes have been proposed as therapeutic targets. Pharmacologic inhibition of these targets could create a synthetic lethal interaction with *TP53* mutations if combined with a DNA damaging agent

applications of cancer genetics, among the most exciting is the use of recurrent genetic alterations to guide the development of new drugs.

A cancer that represents a relatively simple paradigm for gene-based, rational design of anti-cancer therapy is chronic myeloid leukemia (CML). CML is a disease that was historically very difficult to treat. Interferon-based treatments resulted in a life expectancy of 4–6 years after diagnosis. The use of a molecularly-targeted therapeutic has transformed CML to a chronic illness.

Like many cancers, untreated CML evolves through a series of discrete stages. A stable, chronic phase of the disease is characterized by excess numbers of myeloid cells that differentiate normally. Within 4–6 years, the disease passes through an accelerated stage and then enters a terminal stage known as *blast crisis*. Blast crisis is an acute leukemia that was refractory to older conventional treatments and therefore invariably fatal.

More than 95 % of CML cases exhibit the reciprocal translocation between chromosomes 9 and 22 that creates the *BCR-ABL* oncogene (Chap. 2). The *BCR-ABL* fusion protein is constitutively expressed and as a result, the tyrosine kinase encoded by *ABL* is highly active in CML cells. Dysregulated ABL activity causes the cancer phenotype of CML. Inhibition of ABL catalytic activity is an effective strategy for CML therapy.

At the dawn of the cancer gene revolution it was already apparent that protein kinases play central roles in cancer. Accordingly, pharmaceutical companies had developed numerous specific inhibitors of these diverse enzymes and tested them as potential anticancer agents. One compound under investigation was an inhibitor of the platelet-derived growth factor receptor (PDGF-R). This compound, designated imatinib mesylate (often referred to simply as imatinib, alternatively known as STI571 and marketed as Gleevec) was subsequently found to also potently inhibit the ABL tyrosine kinase (Fig. 8.5). It was experimentally demonstrated that imatinib could specifically block the proliferation of cells expressing the *BCR-ABL* oncogene. These preclinical studies suggested that imatinib might show efficacy in the treatment of patients with CML.

The clinical trials of imatinib, reported in 2001, were a striking success. Nearly all of the *BCR-ABL*-positive CML patients that were in the chronic phase of the disease achieved long-term remission after imatinib therapy. The patients selected for these trials had previously failed other therapeutic regimens, making the rate of response all the more impressive. Even patients in the midst of blast crisis were found to benefit from imatinib therapy. Unfortunately, a majority of these patients

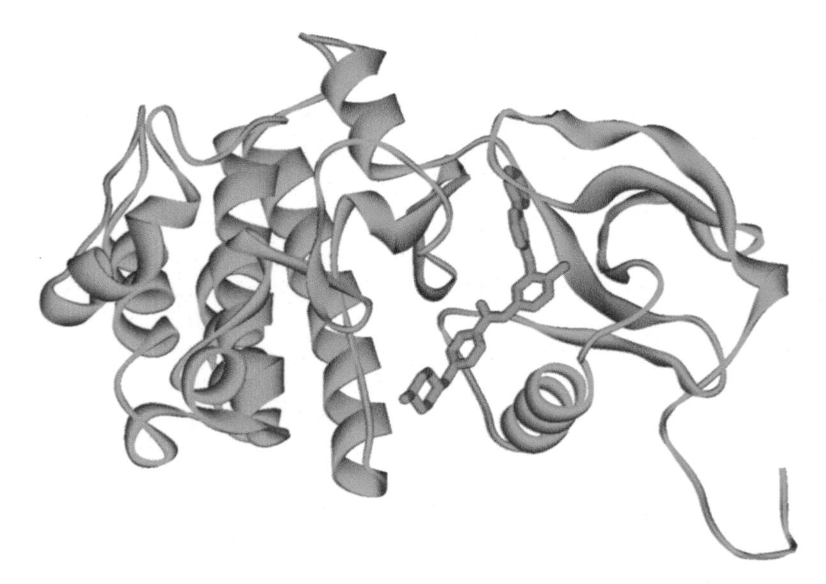

Fig. 8.5 Inhibition of the ABL tyrosine kinase by imatinib mesylate. This structural representation demonstrates how the imatinib molecule (*red*) fits into the nucleotide binding pocket of ABL (*green*)

experienced eventual recurrence of disease. Unlike other forms of cancer therapy, imatinib was associated with only minimal toxicity; only a small percentage of the patients in the trial reported adverse effects and these were generally mild in nature. The high rate of remission and the low toxicity of imatinib were unprecedented for an experimental cancer drug.

In several respects, CML presents an ideal challenge for molecularly-targeted therapeutic. CML was among the first cancers to be associated with a defined genetic alteration that is pathognomonic. The *BCR-ABL* gene is present in the vast majority of CML patients and underlies the cancer phenotype. CML cells require constitutive ABL activity to maintain their highly proliferative state. Not only is BCR-ABL a thoroughly validated target, it is also an enzyme that is inherently "druggable", ie. a small, diffusible molecular can block ATP-binding and thus inhibit the catalytic moiety. As the clinical trials of imatinib have demonstrated, the systemic inhibition of ABL and PDGF-R have little effect on normal proliferating cell populations.

In addition to PDGF-R and ABL, imatinib also inhibits the protein tyrosine kinase encoded by the *KIT* oncogene. Oncogenic mutations in *KIT* drive a relatively rare type of cancer known as the *gastrointestinal stroma tumor* (GIST), a cancer that arises from the mesenchymal tissues of the gut wall. Imatinib administered to patients with metastatic GISTs has resulted in dramatic regression of disease.

The successful development of imatinib was a watershed event in experimental cancer therapeutics. Most importantly, imatinib provides a powerful treatment for a cancer that recently had been considered incurable. From a research standpoint, imatinib provides a paradigm for the design of specific forms of therapy based on the genetics of a cancer. Forty one years elapsed from the discovery of the Philadelphia chromosome to the approval of imatinib by the US Food and Drug Administration. The interval between cancer gene discovery and the use of an agent that can target that gene product has recently become significantly shorter.

Unfortunately, the success in treating CML with imatinib is not readily replicated in other types of cancer. BCR-ABL is a well-validated molecular target. Other cancers have molecular origins that are substantially more complex than those of CML; in essence, many cancers are a spectrum of genetically diverse tumors that arise at a common site. The gains-of-function that result from the activation of oncogenes such as *BCR-ABL* can in some cases be directly targeted by small molecules or antibodies. More theoretically complex synthetic lethal approaches are required for targeting the losses of tumor suppressor genes. This difference is critical because in most cancers tumor suppressor genes are the more prominent feature in the genomic landscape. There are both theoretical and practical obstacles to the design of specific therapeutic strategies for some of the most common cancers. Nonetheless, the success of imatinib demonstrates that cancer genes can inform the development of specific approaches to treatment.

Clonal Evolution of Therapeutic Resistance

The term 'magic bullet' was originally coined in the 1800s by the bacteriologist Paul Ehrlich to describe a drug that would specifically target pathogenic microorganisms. This term has since been applied to drugs, such as imatinib, that can target cancer cells harboring specific cancer genes. A magic bullet for cancer is a tantalizing concept. For several forms of cancer, this concept has become a near-reality. New drugs based on our understanding of cancer genetics have revolutionized the approach to treating many cancers, and saved or extended patients' lives. Our deeper understanding of the evolutionary forces that shape tumor growth and the effects of tumor heterogeneity provides some sense of the limitations that will likely be encountered.

Targeted therapies such as imatinib are directed against the proteins encoded by cancer genes. The clinical responses to imatinib are therefore closely linked to the original mutation in the target cancer gene. After prolonged therapy, this response is often reversed by secondary mutations in the subclones that emerge after the initiation of therapy.

The primary mutation in an activating oncogene can largely determine the response to a targeted therapeutic. In patients with gastrointestinal stromal tumors (GISTs), several different somatic *KIT* mutations underlie distinct responses to imatinib. Tumors harboring mutations in exon 11 of *KIT* are more sensitive to imatinib than are tumors with mutations in *KIT* exon 9, for example. As a result, patients whose tumors contain exon 11 *KIT* mutations remain disease-free for a longer period and have a greater survival after therapy than those whose tumors express the an exon 9 *KIT* mutant. Thus, the *KIT* alleleotype can be used to predict the initial clinical response of GIST patients to imatinib.

Despite the striking success of imatinib as a therapeutic agent against CML and GIST, many patients eventually become resistant to the effects of the drug and suffer relapse. In such cases, sequence analysis of the target gene, (*BCR-ABL* in CML and *KIT* in GIST) often reveals mutations that preserve oncogenic activity but disrupt the inhibitory binding of imatinib.

In leukemias, the cells from newly arising clones are mixed with cells from precursor clones and normal cells. For this reason, the process by which secondary mutations develop into drug-resistant cancer is more readily studied in a solid tumor, such as a GIST, in which cancer cells grow in clonally-derived metastatic foci that can be monitored and sampled. GISTs that harbor *KIT* mutations tend to respond dramatically to the effects of imatinib. However, many patients suffer relapse and develop new metastatic foci with several years of treatment. Analysis of these metastatic tumors has revealed a recurrent mutation within the region of *KIT* that encodes the first portion of the tyrosine kinase domain. A T→C transition at position 1982 results in an amino acid substitution, V654A. The V654A missense mutation is detected at the time of relapse, on the same allele that harbors the original, primary mutation (Fig. 8.6). Secondary mutations in *KIT* within exons 13, 14 and 17 that similarly block the interaction of *KIT* with imatinib have also been described.

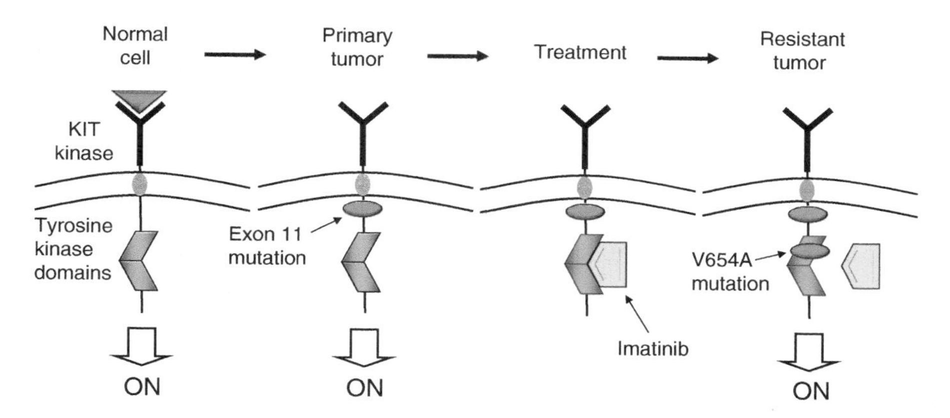

Fig. 8.6 A secondary *KIT* mutation causes imatinib resistance. In normal cells, the transmembrane KIT receptor responds normally to ligand (*red triangle*). A frequently-observed mutation of *KIT* within exon 11 causes ligand-independent activation of the KIT receptor and drives the growth of GISTs. Imatinib (*yellow*) binds within two tyrosine kinase domains (*blue*) that span amino acids 598–694 and 771–924, causing a therapeutic response. A secondary mutation affecting codon 654 disrupts the binding of the imatinib molecule, and causes drug-resistant tumor growth

A newer agent called sunitinib (marketed as Sutent) also targets KIT. GISTs that evolve to become resistant to imatinib often retain sensitivity to sunitinib because this molecule interacts with KIT in a distinct manner. Sunitinib also exhibits inhibitor activity against the RTKs encoded by *RET* and *FLT3*, and the receptors for the vascular endothelial growth factors. Accordingly, sunitinib has been approved or tested for use in a broad range of malignancies.

Most common tumors are genetically heterogeneous. Many mutations arise even before the first clonal expansion of a developing neoplasm, and additional mutations arise as the tumor evolves. Understanding tumor heterogeneity as a repository for new phenotypes provides a framework for understanding the evolution of drug resistance. Treatment of a cancer with a therapeutic agent causes a new form of selective pressure. As demonstrated by the emergence of imatinib-resistant metastases in GIST, the selective pressure provided by a gene-specific drug can result in the expansion of clonal populations that harbor additional mutations in the target gene. The approach of switching to an alternative therapeutic that is specific to the same target, or another target in the same pathway, is essentially a game of cat and mouse.

Targeting *EGFR* Mutations

Another compelling target for cancer gene-specific therapy is the protein tyrosine kinase encoded by *EGFR*. *EGFR* is activated by mutations in about 10 % of non-small cell lung cancers (NSCLC), a type of tumor that is common and refractory to conventional therapy. Highly selective small-molecule inhibitors of the EGFR kinase have been developed by the pharmaceutical industry as targeted therapies for *EGFR*-mutant cancers. The prototype inhibitor is a drug called gefitinib.

Clinical trials were designed to test whether gefitinib could effectively treat metastatic NSCLC, particularly in cases where other forms of therapy had failed. Gefitinib was originally designed to inhibit wild type EGFR. Many tumors that retain wild type *EGFR* nonetheless overexpress wild type protein as a result of gene amplification, so it was initially believed that gefitinib might elicit responses in many patients. In fact, the majority of NSCLC patients did not respond to gefitinib treatment. The 10 % of patients with rapid and in many cases dramatically positive responses to gefitinib had tumors that were *EGFR*-mutant. For reasons that are not apparent, these *EGFR*-mutant gefitinib responders were disproportionately women, patients who had never smoked, patients with the adenocarcinoma type of NSCLC, and patients with Asian heritage.

The *EGFR* mutations detected in gefitinib responders included small, in-frame deletions or missense mutations around the domain that encodes a bi-lobed ATP-binding pocket. These activating mutations cause the repositioning of critical residues that are involved in ATP-binding, thereby stabilizing both the binding of ATP and the binding of gefitinib. Accordingly, *EGFR* mutations that increase EGFR catalytic activity and autophosphorylation simultaneously increase the affinity of EGFR for gefitinib. This increase in affinity was unexpected, as gefitinib had originally been designed to inhibit overexpressed, wild type EGFR. Structural studies were able to explain why patients with tumors that harbor *EGFR* mutations responded to gefitinib and those with wild type alleles did not.

Cell-based studies have suggested that specific *EGFR* mutations can further predict the gefitinib sensitivity. For example, the introduction of an exon 20 insertion mutant makes a cancer cell 100-fold more gefitinib-resistant compared with cells that express the more common deletions in exon 19 and point mutations in exon 21.

Many NSCLC patients who initially respond to gefinitib therapy unfortunately go on to develop gefitinib-resistant disease. A secondary mutation affecting the amino acid at position 790 (*EGFR* T790M) renders expanded cell clones resistant to the inhibitory effect of gefinitib. The *EGFR* T790M mutation can also be found as a primary mutation in some patients not treated with gefitinib. Thus, the selective expansion of resistant clones leads to disease recurrence, similar to what has been observed following the use of the targeted therapeutic imatinib in the treatment of CML and GIST.

The evolution of drug resistance presents a major obstacle to achieving durable responses to molecularly targeted therapies. One solution may lie in using combinations of drugs in the same class. Two different inhibitors of the ABL tyrosine kinase, named dasatanib and nilotinib, have shown promise in treating CML patients who initially responded to imatinib and subsequently relapsed. These drugs appear to interact with ABL in a slightly different way than imatinib, and therefore can block the growth of cells harboring *BCR-ABL* alleles that contain a secondary mutation. In a similar manner, inhibitors directed against different structural aspects of the EGFR tyrosine kinase can inhibit the protein encoded by the T790M *EFGR* mutant.

Understanding how a therapeutic target functions within a delineated cellular pathway is important to predicting its effectiveness. In the case of EGFR inhibitors, the rate of response can be reliably predicted by the mutational status of *KRAS*. The oncogenic RAS signaling pathway is directly activated by EGFR (see Chap. 6). Mutational activation of *KRAS* causes constitutive activation of the downstream pathway, thereby rendering the upstream activity of EGFR functionally irrelevant. The recurrent mutations in *KRAS* that occur in about one third of NSCLCs thus represent a biomarker of resistance to EGFR inhibitors. Patients are now tested for *KRAS* mutations before such therapy is initiated.

Antibody-Mediated Inhibition of Receptor Tyrosine Kinases

Small molecule inhibitors have proven effective at blocking the catalytic activity of mutant receptor tyrosine kinases, as illustrated by imatinib and gefitinib. Alternatively, when a receptor tyrosine kinase (RTK) is oncogenically activated by gene amplification, a reduction of downstream pathway activation can be achieved by targeting the extracellular RTK domains, known as *ectodomains*. Therapeutic antibodies specifically directed against ectodomains can either interfere with ligand binding or inhibit receptor dimerization. Both of these strategies result in reduced receptor tyrosine kinase activity, leading to reduced cell proliferation and survival. Specific monoclonal antibodies have been developed against several RTKs, including the frequently amplified *EGFR* and *ERBB2* (formerly designated *HER2*). Such types of therapeutic agents belong to a broad category known as *biological therapeutics*, so named to contrast them with small molecules synthesized by chemical approaches.

Several forms of antibody therapy are employed in the clinic. Cetuximab (also known by the trade name Erbitux) is a therapeutic monoclonal antibody that binds to the ectodomain of EGFR with high affinity. The association of cetuximab with EGFR blocks ligand binding and thus prevents activation of EGFR tyrosine kinase activity.

In contrast to EGFR, ERBB2 is a RTK that has no known ligand, but rather is activated by forming complexes with other members of the ERBB family of receptors. Trastuzumab (marketed as Herceptin) is a monoclonal antibody that avidly binds to the extracellular segment of ERBB2 and potently inhibits the protein-protein interactions that result in ERBB2 activation. Approved by the Food and Drug Administration in 1998, trastuzumab was the first agent designed to target a specific genetic alteration: *ERBB2* amplification in breast cancer. (Imatinib was approved for use in 2001.)

Cetuximab has has shown efficacy in the treatment of some patients with colorectal cancer, head and neck cancer and several other types of solid tumors. Trastuzumab has proven to be useful for the treatment of breast cancers that overexpress ERBB2. Overall, monoclonal antibodies have been found to induce growth arrest and cell death in tumor cells. For some types of cancers, the combination of monoclonal antibody therapy with small molecule kinase inhibitors, and also with traditional forms of growth inhibitory therapy, have proven to be synergistic.

One obstacle that arises with the use of antibodies as drugs is the immune response that would be triggered by foreign proteins. Monoclonal antibodies used for research purposes are most commonly raised in mice. To circumvent problems of cross-species immunogenicity, antibodies used for therapy are engineered to contain protein regions encoded by human genes. Such antibodies are said to be *humanized*. Trastuzumab is an example of a humanized antibody. Cetuximab is a *chimeric* monoclonal antibody, in which the variable regions are derived from mouse genes, while the constant regions of the antibody molecule are derived from human genes. The inclusion of human gene sequences significantly lowers the immunogenicity of therapeutic antibodies.

Inhibiting Hedgehog Signaling

Mutations that inactivate the tumor suppressor *PTCH1* cause the ligand-independent activation of the G-protein-coupled receptor-like transmembrane protein SMO, and trigger a signaling cascade that ultimately stimulates transcription by the GLI proteins (Chap. 6). Efforts to target the Hedgehog pathway have been hampered by an incomplete understanding of exactly how it works, but boosted by an unusual observation that indirectly led to an approved anti-cancer therapy that suppresses Hedgehog signals.

The repression of SMO by PTCH1 was originally defined genetically, in model organisms (Chap. 3). The biochemical basis of the PTCH1-SMO interaction remains an enigma, as does the mechanism of SMO activation. SMO is therefore unlike many cancer targets in that there is not an obvious enzymatic active site or other functional feature that could be targeted with a custom-designed small molecule. Instead, the prototypical SMO inhibitor emerged from an investigation into a curious birth defect among sheep raised on a farm in Idaho. Sheep that grazed on wild corn lily were observed to give birth to one-eyed lambs (Fig. 8.7), a developmental abnormality known as *cyclopia*. This birth defect eventually traced to a natural compound extracted from the corn lily that was designated cyclopamine.

Hedgehog ligand is a developmental morphogen, required for the bilateral symmetry of neural tissues, including the brain and the eyes. The disruption of normal Hedgehog signaling during development leads to severe abnormalities that are collectively termed *holoprosencephaly*. Cyclopia is an externally apparent manifestation of this condition in its most extreme form. Holoprosencephaly in humans occurs at a low frequency in both live births and spontaneous abortions; some of these defects have been linked to mutations in the genes that populate the Hedgehog pathway, including *SHH*. The ingestion of cyclopamine by pregnant sheep, and the resultant inhibition of Hedgehog signaling, was thus the underlying cause of cyclopia in their offspring. This discovery revealed the possibility that a small molecule such as cyclopamine might effectively inhibit the growth of Hedgehog-dependent cancers.

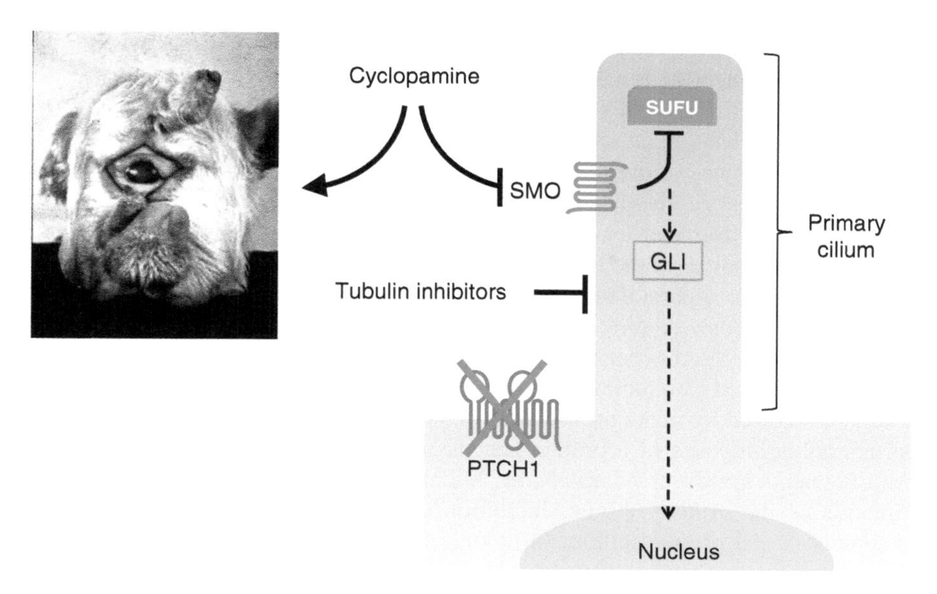

Fig. 8.7 Targeting the Hedgehog pathway. A means of suppressing Hedgehog signals was suggested by the observation that cyclopamine, a natural compound derived from the wild corn lily, was the cause of cyclopia in fetal lambs (*inset photo*). SMO is constitutively active in tumors that harbor inactivating mutations in *PTCH1*. Cyclopamine directly binds and inhibits SMO, and thereby prevents the signaling cascade that ultimately leads to the translocation of GLI to the cell nucleus. Compounds that can similarly engage SMO have been developed as anti-cancer therapeutics. An alternative approach to Hedgehog pathway inhibition is to block the polymerization of tubulin, which is required for the assembly of the primary cilium. The simultaneous use of SMO inhibitors and tubulin inhibitors is a prospective strategy to lower the probability of recurrence

Molecular analysis of cyclopamine and other naturally-occurring inhibitors of Hedgehog signaling revealed that these compounds reversibly bind to SMO and cause a conformational change that result in increased activity. The development of cyclopamine as a drug was abandoned because of its poor solubility, low potency, short half-life, and high toxicity that made it poorly suited for clinical use. However, the pharmacodynamic characterization of cyclopamine inspired chemical screening efforts that ultimately identified novel SMO inhibitors that were better suited to further development. Thus, SMO was revealed to be a highly druggable target.

The first Hedgehog inhibitor, a small molecule called vismodegib (marketed as Erivedge) was approved in 2012 for the treatment of basal cell carcinoma of the skin. Basal cell carcinoma is prominent feature of basal cell nevus syndrome (also known as Gorlin syndrome, see Chap. 3). Both heritable and sporadic lesions are generally curable by surgery, but occasionally tumor cells metastasize to other sites. These lesions characteristically harbor inactivating *PTCH1* mutations, and are therefore highly dependent on SMO activity. Vismodegib and cyclopamine bind the same site on SMO, but the former drug is less toxic and is better suited for clinical use. A new SMO antagonist called sonidegib (marketed as Odomzo) was approved for treatment of basal cell carcinoma in 2015.

Vismodegib was reported to elicit marked responses when used off-label for the treatment of a metastatic medulloblastoma that harbored an inactivating *PTCH1* mutation. Unfortunately, this systemic response was not durable; recurrent tumors harbored secondary mutations in *SMO* that altered the vismodegib binding site. Thus, the emergence of drug-resistance tumor cell clones may well limit the long-term effectiveness of vismodegib against many Hedgehog-dependent tumors. This phenomenon of drug resistance caused by a secondary mutation is a problem common to most if not all of the molecularly targeted anti-cancer therapeutics.

A conceivable approach to reducing the probability of disease recurrence would be to simultaneously employ a second drug that inhibits Hedgehog signaling via a different site on SMO or an entirely distinct target in the pathway. A strategy that has been proposed is to inhibit the formation of the primary cilium, a signaling hub that is elaborated by many proliferating cells (see Chap. 6). The primary cilium is structurally composed of a protein called tubulin. Tubulin molecules polymerize into filaments known as *microtubules*. Microtubules are intrinsic to the form and function of the primary cilium. Inhibition of tubulin polymerization blocks the assembly of the primary cilium (a process known as *ciliogenesis*) and therefore leads to markedly decreased levels of Hedgehog activity.

Tubulin inhibitors can be safely used in humans, and in fact have been employed for decades as anti-parasitic agents. A class of drugs related to the heterocyclic aromatic compound benzimidazole can bind avidly to the tubulin proteins in the gut of infectious roundworms and thereby prevent them from absorbing nutrients. Serendipitously, a benzimidazole called mebendazole has been observed to be active against several types of cancer, both in the laboratory and in the clinic. At the cellular level, mebendazole has multiple cellular effects that include the suppression of ciliogenesis. Recent studies have shown that mebendazole can suppress Hedgehog signaling and impede the growth of tumors, even those that harbor mutations in *SMO* associated with vismodegib resistance. Clinical trials are currently under way to determine whether this well-tolerated anti-parasitic compound might find a new purpose as an anti-cancer agent.

A Pipeline from Genetically-Defined Targets to Targeted Therapies

The first generation of targeted cancer therapeutics paved the way for the ongoing development of small molecules and biologics that can be deployed against a broader range of cancers. New agents target several pathways that are recurrently dysregulated in growing tumors.

Mutations in *KRAS* occur in nearly 15 % of all human cancers. While efforts to develop useful inhibitors of mutant KRAS proteins have not yet been successful, a broader view of the RAS pathway suggests several alternative targets. The RAS pathway can be inhibited by the upstream blockade of EGFR, which is frequently overexpressed or less often altered by mutations. The activation of the proto-oncogene *ALK* by gene fusion can similarly trigger downstream RAS signaling. A drug called crizotenib (marketed as Xalkori) potently inhibits the receptor tyrosine kinase activity of ALK and thus prevents RAS activation. Crizotenib is effective in ALK-positive non-small cell lung cancers, which harbor the *EML4-ALK* fusion gene.

Another strategy for blocking RAS signals is the downstream inhibition of BRAF. The *BRAF* gene is mutated in about one half of melanomas and in several other cancers. A molecule called vemurafenib (marketed as Zelboraf) has been developed to specifically inhibit the BRAF protein encoded by the highly prevalent V600E mutant. This agent prevents the activation of the downstream MAPK pathway in cells with the V600E *BRAF* mutation, and thereby blocks the proliferation of cells and experimental tumors. In patients, vemurafenib has been shown to induce complete or partial tumor regression of late stage melanomas that harbor the *BRAF* V600E mutation. In some cases, vemurafenib resistance is caused by secondary mutations in *NRAS* that reactivate the RAS pathway.

Several molecular targets are presented by the complex signaling pathways orchestrated by mTOR. The mTOR protein itself was originally discovered and named as the cellular target of rapamycin (also known as sirolimus and marketed as Rapamune). Rapamycin was initially characterized as a prospective antifungal compound that could block the cell's ability to generate energy for growth, and was subsequently found to have potent immunosuppressive and antiproliferative properties. A rapamycin derivative called everolimus is approved for use in advanced kidney cancers and pancreatic neuroendocrine tumors.

In addition to its stimulatory effect on cellular energy production, mTOR also promotes angiogenesis via the downstream regulation of the transcription factor HIF1α. The HIF1α-induced protein VEGFA can be blocked by a recombinant humanized antibody called bevacizumab (marketed as Avastin). Bevacizumab belongs to a new class of drugs called *angiogenesis inhibitors*, and has been approved for use in combination with conventional drugs for the treatment of advanced colorectal cancer, non-small cell lung cancer, kidney cancer, ovarian cancer, and a type of highly lethal brain tumor called glioblastoma multiforme. A humanized monoclonal antibody called ramucirumab (marketed as Cyramza) is directed against the ectodomain of the receptor tyrosine kinase that interacts with VEGFA. Ramucirumab was approved in 2014 for the treatment of advanced cancers in the stomach and esophagus. The small molecule KIT inhibitor sunitinib also targets this receptor and thereby inhibits angiogenesis.

Inflammation is a risk factor for cancer development as well as a component of most established tumors (see Chap. 1). STAT signaling is highly responsive to inflammatory cytokines. In some malignancies, this pathway is frequently activated by oncogenic mutations in the genes that encode the Janus kinases (JAKs), which function downstream of STAT. The drug ruxolitinib (marketed as Jakavi) is designed to inhibit JAK signaling, and is approved for use in myeloproliferative disorders. Recent studies have suggested that ruxolitinib may improve survival in patients with metastatic pancreatic cancer, a disease characterized by high levels of inflammation and a microenvironment that is rich in cytokines.

For every successful drug ultimately approved for use in cancer, there are numerous failures. Notably absent in the current anti-cancer armamentarium are agents that can effectively target alterations in the PIK3CA/AKT or the WNT/APC pathway. Several agents have been formulated to inhibit the AKT kinase, which functions downstream of PIK3CA. These compounds showed promise in early studies but thus far all have failed in the later stages of development. Like KRAS, PIK3CA is a tantalizing target that has been difficult to hit. Unlike the highly prevalent V600E mutation in *BRAF*, the mutations in *PIK3CA* occur in several hotspots and encode functionally diverse proteins. In the WNT/APC pathway, the major interactions between upstream players are mediated by protein-protein interactions rather than RTKs; such interactions have proven to be more difficult to inhibit with small molecules. Many inhibitors have been designed against the downstream kinase GSK3β, but none has yet been validated in late-stage clinical trials.

Neoantigens Are Recognized by the Immune System

The immune system plays a critical role in the body's response to a growing neoplasm. During the early stages of tumor growth, evolving tumor cells manage to evade surveillance by the adaptive immune system, particularly T-cells, and continue to grow in a relatively immune-privileged state. Among the most exciting development in cancer therapy are drugs that can unleash the immune system against advanced cancers. The complex interactions between cancer cells and the cells of the immune system are well beyond the scope of this text. However, there is one important facet of immune reactivity of tumors that is highly dependent on the characteristics of the cancer genome. Under conditions created by a new class of drugs, mutations can render a cell detectable by the immune system.

Cancer presents a unique challenge to the immune system, the basic function of which is to discriminate between 'self' (normal cells) and 'non-self' (pathogens or cells that are antigenically unfamiliar). T-cells, the effectors of cell-mediated immunity, strike a balance between reactivity and tolerance based on a plethora of stimulatory and inhibitory signals. Normal cells are not recognized and attacked by the immune system because a complex network of inhibitory pathways keeps immune cells in check, and thereby maintains self-tolerance. These inhibitory networks are known as *immune checkpoints. (These are mechanistically unrelated to the cell cycle checkpoints described in Chap. 6)*. Tumor cells activate immune checkpoints despite the fact that they express 'non-self' antigens.

Many of the immune checkpoint pathways are initiated at the interface between T-cells and the cells that stimulate them with antigens, known as antigen presenting cells (APCs). The pathways that allow T-cells to tolerate a presented antigen are mediated at the cell surface by ligand-receptor interactions. Prominent among the inhibitory ligands on APCs are PDL-1 and CD-80/86. These ligands interact with their respective receptors PD1 and CTLA4, which reside on the surface of T-cells. Therapeutic antibodies have been developed that avidly bind CTLA4 or PD1 and which can disrupt their inhibitory interactions with their respective ligands. These antibodies thus allow T-cells to be activated by antigens derived from cancer cells.

A T-cell can detect an abnormal cell when foreign proteins are presented to it by an APC. The mutations harbored by a tumor serve to distinguish the tumor cells as 'non-self'. The genetic mutations in protein-coding genes harbored by cancer cells create new antigens, known as *neoantigens*. When the immune checkpoint is blocked with anti-CTLA4 or anti-PD1 antibodies, T-cells are able to sense neoantigens and attack the cells of the tumor.

The effectiveness of immune checkpoint blockade therapy is highly dependent on the extent that antigen profile of a tumor differs from that of normal cells, an attribute known as tumor *immunogenicity*. Recent studies have demonstrated that tumors with large numbers of mutations – and therefore a large number of neoantigens – have greater responses than tumors with fewer mutations. Thus, melanomas, lung cancers and mismatch-repair deficient colorectal cancers tend to exhibit heightened responses to immune checkpoint blockade therapy. Even within a specific cancer type, tumors with more neoantigens provoke a more effective T-cell response following administration of an immune checkpoint inhibitor.

An anti-CTLA4 antibody called ipilimumab (marketed as Yervoy) is the first approved anti-cancer therapeutic that inhibits the immune checkpoint and unleashes T-cell activity. Ipilumumab has been approved for use in patients with late stage melanoma. About 20 % of patients respond to immune checkpoint blockade caused by ipilimumab. DNA sequence analysis has revealed that the tumors with the greatest numbers of mutations respond most dramatically. Removing the natural restraints on the immune system is not without risk, and severe adverse effects have been reported in some patients. Early evidence suggests that new antibodies that selectively target PD1, currently in development, may be more tolerable.

In most common tumors, there are many more passenger mutations than driver mutations. This is certainly true in melanomas, most of which are highly exposed to the mutagenic effects of ultraviolet light, and mismatch repair-deficient colorectal cancers, which typically accumulate thousands of mutations over generations of error-prone cell division. Passenger mutations do not provide a selective growth advantage to evolving tumors and do not contribute to cancer cell phenotypes. But when they occur in protein-coding regions of the genome, passenger mutations can generate novel proteins that are recognized as neoantigens by the immune system.

Neoantigens are a major determinant of the efficacy of immune checkpoint blockade. Because these proteins define the immunogenicity of a tumor, neoantigens also factor into efforts to harness the power of the immune system against evolving tumors by vaccination. The use of mutation-defined neoantigens as components of anti-cancer vaccines represents an exciting goal at the horizon of cancer research.

The Future of Oncology

Cancer genes are the cause of cancer, but they also define vulnerabilities in cancer cells. Drugs directed against specific targets have demonstrated effectiveness in treating cancers that had responded poorly to older modes of therapy. The comprehensive analysis of cancer genomes has provided insights and possible solutions to treatment failures. These experiences have generated a great deal of optimism surrounding the feasibility of rationally designed, targeted therapy. The foundation of this new approach to treating cancer patients is an understanding of cancer genetics.

Several simple principles underlie efforts to prevent, detect and cure cancers:

Germline cancer genes facilitate risk assessment. An understanding of germline cancer genes allows high-risk groups to be appropriately screened, and at-risk individuals to be more closely monitored.

Cancer genes are quantitative biomarkers of cancer. Cancer cells can be detected by virtue of the genes they harbor. The release of cancer DNA into bodily fluids provides an avenue for highly sensitive and quantitative methods of early detection.

Recurrent genetic alterations define molecular targets. The successful therapy of CML with imatinib provides a paradigm for targeting an oncogene-encoded protein required for cell survival. This highly effective approach requires both a target that is common in a given type of cancer and a specific inhibitor that can engage that target in a way that selectively impedes cancer cell growth. Because targeted therapy depends upon the specific molecular interaction between a drug and a protein, distinct mutations within a target gene can affect efficacy. This principle is vividly illustrated by the mutations in *EGFR* that affect responses to gefitinib. Industrial pipelines are now generating new drugs that are collectively projected to have a significant impact on cancer mortality.

Secondary mutations cause the development of therapeutic resistance. Targeted therapeutics are a source of selective pressure that drives ongoing clonal evolution. Secondary mutations that prevent inhibitor binding but preserve oncoprotein function provide a significant selective advantage, and lead to recurrence.

Combination therapy is a strategy for overcoming resistance. Clonal evolution in essence creates a moving target. Fortunately, the use of multiple agents that interact with a single target in different ways, or those that interact with multiple targets, can circumvent this problem. As cancers evolve, so do the therapeutic strategies to defeat them.

Older agents that induce DNA damage and block DNA replication, and which are often employed before or after surgery, are the current mainstays of therapy for the majority of cancers and will continue to be important for the foreseeable future. The use of new molecularly targeted therapeutics to treat cancers with defined genetic alterations is a significant departure from more general growth inhibitory strategies that predate the cancer gene theory. The modulation of the immune system is an entirely new approach that also exploits the genetic lesions accumulated and amplified by growing cancers.

Continued improvements in cancer survival will likely emerge from the combined use of these different types of drugs. The goal will be to identify those at risk, detect cancers at their earliest stages, and to manage later stage cancers like chronic diseases that are ultimately survivable.

Futher Reading

Amakye D, Jagani Z, Dorsch M (2013) Unraveling the therapeutic potential of the Hedgehog pathway in cancer. Nat Med 19:1410–1422

Ashworth A (2008) A synthetic lethal therapeutic approach: poly(ADP) ribose polymerase inhibitors for the treatment of cancers deficient in DNA double-strand break repair. JCO 26:3785–3790

Azam M, Latek RR, Daley GQ (2003) Mechanisms of autoinhibition and STI-571/imatinib resistance revealed by mutagenesis of BCR-ABL. Cell 112:831–843

Bettegowda C et al (2014) Detection of circulating tumor DNA in early- and late-stage human Malignancies. Sci Transl Med 6:224ra24

Bianchi DW et al (2015) Noninvasive prenatal testing and incidental detection of Occult Maternal Malignancies. JAMA 314:162–169

Chin L, Andersen JN, Futreal PA (2011) Cancer genomics: from discovery science to personalized medicine. Nat Med 17:297–303

Domchek SM, Weber BL (2006) Clinical management of BRCA1 and BRCA2 mutation carriers. Oncogene 25:5825–5831

Domchek S, Weber BL (2008) Genetic variants of uncertain significance: flies in the ointment. J Clin Oncol 26:16–17

Druker BJ (2002) Perspectives on the development of a molecularly targeted agent. Cancer Cell 1:31–36

Easton DF et al (2015) Gene-panel sequencing and the prediction of breast-cancer risk. NEJM 372:2243–2257

Greulich H et al (2005) Oncogenic transformation by inhibitor-sensitive and -resistant EGFR mutants. PLoS Med 2:e313

Gross AM et al (2014) Multi-tiered genomic analysis of head and neck cancer ties *TP53* mutation to 3p loss. Nat Genet 46:939–943

Guttmacher AE, Collins FS (2005) Realizing the promise of genomics in biomedical research. JAMA 294:1399–1402

Herbst RS, Fukuoka M, Baselga J (2004) Gefitinib-a novel targeted approach to treating cancer. Nat Rev Cancer 4:956–965

Hu YC, Sidransky D, Ahrendt SA (2002) Molecular detection approaches for smoking associated tumors. Oncogene 21:7289–7297

Hynes NE, Lane HA (2005) ERBB receptors and cancer: the complexity of targeted inhibitors. Nat Rev Cancer 5:341–354

Kelley SK, Ashkenazi A (2004) Targeting death receptors in cancer with Apo2L/TRAIL. Curr Opin Pharmacol 4:333–339

Kinde I et al (2013) Evaluation of DNA from the Papanicolaou test to detect ovarian and endometrial cancers. Sci Transl Med 167:167ra4

Krause DS, Van Etten RA (2005) Tyrosine kinases as targets for cancer therapy. N Engl J Med 353:172–187

Lacroix M (2006) Significance, detection and markers of disseminated breast cancer cells. Endocr Relat Cancer 13:1033–1067
Larsen AR et al (2015) Repurposing the antihelmintic mebendazole as a Hedgehog inhibitor. Mol Cancer Ther 14:3–13
Mao L et al (1994) Microsatellite alterations as clonal markers for the detection of human cancer. Proc Natl Acad Sci U S A 91:9871–9875
Masica DL et al (2015) Predicting survival in head and neck squamous cell carcinoma from TP53 mutation. Hum Genet 134:497–507
Mills NE et al (1995) Detection of K-ras oncogene mutations in bronchoalveolar lavage fluid for lung cancer diagnosis. J Natl Cancer Inst 87:1056–1060
Morgensztern D, Govindan R (2007) Is there a role for cetuximab in non small cell lung cancer? Clin Cancer Res 13:4602s–4605s
Nahta R, Esteva FJ (2007) Trastuzumab: triumphs and tribulations. Oncogene 26:3637–3643
Ng JMY, Curran T (2011) The Hedgehog's tale: developing strategies for targeting cancer. Nat Rev Cancer 11:493–501
Pardoll DM (2012) The blockade of immune checkpoints in cancer immunotherapy. Nat Rev Cancer 12:252–264
Petitjean A et al (2007) TP53 mutations in human cancers: functional selection and impact on cancer prognosis and outcomes. Oncogene 26:2157–2165
Polyak K, Garber J (2011) Targeting the missing links for cancer therapy. Nat Med 17:283–284
Schindler T et al (2000) Structural mechanism for STI-571 inhibition of abelson tyrosine kinase. Science 289:1938–1942
Schwartz RS (2002) A needle in a haystack of genes. N Engl J Med 346:302–304
Sharma SV, Bell DW, Settleman J, Haber DA (2007) Epidermal growth factor receptor mutations in lung cancer. Nat Rev Cancer 7:169–181
Smith BD (2011) Imatinib for chronic myeloid leukemia: the impact of its effectiveness and long-term side effects. JNCI 103:2–4
Trepanier A et al (2004) Genetic cancer risk assessment and counseling: recommendations of the national society of genetic counselors. J Genet Couns 13:83–114
Wang S, El-Deiry WS (2003) TRAIL and apoptosis induction by TNF-family death receptors. Oncogene 22:8628–8633
Wexler NS (1992) The Tiresias complex: Huntington's disease as a paradigm of testing for late-onset disorders. FASEB J 6:2820–2825

Index

F. Bunz, *Principles of Cancer Genetics*, DOI 10.1007/978-94-017-7484-0

Printed by Printforce, the Netherlands